The New Handbook of Health and Preventive Medicine

The New Handbook of Health and Preventive Medicine

Kurt Butler and
Lynn Rayner, M.D.

PROMETHEUS BOOKS
BUFFALO, NEW YORK

THE NEW HANDBOOK OF HEALTH AND PREVENTIVE MEDICINE.

Inquiries should be addressed to : Prometheus Books, 700 E. Amherst St., Buffalo, New York 14215, 716-837-2475.

94 93 92 91 90   5 4 3 2 1

Drawings: Diana Thewlis

Library of Congress Cataloging-in-Publication Data

Butler, Kurt.
The new handbook of health and preventive medicine / by Kurt Butler and Lynn Rayner.
p. cm.
ISBN 9780879755812
1. Medicine, Popular. 2. Medicine, Preventive. 3. Health.
I. Rayner, Lynn. II. Title.
RC81.B964 1990
613—dc20   90-32513
CIP

Acknowledgments

Our profound thanks go to Alicia Leonhard and John Mickey, M.D., for their multifaceted assistance in the preparation of this work. Their generous help with research, writing, and manuscript preparation made our work much easier.

Contents

Introduction

For most of our existence human beings have regarded diseases as acts of angry gods, the will of God, or simply fate. Only in very recent times have epidemics and chronic illnesses been demystified and explained. The more we have learned about health and disease, the less fatalistic we have become. It is now clear that many serious diseases can be prevented or delayed for many years. By making the right choices in several key areas of living, we can live longer, healthier lives. We can also save enormous amounts of money as individuals and as a society.

The purpose of this book is to help you make the right choices on personal, family, and community levels. We all make decisions about diet, exercise, drugs, vaccinations, and the like that often affect not only ourselves but our children and our neighbors. The more we base these decisions on facts, the better off everyone is.

There are, of course, still many disorders that are not well understood and cannot be prevented or even adequately treated at this time; they still seem to be acts of fate. Moreover, no matter how far medical science progresses and no matter how careful we are, we will still all die. The best we can hope for, the ideal we should aim for, is to be in excellent health for eight or nine decades, and then die painlessly while sleeping. Only a few of us will be this fortunate, but by applying the principles of preventive medicine we can more closely approach the ideal. This book, then, is not about absolutes, but about risk factors; we cannot make guarantees, but we can help improve your chances of staying healthy for as long as your genes will allow.

How to Use This Book

The subjects discussed in this book are loosely arranged from prevention and self-care to consulting and cooperating with a physician. The order of both the sections and the material within them reflects this arrangement.

Section One, "Healthy Habits," focuses on proper eating and exercise as general health-promoting factors. Although health professionals provide information about these things, individuals are responsible for the application of the information: these are things you do for yourself.

Section Two, "Common Diseases—A Preventive Approach," tells you what you need to know about the most important diseases and disorders, those you are most likely to encounter in yourself or loved ones, and may be able to prevent, delay, or control. These are the health problems the average educated person should know something about. We should understand their impact on individuals and society; we should know which of them we are at risk for and what we can do. For easy reference the diseases are listed at the beginning of the section in the order of their appearance. Each subchapter moves from general information to prevention, self-care, and consulting a physician.

Section Three, "Self-Care and Rational Use of the Health Care System," focuses on symptoms and examinations commonly needed. No matter how well we apply the principles of prevention discussed in Sections One and Two, we will all get sick or injured at some time, and we won't always be able to heal ourselves. Moreover, we all need vaccinations and health monitoring. This section is a guide to dealing with symptoms, by self-care when appropriate and by seeking medical help when necessary. It also summarizes key points about vaccinations and various health examinations needed by different people.

Section Four, "Drugs and Health," will help you understand and properly use (or avoid) most of the drugs you will ever encounter. There are four main categories: nonprescription or OTC (over-the-counter) drugs; herbal drugs; addicting and "recreational" drugs; and prescription drugs, including vaccinations. The section moves from drugs likely to be self-prescribed and administered to a general discussion of prescription drug use.

Please Note: Health maintenance is an evolving science; advice is always subject to revision based on more knowledge. The information we provide is for general educational purposes and should not be construed as prescriptions for individuals. You should always take your physician's advice if it seems to contradict what we present here. If the contradiction is glaring, however, you may want to seek a second opinion.

Section One
HEALTHY HABITS

Healthy Habits

The old cliche is true: Human beings are creatures of habit. We tend to do pretty much the same things every day, from one week to the next. We shop at the same stores, buy the same foods, and take the same route to work or school. We exercise about the same time each day or each weekend. Habits come naturally to us; they simplify life and make our efforts more efficient. The problem with habits is that bad ones are as easily established as good ones, perhaps more so. Knowledge and understanding, however, can nudge and guide us toward better ones. This section focuses on the daily habits most likely to affect our health, eating, and physical activity. Poor nutrition and under- or overexercise can have serious consequences. The information and advice herein should motivate you and help you to develop and maintain good eating and exercise habits.

A Note on Psychosocial Hygiene and Safety

We must acknowledge here that behavioral factors other than eating and exercise can affect our health. Isolation and loneliness, for example, predispose people to alcoholism and other drug abuse, depression, poor eating habits, and suicide. Pregnant women tend to have more complications if they are isolated than if they have supportive friendships. Loneliness in infants and children can be devastating, especially if compounded by physical abuse. For example, hostile and violent behavior often has its roots in "love deficiency" in infancy: infants should be caressed and carried a lot, and shown a great deal of affection. Otherwise they are more likely to grow up angry, with a sense of deprivation and alienation that leads to self-destructive and antisocial behavior.

Stress is another important factor in health, though it is difficult to quantify. It's hard to even define because one person's source of severe stress, say, loud heavy metal music or becoming a parent, may be another person's source of bliss. But there are some universal stressors. Consider, for example, prolonged exposure to extreme hot or cold, absolute sleep deprivation, exercising or working to exhaustion, and prolonged pain or fear. All these can cause or aggravate peptic ulcers, asthma, hypertension, headaches, anxiety disorders, chronic back pain, and menstrual disorders. They can even impair immune functions and increase the risk of some infections.

Now consider some of the more common sources of stress, such as doing a difficult and unpleasant job all day, prolonged exposure to loud noise, losing a job, losing a spouse by divorce or death, or having to move. Like the physical stressors above, these can be accompanied by hormonal and nervous system changes that can aggravate health problems. Learning to recognize stress is important so we can avoid stressors or modify our response to them. If we learn to relax and consciously practice relaxation on a daily basis, we can reduce the impact of stress on our health.

Relaxation for Stress Reduction

Everyone relaxes just before and during sleep, but it is useful to be able to relax at will and without necessarily getting sleepy. If you have trouble relaxing, feel wound up all day, and tend to overreact to daily aggravations, try this exercise. While sitting or lying, close your eyes, be still, and imagine yourself floating in a clear pool, serene and totally comfortable. Take a few slow, deep breaths and go limp, melting into the bed or chair. Now breathe normally and with every exhalation repeat to yourself, "relax." If you take a few minutes to do this two or three times a day some stress-related symptoms may start to fade away, and you may work more efficiently. Another good way to relax and relieve stress is to laugh. If you don't laugh often perhaps you need to develop your sense of humor and try to get more pleasure from daily life.

The Pleasure Principle

It's important to eat nutritious food, but it's also important to enjoy your meals. A perfectly prepared and perfectly balanced meal served in an atmosphere of anxiety or anger is more likely to cause indigestion than to nourish. Likewise, it's important to encourage children to be active, but a strict exercise schedule grimly adhered to can turn kids off and make them couch potatoes. It's more important to have fun being active than to do any particular exercises or be involved in certain sports.

Safety Awareness

Another important aspect of health maintainence that this book doesn't cover in detail is accident prevention. Some of the most important causes of preventable injuries and deaths are: driving while intoxicated; otherwise unsafe driving; not wearing seat belts; motorcyclists and bicyclists not wearing helmets; pedestrian carelessness among vehicular traffic; falls (by the elderly); suffocation (among infants); careless use and storage of guns; irresponsible dog owners; careless use of lawn mowers, ladders, and other home tools; drowning; fires (most often caused by smoking, children playing with matches, and defective electrical wiring and appliances); carelessness with hot water, food, and utensils (resulting in burns); and careless handling and storage of household chemicals.

These things kill and maim hundreds of thousands of people every year. Efforts to prevent injuries and death from them are as important as efforts to prevent heart disease and cancer. We mention them to help readers keep matters in perspective. Some people get obsessed with details of their diets but neglect to wear seat belts, bicycle helmets, or safety goggles while hammering nails. Some worry about tiny traces of pesticides in baby food but leave their infants alone in a bathtub or near a swimming pool while they answer the phone.

Therefore, while further elaboration on psychosocial and safety factors is beyond the scope of this book, we suggest that such factors be carefully considered by those interested in maintaining their health and that of their families. We mention them here because they are, to a large extent, matters of habit. Safety consciousness in driving, working, playing, cooking, and all other activities reduces our risk of injury. Cheerfulness, friendliness, considerate and loving behavior, a sense of humor, and relaxation can also be habits, and they can also help maintain good health.

Good Nutrition for Health and Pleasure

Nutrition Science and Superstition

The empirical science of nutrition, the study of foods and their effects on health, must be many thousands of years old. Early humans tried various plant, animal, and mineral matter and learned what was poisonous and what was edible, tasty, and filling, and perhaps even what promoted growth in their children. The nutritious plants were cultivated and the animals domesticated; the science of nutrition grew hand-in-hand with the science of agriculture.

Early medical science was helped along when certain foods were found to prevent or cure certain disorders. For example, Hippocrates advocated liver for night blindness, which we now know works when the problem is caused by vitamin A deficiency. In 1753 James Lind, a Scottish naval surgeon, published his famous report of experiments done in the British Navy proving that lemons and oranges prevented and cured scurvy. This disease had been written about as early as 1500 B.C. and was one of the most mysterious and feared in all Europe.

Nutritional science remained strictly empirical and rudimentary until the development of modern chemistry and biochemistry within the past two hundred years. Among the earliest nutrients recognized and chemically identified were proteins, carbohydrates (starch, glycogen, and sugars), fats, and minerals like calcium and iodine. By the early 1900s scientists were doing animal studies in labs around the world and filling in bits of the giant puzzle.

As chemical techniques developed, it became clear that animals could not survive on artificial mixtures of purified carbohydrates, proteins, fats, and minerals. As various extracts of different foods were withheld or fed to animals and their growth and health studied, clear patterns emerged. Removing certain elements from the foods caused certain symptoms, although the amounts were so small that their removal did not significantly affect the weight or caloric value of the foods. Gradually these factors, the vitamins and trace minerals, have been identified and their biochemical roles sketched out. Besides adequate calories and water, there are now about forty-five substances known to be required in the diet for health.

The scientific study of foods, nutrients, and their effects on health has resulted in a consensus, with healthy debate on fine points, among experts. The recommendations of the National Research Council (which publishes the Recommended Dietary Allowances), the American Heart Association, the American Cancer Society, the Surgeon General, the Department of Agriculture, and other responsible agencies and authorities are all essentially the same.

However, while nutrition science has made steady progress, nutrition superstition and quackery have held their own. Dietary hogwash has become an American staple. The business of peddling nutrition misinformation and worthless and dangerous supplements has never been better. Just check the bestseller lists for the past twenty years, watch Phil Donahue, or take a look at the thousands of bottles of Megathis and Superthat at "health food" stores, drug stores, and even some supermarkets and sporting goods stores. The promoters of these diets, pills, and powders peddle their wares with a religious zeal that many find persuasive. In fact, many people have a sort of religious faith in the nutrition philosophy they have converted to, whether it be macrobiotics, fruitarianism, or megavitamins.

We have good news for you: You don't need to read those silly books, convert to a nutrition religion, or buy those expensive pills and powders. Understanding proper nutrition is simple, and good food is widely available and inexpensive.

The U.S. Senate Recommendations

The diet of the nation is so important to national health, health care costs, and agricultural policies that the United States Senate has taken an intense interest in it. In 1977 the Select Committee on Nutrition and Human Needs (the McGovern Committee) held extensive hearings and issued its conclusions in the now-famous *Dietary Goals for the United States.* As Professor D. M. Hegsted of the Harvard School of Public Health told the McGovern Committee, the increasingly rich diet (high in fats, cholesterol, and sugar) "which affluent people generally consume, is everywhere associated with a similar disease pattern—high rates of ischemic heart disease, certain forms of cancer, diabetes and obesity. These are the major causes of death and disease. . . . They are epidemic in our population. We cannot afford to temporize." The changes favored by the Senate committee were:

- increased consumption of whole grains, vegetables, fruits, fish, and poultry;
- decreased consumption of fatty meats, whole dairy products, eggs and high-cholesterol foods, with a partial substitution of polyunsaturated fat for saturated fat;
- decreased consumption of sugar and salt.

These recommendations were widely publicized and it's now clear that they have been adopted to some extent by many Americans. National consumption of fatty meats, eggs, and whole dairy products has gone down, while consumption of fruits and vegetables has gone up. This trend, along with the general decrease in smoking, may be partly responsible for the gradual improvement in our cardiovascular health; fewer people are dying from heart attacks and strokes. Nevertheless, preventable cardiovascular diseases are still, by far, the most common causes of premature death and disability in the United States, and poor diet has a lot to do with that.

The Ideal Diet

Our concept of the ideal diet is based on the consensus among responsible scientists and agencies. It can be stated very simply:

Eat a wide variety of foods from the starch, produce, protein, and calcium groups. Limit or avoid fatty and high-cholesterol meat, eggs, charcoal-broiled or smoked meat and fish, burned foods, reheated cooking oil, sugary snacks, pickled vegetables, alcohol, and excessive salt if it tends to raise your blood pressure or aggravate other health problems. Eat enough to maintain normal weight and no more.

More specifically, we recommend daily consumption of:

Starch. Four or more servings of whole grain foods such as oatmeal, brown rice, corn, buckwheat, millet, whole wheat, cracked wheat, or breads and cereals made from them, or similar unrefined starchy foods such as potatoes and yams.

Produce. Five or more servings of a variety of dark green and yellow vegetables, citrus fruits, and tomatoes, preferably fresh.

Protein. Two or more servings of fish, seeds, beans, nuts (fresh and free of added oils and salts), poultry, eggs, or lean meat. Fish is generally superior to pork, lamb, eggs, and beef. It has higher quality protein, less of the undesirable fats, and more of the unsaturated oils believed to help lower cholesterol levels. Poultry is intermediate in value since it has less undesirable fat but more cholesterol than most meats. Minimize smoked flesh foods of all kinds. They often have high levels of carcinogens.

Calcium. Two to four glasses of milk or the equivalent in cheese, yogurt, almonds (not oiled or salted), sesame seed butter, leafy greens, broccoli, tofu made with calcium, or other high-calcium foods. The dairy products should be mostly nonfat or low-fat for most people. Lactase-deficient persons who want to drink milk can buy lactase (the enzyme necessary to digest milk) and add it to milk. Most lactase-deficient people can tolerate substantial amounts of yogurt unless lactose has been added (check the label).

Variety Is Important

We are fortunate to have available a huge variety of wonderful foods, each of which is a complex mixture of many nutrients. To plan healthy menus for yourself and your family all you have to do is plan meals with items from each of the four groups. If you shop without planning meals ahead, just see that your basket has a mix of items from each food group. When you get all your raw ingredients for a meal out ask yourself whether they include a reasonable proportion from each of the groups. And think variety. Especially get lots of different kinds of fruits, vegetables, beans, and grains. Moderate amounts of nuts, seeds, and peanuts are also good. Variety assures you not only more enjoyable eating, but better nutrition, especially of trace nutrients.

This is where we sharply disagree with the "health food" industry, which has it all backwards. We believe good nutrition comes from real foods, not pills and powders of isolated nutrients; and good medicines come in precise doses of known components (preferably isolated components in most cases). Good nutrition is a shotgun affair; good medicine is, as much as possible, a precision affair. The "health food" industry, however, promotes specific nutrients in pill form and medicines in the form of various leafs, roots, and other whole plant matter as well as crude extracts. Of course, nutrition supplements are sometimes valuable, even life-saving for the malnourished; and some herbs are beneficial and practical. But, in general, it's far better to eat your nutrients in the food form and take your medicines in the pill form, rather than the other way around.

Should You Take Supplements?

If you follow these guidelines you don't need to even think about vitamins, minerals, and other nutrients, or worry whether you're getting enough. They will take care of themselves. Below we will present the nutrients in detail to set some facts straight, dispel some myths, and reinforce our guidelines—not because you need to check your diet on a daily basis for individual nutrients.

If you aren't confident in your diet and don't believe you are getting adequate nutrition from your food, it won't hurt to take a multivitamin and mineral supplement. If you do, take one with moderate amounts of each required nutrient, about 100 percent of the RDA. Avoid those with excessive amounts (more than 100 percent of the RDA) of vitamins A and D, niacin, vitamin B-6, and zinc (for reasons discussed in the pages ahead).

The Meaning of the RDAs

The Food and Nutrition Board of the National Research Council (NRC) periodically publishes a revised set of Recommended Dietary Allowances (RDAs) based on the latest information from thousands of studies around the world. The RDAs are considered to be adequate for practically all healthy people, but are not necessarily applicable to those with infections, metabolic disorders, chronic diseases, or in special situations like premature birth or drug abuse. The RDAs have been established for almost half of the known required nutrients. They are calculated, using several safety factors to ensure adequacy, for close to 100 percent of the healthy population, and are substantially higher than the World Health Organization standards for most nutrients. Most people will not develop deficiency symptoms unless their intake falls below two-thirds the RDA of a nutrient for several weeks. (See Appendix A for RDA tables.)

RDAs and food value tables are commonly used by nutritionists to determine whether nutrient intake by groups and individuals is adequate, borderline, or inadequate. Following a dietary recall, the intake of protein, amino acids, vitamins, and minerals is estimated. If necessary, dietary changes or supplements are then suggested.

The RDAs are often abused by food manufacturers to make inflated nutritional claims about their products. NRC publications caution that the RDAs are based on a diet including a variety of common foods in order to provide sufficient amounts of the nutrients for which RDAs have not been determined. The reasonable assumption here has been that if we eat a variety of common, whole, natural foods with their large mix of nutrients, such that the RDAs for half the nutrients are met, the requirement for the other half will probably also be met.

However, processing food often removes trace minerals, amino acids, fibers, and components for which no RDA has yet been set. The manufacturers then add a few of the "popular" nutrients (those for which RDAs are known), and call the product "enriched." By "a variety of common foods" the NRC Committee on Dietary Allowances does not mean a diet of "enriched" Snacky Poppies, Lunchy Munchies, and Snow White Rice. One could meet almost all the RDAs by eating nothing but a fortified low-fiber, high-salt, high-sugar, high-fat breakfast cereal with fortified milk, but it would be a very poor diet. Clearly the RDAs alone, without consideration of the food itself, cannot be taken as gospel. Nevertheless, applied with proper understanding and qualifications, the RDAs provide reasonable estimates of the adequacy of nutrient intake.

Infant Nutrition

The guidelines above are generally valid for almost everyone. Infants, however, are obviously a special case. Here's a look at infant nutrition.

Breast-feeding for at least the first several months is the preferred source of infant nutrition in most cases. In the 1940s about 65 percent of United States infants were breast-fed, but in the late sixties only 15 percent were nursed. More recently breast-feeding has made a comeback and more than half of American infants are breast-fed. The American Academy of Pediatrics and the Canadian Pediatric Society have issued a joint statement strongly encouraging physicians to recommend breast-feeding. Given with care, formula and solid food can be very nutritious, but breast-feeding is considered generally superior for the following reasons:

- At birth the infant emerges from an almost germ-free environment into a world teeming with bacteria as well as viruses, fungi, and other infectious organisms. The immune system at birth is not well developed, and the infant is especially susceptible to intestinal and respiratory infections and to allergy development for about a year. Fortunately colostrum, a watery yellowish fluid released by the breast during the first few days after birth, and mother's milk itself are rich in the antibodies the infant lacks. Colostrum and mother's milk are also very rich in infection-fighting white blood cells, particularly the very efficient "killer" macrophages. The incidence of respiratory, intestinal, ear, and other infections is generally much lower among breast-fed infants.

- Widespread bottle-feeding in developing countries, where sanitation is poor and formulas are often diluted for economy, has contributed to high infant mortality rates. Some countries have declared baby bottles a health hazard and banned their sale without a health worker's prescription.
- Breast-feeding provides substantial protection from allergic problems. The very young intestinal wall does not always manage to absorb only digested nutrients and keep out large protein fragments. When such undigested molecules are absorbed sensitization may occur, in which case allergic problems with that food will appear in the future.
- The psychological benefits to the infant and mother of early, close, prolonged contact are enhanced by nursing.
- Breast-feeding may provide some protection from obesity because infants tend to stop when they are full, and are not encouraged to continue beyond the point of satisfaction. With bottle-feeding the infant is often urged to finish what has been prepared. Breast-feeding is also a great help in controlling the weight of the mother, since it can use about 1,000 calories a day and speeds maternal recovery by stimulating the uterus to recover its tone and shape.
- The protein, mineral, and fat composition of mother's milk is quite different from cow's milk. The protein content of cow's milk is so high that it is dangerous to feed to an infant without dilution. Indeed, cow's milk should not be given for at least six months or, preferably, one year. Human milk has more unsaturated fatty acids (like vegetable oils) and less of the saturated fatty acids. However, most commercial milk-based formulas are modified to resemble mother's milk in these respects. The iron in mother's milk is better absorbed and capable of meeting the infant's needs for at least the first six months of life.
- Breast-feeding is better for dental development. Though it is not clear why, children who are breast-fed for at least six months are less likely to have malocclusions due to crooked teeth and jaws.
- Breast-feeding is generally less expensive than bottle-feeding. It is also much more convenient, since it does not require bottles, cans, sterilization, equipment, and so on.

 Breast-feeding is not adequate, of course, when the mother is malnourished. She should have a balanced diet of whole, natural foods without excessive supplements. Vegetarians should be certain to get adequate vitamin B-12, either from dairy products or supplements.

Many drugs taken by the mother are excreted in her milk and may be harmful to the infant. Especially important to avoid while breast-feeding are: oral contraceptives, reserpine, atropine, steroid hormones, diuretics, anticoagulants, antithyroid drugs, barbiturates, and various anticancer drugs. Marijuana, alcohol, caffeine, cigarettes, narcotics, tranquilizers, and laxatives should also be avoided or minimized.

Certain foods eaten by a mother may cause colic in a nursing infant. Milk, garlic, onions, and vegetables from the cabbage family are common culprits, but this is highly variable.

When to start solid foods is a much-debated subject; no hard rules can be given. Solid feeding too early may increase the susceptibility to allergies, but most infants have low iron reserves, and mother's milk does not supply as much iron as some solid foods. A safe bet is to exclusively breast-feed for about three to seven months, and then start giving small amounts of solids, especially iron-rich foods, including iron-fortified cereals. There is no need to buy prepared baby food. Most regular family fare, preferably unsalted and without strong seasonings, can be pureed.

As teeth develop, larger, chewy morsels can be given. However, care must be taken not to serve food that can be choked on. Be especially careful with hot dogs, candies, nuts, grapes, beans, and apples. These should be mashed, cut, or broken into safer forms.

Infants under one year of age should *not* be fed honey. Even "pure" or "filtered" honey often contains botulism spores that can produce the deadly toxin in infants.

Children of parents with many allergies should not be given cow's milk, eggs, nuts, peanuts, chocolate, citrus fruit or juice, wheat, or other commonly allergenic foods for the first year.

Infants and Fat

The growing concern of Americans about dietary fat and its relation to heart disease has caused some parents to put their children on low-fat diets at a very young age. They give their kids diluted formula and juices, low-fat milk, very little fat and oil, and lots of starch. The result is often a malnourished child with poor weight gain and slow growth. Babies' brains need fat for proper development, and they often can't get enough from such limited fare. Fats should not be limited before age two without consulting a physician. Skim milk should not be given before eighteen months.

Do Infants Need Supplements?

In general, no, but this should be discussed with your pediatrician or a dietician. The most important exception is fluoride, small doses of which should be given if the family's drinking water is fluoride poor. In areas with high levels of fluoride, supplements should not be given. Your dentist, local water board, or city councilmember can tell you whether your drinking water has fluoride.

Fruit Juice and Children

Infants and toddlers are often given far too much fruit juice, as much as one to four quarts each day. The juice supplies too much sugar, including sorbitol, which can cause diarrhea and stomach cramps in large amounts. Apple juice is the worst in this respect. The juice habit often leads to chronic diarrhea and malnutrition. Juice should be limited to a couple cups of each day.

Major Nutrient Categories

Carbohydrates

Carbohydrates are simple sugars, like glucose and fructose; double sugars, like sucrose and lactose; and polysugars, like starch and glycogen. They are made of carbon, hydrogen, and oxygen, and yield (or store) 4 calories of energy per gram. The polysugars and double sugars must be broken down into simple sugars before they can be absorbed into the blood. (The indigestible carbohydrate cellulose is discussed with fibers, below.)

SIMPLE SUGARS

Fructose is present in many fruits and in honey. It is the sweetest of all sugars and is commonly used in soft drinks and candies. Fructose is heavily promoted by the "health food" industry as a miracle food that provides instant energy, and cures insomnia, anxiety, and other problems. This is all nonsense. Its only advantage over sucrose is more sweetening "power" per calorie (about 50 percent) when not heated. This is a minor advantage since the cost of fructose is usually several times the cost of sucrose.

Galactose, the least sweet of the common sugars, is one component of the double sugar lactose (milk sugar); the other component is glucose.

Glucose is the basic fuel of the body, the carbohydrate that is freely soluble in blood and cell fluids and available to all tissues for their energy needs. Only small amounts of actual glucose are ingested, but all foodstuffs except fatty acids are converted to glucose before being used for energy. Blood sugar levels refer to blood glucose.

DOUBLE SUGARS

Lactose is milk sugar, the major carbohydrate provided by mammals to their infant offspring and a major source of energy for milk drinkers. Lactose is digested to glucose and galactose by the enzyme lactase before it is absorbed into the blood. Many people, especially blacks and Asians, gradually lose their lactase, and therefore their ability to digest lactose, as they mature. Too much lactose can cause gas, bloating, cramps, and diarrhea.

Maltose is a sugar formed when starch is partly digested, such as when grains are sprouted or corn starch is partly hydrolyzed. A molecule of maltose consists of two molecules of glucose linked together. Small amounts occur naturally, but most maltose used in food is made from starch. It is somewhat less sweet than sucrose, and is used in malted milk, some breakfast cereals, and other products.

Sucrose is common table sugar, the sweetest of the double sugars. In digestion it is broken down to glucose and fructose, which are absorbed into the blood and either used for energy or stored as glycogen or fat. Sucrose is very widespread in plants and reaches high concentrations in the sweeter fruits, which frequently also contain fructose and glucose from broken down sucrose. Most table sugar is extracted from sugar cane and sugar beets.

SUGAR—VILLAIN OR SCAPEGOAT?

In recent years common sugar, or sucrose, has taken a terrific beating in the "health food" press. Books and articles accuse it of causing a list of diseases a mile long, including heart disease, ulcers, hypoglycemia, diabetes, and insanity. Many people now shy away from sugar as if it were a poison. But is it?

The natural foods with high concentrations of sugar, far from poisoning us, are among the most nutritious. Sweet fruits and vegetables are generally excellent sources of vitamins, minerals, and fiber. Moreover, the popular tirades against sugar do not hold up very well under scrutiny. William Dufty's *Sugar Blues,* for example, describes how he lost weight, got rid of his hemorrhoids, and generally felt better after giving up sugar. He also gave up cocaine, caffeine, and aspirin and started to exercise at the same time, but still blames his previous health problems on sugar.

The problem with sugars is that food manufacturers use them to make candies and other snacks and desserts that are almost invariably less nutritious than nature's sweet treats. They have fewer vitamins (unless fortified), minerals, trace elements, and fiber, and more oils and fats. They usually stick to the teeth more than the natural foods, and so tend to cause tooth decay.

POLYSUGARS

Starch is formed by branched chains of glucose molecules and is the energy store in seeds (including beans and grains) and tubers (potatoes and such). When moistened and heated, the starch granules absorb water, swell, and burst, rendering the starch more digestible. It is broken down into glucose, which is absorbed into the blood. High-starch foods include grains such as rice, wheat, and corn, and beans, peas, potatoes, yams, tapioca, and poi.

Starchy foods have long been erroneously considered "fattening" and generally not very wholesome. It is now clear that the problem is not bread and potatoes but the butter and sour cream we put on them. Most Americans would do well to include more starchy vegetables, grains, and beans in their diet without excessive butter, oils, and salt. However, eating mostly refined grains like white rice and bread promotes constipation and hemorrhoids because the fiber has been removed.

Glycogen is animal starch, the stored form of glucose in the liver and muscles. It is essentially identical to starch, but the chains of glucose are shorter and the molecule is more highly branched than starch. It is broken down into glucose as needed for energy. Only small amounts are present in most meats, but oysters and other shellfish may contain up to 5 percent of their weight in glycogen.

FIBERS

Cellulose, hemicellulose, pectin, lignin, and other structural components of plants are frequently present in fruits, vegetables, grains, and beans. They are important in the diet because they swell with water and provide the roughage that stimulates peristalsis, keeping the contents of the intestines moving along. As intestinal bacteria multiply on the fiber, a gelatinous mass is formed and laxative compounds are generated. A high-fiber diet helps prevent constipation, hemorrhoids, diverticular disease, and possibly appendicitis. Moreover, by increasing transit speed, fiber decreases the contact of carcinogens generated in the bowels with the intestinal wall, and may thereby decrease the risk of bowel cancer.

Fiber in the diet helps diabetics and the obese by slowing the speed of eating and digestion, moderating the insulin response, and increasing the satiety value of the food, thereby inhibiting overeating. Fiber may also help prevent atherosclerosis by decreasing cholesterol absorption. Adding carrots, beans, and certain whole grains and their brans to your diet may decrease blood cholesterol levels.

Who Needs Fiber Supplements? If you eat plenty of whole grains, vegetables, and fruits, extra fiber is not necessary and may even be harmful. If you do eat wheat, oat, corn, or rice bran be sure to drink plenty of water, as the fiber could dry out and block your intestine. Excessive fiber supplementation can also cause flatulence, bowel rumblings, frequent defecation, constant awareness of bowel activity, and possibly excessive excretion of calcium, zinc, iron, and other minerals.

COMPLEX CARBOHYDRATES

This faddish term has become quite popular in recent years; even ads for breakfast cereals use it. It simply refers to grains, potatoes, and the like—that is, starchy foods. It's accurate, but pretentious; why not simply say "starchy foods"?

Fats

Fats, like carbohydrates, are made of carbon, hydrogen, and oxygen, but they take additional oxygen to metabolize and they pack more energy than carbohydrates. One gram of fat is good for 9 calories, while one gram of carbohydrate or protein releases only 4 calories when oxidized. Fats are the most fattening components of foods because smaller amounts of them fulfill our energy needs.

The nature of a fat is determined by the nature of the bonds between the carbons. If all the bonds are single, meaning no more hydrogen can be accepted, the fat is said to be *saturated* and is solid at room temperature. If one double bond is present the fat is *monounsaturated.* If the fat has two or more double bonds it is said to be *polyunsaturated,* and is liquid (oil) at room temperature. Food oils and fats are generally blends of polyunsaturated, monounsaturated, and saturated fatty acids. Animal fats are mostly saturated and vegetable fats are mostly unsaturated. Vegetable oils are made into semisolid margarines by hydrogenation—hydrogen is added until the oil becomes saturated. Saturated fats tend to raise cholesterol levels, which increases the risk of heart disease, so efforts to decrease fat intake generally concentrate on animal fats.

For some thirty years now Americans have been advised to replace some of their saturated fats with polyunsaturated fats, like those from safflower oil and corn oil, to reduce cholesterol levels. This is still good advice, but it may be even better to use monounsaturated fats, like those from olive oil and canola oil. The reason is that polyunsaturates tend to lower HDL-cholesterol (the "good cholesterol") while monounsaturates do not.

Linoleic acid, an essential nutrient, is a component of many fats and oils in both plants and animals. It is required for the production of the structural fats of cellular membranes, for regulating cholesterol metabolism, and for the synthesis of prostaglandins, which regulate many physiological functions throughout the body.

Deficiency of linoleic acid is very rare, but has occurred in hospitalized patients fed intravenous solutions without any fat and in infants fed fat-free formulas. The first obvious symptom is dry and flaking skin. Borderline deficiency, detectable by blood test, inhibits the transport, breakdown, and excretion of cholesterol.

The requirement for linoleic acid is about 2 percent (3 percent for infants) of total caloric intake. Most Americans consume at least twice this amount. The most concentrated sources are various nuts, seeds, and vegetables and their oils, especially corn and soybean oils. Margarine, olive oil, and shortening are fair sources. Coconut has no linoleic acid.

The functions of fats in the diet are to provide linoleic acid, to promote absorption of the fat-soluble vitamins A, D, E, and K, to provide a concentrated source of energy, to make food tasty, and to promote satiety, that is, to make food satisfying. A diet too low in fat may be low in the fat-soluble nutrients and in calories, which is especially hazardous to children. Most people find meals with very little fat (less than 10 percent of total calories) less palatable and less satisfying than those with more.

How fatty is your diet? Although the trend has been away from fatty meats, eggs, and dairy products, most Americans still eat too much fat. The average diet is 35 to 40 percent fat. Because of the association of high-fat diets with cardiovascular disease, some cancers, obesity, and other problems, experts agree that this is too much fat intake and should be reduced. There is an ongoing debate on how much fat would be best, with estimates ranging from 10 to 30 percent; 20 to 30 percent is probably about right for most people, though persons at high risk for atherosclerosis might go a little lower.

Keep in mind that these figures refer to percentage of calories, not percentage of weight. Ambiguity and confusion about this has led to widespread deception of consumers by major food manufacturers: assorted high-fat meats are marketed as "low-fat" and "90% fat-free." The claims may be true in reference to weight, but, since the products may have more than 60 percent water, grossly false in reference to calories. They may really be 75 percent or more fat.

High fat foods include butter, margarine, and oils; whole milk, cheese, and other dairy products; most red meats, especially bacon and sausages; nuts, seeds, and peanuts. Significant amounts of "hidden" fats are contributed by foods usually thought of as carbohydrate foods such as doughnuts, pies, cakes, and other pastries, as well as many candies.

It's easy for experts to advise people to keep total fat intake around a certain percentage, but it's not always easy to figure out the percentage of fat in your diet. Unless you actually weigh or measure and log everything you eat, know exactly how much fat is in everything you eat, and do some calculations, you can't be sure. If you really must know (because of obesity, diabetes, hypertension, or any other reason) a registered dietician can be a big help. Before you go to an appointment make a careful log of everything you eat for at least three days. Your record won't be perfect, but it will give the dietician a good idea of your eating habits, and this may save you some consulting time and cost.

You can estimate the fat percentage in a given food if you know the amount of fat and calories in a given serving. Multiply the grams of fat by 9, divide the result by the total number of calories, and multiply the result by 100. This gives you the fat percentage of the food. If you know your total daily calorie and fat intake, you can calculate the percentage of fat in your diet. But, again, a dietician can be a big help.

Cholesterol is not really a fat but a complex alcohol that occurs in foods from animals. It is important as a precursor of vitamin D, sex hormones, and other substances, but the liver makes it; it is not required in the diet. High blood levels are associated with atherosclerosis and heart disease. While dietary cholesterol tends to suppress one's own liver production to some extent, it nevertheless contributes to blood cholesterol and should be minimized in the diets of those with a tendency to abnormal blood lipids.

Protein

When we ingest proteins they are digested down to amino acids, small nitrogen-containing molecules that are absorbed into the blood. Our cells then reassemble the amino acids into the appropriate proteins such as enzymes, hormones, and muscle fibers. There are twenty-two amino acids, but some can be made from others, so only nine are required in the diet.

If your protein intake is low, the necessary amino acids will not be presented to the cells, the essential proteins will not be made, and symptoms of deficiency will eventually occur. Early signs include poor growth in children, poor nail and hair growth, poor weight gain in pregnancy, fatigue, slow wound healing, and sluggish immune response with increased susceptibility to infections. Later signs include anemia, edema (swelling), muscle wasting, weight loss, and poor digestion.

The RDA for protein ranges from about 10 grams for infants to 75 grams for pregnant women. Nonpregnant women are said to need about 45 grams, men about 55. These include generous safety factors to assure adequacy for those who have higher than average requirements, and for protein of less than perfect quality, that is, protein that does not provide enough of one or more of the essential amino acids. The RDAs also assume adequate calorie intake; if more energy is spent than calories replace, some of the amino acids provided are used for energy rather than building proteins. Amino acids, and therefore protein, supply 4 calories per gram.

Most Americans eat almost twice as much protein as they need, so protein deficiency is not very common. It does occur, though, with gross malnutriton such as in eating disorders, alcoholism, and some fad diets.

Protein Supplements. Concentrated protein powders are commonly advertised as helpful for developing muscles and fitness, but these mixtures of purified soy, milk, and egg proteins are more likely to do harm than good. Like refined grains and sugar, they provide calories without the vitamins, minerals, and fibers that normally accompany them. Unlike the other refined foods, they are very expensive. They also taste bad, though not as terrible as liquid amino acid products, which should be completely avoided. Excessive protein can cause excessive calcium excretion, poor zinc absorption, and possible kidney damage. When substantially higher protein intake is needed, such as after major surgery, injury, or other severe physical stress, it is far preferable to increase the intake of high-quality, high-protein foods.

 Amino Acid Supplements. Several amino acids are sold in pill form and some rather fantastic claims are being made for them. In general, these claims are mere marketing ploys with little evidence to support them. Nevertheless, sometimes amino acid supplements may be useful. Tryptophan, for example, may help in insomnia and chronic pain, and tyrosine may be useful in depression. Studies on these effects are in progress. Because of the potential hazards of amino acids (such as hyperacidity, decreased absorption of the unsupplemented amino acids, and blood disorders) supplements should not be taken for more than a few days without consulting a physician.

Recently tryptophan supplements have been associated with a rare blood disorder. It is not yet clear whether the amino acid or contaminants in the pills are responsible, but the products have been ordered off the market by the Food and Drug Administration.

Vitamins

Humans and other animals cannot live on just proteins, carbohydrates, fats, the macrominerals (calcium, phosphorous, sodium, chloride, potassium, and magnesium), and water. Although these components provide all the calories and more than 99.9 percent of the weight of our foods, there are at least twenty-five other substances that are required in the diet in very tiny amounts. They help keep the metabolic machinery of the cells running by serving as cofactors, or enzyme helpers, in protein synthesis, energy production, and all the other cellular processes of life. About half of them are complex organic molecules and they are called *vitamins.* The rest are simple elements, the trace minerals. The vitamins are discussed in detail in the following pages.

VITAMIN A (RETINOL)

One of the roles of vitamin A is to combine with a protein (opsin) to form the light-sensitive chemical rhodopsin, critical for vision. One of the first symptoms of vitamin A deficiency is night blindness. If deficiency continues after night blindness develops, xerosis (drying) of the conjunctiva (the moist lining of the eyelid) and cornea occur, then corneal distortion and irreversible changes in the retina. The cornea may become ulcerated and the lens may be destroyed, causing blindness. Worldwide, vitamin A deficiency is one of the greatest causes of blindness, affecting many thousands of children each year.

Vitamin A is also necessary for proper growth, resistance to infection, and skin health, probably because of its role in regulating the structure and function of cell membranes. In a deficiency, all the body's mucous membranes, especially those lining the digestive and respiratory tract, degenerate, stop their mucous production, and lose their cilia. Sinus, throat, respiratory, mouth, and ear infections are common results. Tooth and gum health also depend on adequate vitamin A.

Sources. Good sources of vitamin A and beta-carotene, which the body converts to vitamin A, include yellow, orange, and green vegetables and fruits, such as carrots, sweet potatoes, broccoli, melons, squash, corn, pumpkin, peaches, apricots, cherries, prunes, plums, mangoes, papayas, lettuce, chard, green pepper, tomatoes, kale, spinach, and collard greens. Liver, egg yolks, butter, fish, and fish oils are also rich sources. Whole and fortified milk are fair sources.

The vitamin A content of these foods varies enormously, so there is no point in measuring portions and consulting tables to determine adequacy on a daily basis. For example, carrots vary from 2,000 to 12,000 and sweet potatoes from 1,500 to 7,700 International Units (IU) per 100 grams. By eating an average of two or three medium servings a day of a variety of these foods, vitamin A adequacy can be assured. For example, one-half of a medium size yam or mango, or five fresh apricots can supply 6,000 IU, more than adequate for almost everyone.

Who Needs Supplements? If you don't eat several of the above foods on a regular basis, you might benefit from vitamin A supplements. An average of 5,000 IU a day is more than adequate for most healthy people. However, some serious diseases such as cancer, chronic infections, hepatitis, cirrhosis of the liver, and kidney and prostate diseases often cause massive urinary excretion of vitamin A; a higher intake is then in order. Blood tests can determine the need in such cases.

Those who eat more foods with vitamin A and beta-carotene appear to be less susceptible to lung cancer than those who eat less, but there is no evidence of further benefit from massive doses of supplements. In fact, the vitamin and carotene may not even be responsible for the effect, or they may be only partly responsible. The studies support eating carrots and other vegetables as well as fruits, not taking pills with only one component of the foods.

Hazards. Excessive vitamin A can be toxic to the brain, liver, skin, muscles, and bones. Symptoms can include severe headaches, nausea, vomiting, diarrhea, jaundice, fatigue, lethargy, weight loss, abdominal pain, insomnia, restlessness, brittle nails, hair loss, constipation, irregular menses, emotional distress, mouth fissures, bulging eyeballs, and rough, dry, scaly skin. Bone decalcification, fragility, and pain may also occur. In extreme cases recovery can take months.

The amount constituting a toxic dose of vitamin A varies a great deal. Healthy adults may develop symptoms on a regular total intake of 50,000 IU per day. But liver disease or regular alcohol intake can reduce the toxic dose substantially; in these cases supplements should not be taken without consulting a physician. Infants have developed severe symptoms after one month of 25,000 IU per day. Pregnant women are taking a chance at 20,000 IU a day, which could deform the fetus. There is no benefit to such high levels.

Excessive intake of beta-carotene from huge amounts of vegetables, like a quart or two of carrot juice a day, can cause the skin to turn yellow-orange, a benign effect. The potential for toxicity is much less than with vitamin A itself.

VITAMIN B-1 (THIAMIN)

Thiamin, the antiberiberi factor, is a required cofactor in several energy-producing reactions and is especially important in sugar and amino acid metabolism. Deficiency symptoms include muscle wasting, lassitude, weakness, numbness, paralysis, loss of appetite, mental disturbances, neuritis, and disturbed heart function.

Studies have shown an association of low blood thiamin with a wide variety of so-called functional or neurotic symptoms, such as sleep disturbances, night terrors, depression, dizziness, headaches, chronic fatigue, and loss of appetite. People with these problems often eat no breakfast, snack on soda pop and candies, and eat lunches and dinners with low thiamin contents. This borderline beriberi can easily be prevented by proper diet.

Good **sources** include whole grains, nuts, seeds, beans, peanuts, wheat germ, brewer's yeast, potatoes, dairy products, fish, and lean meat.

Who Needs Supplements? Chronic alcoholism and poor eating habits, especially during pregnancy, growth, surgery, illness, and other stresses, are common causes of low and borderline levels. If refined grain products were not fortified, beriberi would probably be widespread. Fortification of alcoholic beverages is advocated by some. This would probably decrease the incidence of serious nervous disorders in alcoholics.

The RDA is .5 milligrams per 1000 calories, or about 1 to 1.5 milligrams per day. Doses a hundred times this, used by some as an insect repellant, are apparently neither effective nor toxic, but subtle effects from long-term use have not been ruled out. Injection of huge doses kills animals by respiratory depression. Rarely, large doses of thiamin in humans have caused serious hypersensitivity reactions resembling anaphylactic shock, a life-threatening physical collapse. Several hundred milligrams may cause drowsiness in some people.

VITAMIN B-2 (RIBOFLAVIN)

Like thiamin, riboflavin is a coenzyme involved in oxidation and energy-releasing reactions in every cell of the body. Deficiency causes poor growth, sore mouth, tongue, and throat, sinus and eye lesions, dimness of vision, burning eyes, general debility, and possibly cataract.

Sources. Riboflavin is very widespread and often found with thiamin. It is present in almost all plant foods, and is more concentrated in milk and less in grains than thiamin. Nuts, leafy vegetables, legumes, and lean meat are good sources. Fruits contribute appreciable amounts. Cooking with baking soda destroys riboflavin.

Who Needs Supplements? The RDA is about 1 to 2 milligrams, and is easily obtained in a varied diet of unrefined foods. Those with generally poor diets are likely to be deficient. Brewer's yeast and wheat germ are excellent concentrated sources. Single doses many hundreds of times the RDA are apparently not toxic, but long-term effects are unknown.

VITAMIN B-3 (NIACIN)

Niacin is a coenzyme involved in energy-producing reactions in the metabolism of carbohydrates, proteins, and fats. Pellagra (which causes the Four Ds: dermatitis, diarrhea, dementia, and eventually death), occurred in some areas of Europe and the southern United States for many years before its nutritional cause, niacin deficiency, was established in 1915 following experiments with volunteer convicts.

Sources. Good sources include whole grains, nuts, seeds, beans, vegetables, fish, lean meat, and eggs. The amino acid tryptophan can be converted to niacin and provide part of the need, so protein foods are generally good sources. Diets with lots of corn and little else are deficient in niacin and tryptophan, and have been a major cause of pellagra.

Who Needs Supplements? The RDA is about 15 to 20 milligrams and it is easily met by a varied diet of natural foods. Niacin is heavily pushed by the megavitamin advocates, mostly on the dubious strength of its use in psychiatry. Even if it were effective in treating psychosis, that would not be evidence that everyone should take huge doses of it every day. Large doses of niacin are also used to lower cholesterol levels.

Hazards. In doses many times the RDA niacin acts as a drug with effects quite different from those of normal doses. One effect is the reduction of serum cholesterol. Doses up to 5 grams per day are used for this purpose, usually without serious side effects. However, like all drugs such doses may be hazardous. Symptoms of excessive intake include flushing, itching, nausea, diarrhea, stomach bleeding, headaches, and changes in blood sugar and uric acid. Large doses of niacin are available without a prescription, but their use should be supervised by your physician.

VITAMIN B-6 (PYRIDOXINE)

Vitamin B-6 is a coenzyme in the energy-producing metabolism of glucose and in the interconversion of amino acids and carbohydrates, which is important in building proteins and body tissue and in breaking amino acids down for energy. Deficiency symptoms include irritability, depression, insomnia, and other personality and mental changes, abnormal electroencephalogram (EEG), poor growth, anemia, mouth sores, seborrhea around the nose and mouth, difficult walking, abnormal tryptophan metabolism, and various other biochemical changes.

Sources. The richest sources are walnuts, peanuts, brewer's yeast, sun-flower seeds, soybeans, wheat germ, bananas, avocados, liver, lean meat, and fish, followed by whole grains, beans, sweet and white potatoes, almonds, and a very wide variety of other natural foods.

Who Needs Supplements? The RDA is 1.5 to 2 milligrams, easily obtained from moderate amounts of whole natural foods, especially if eaten raw. A diet with plenty of the foods mentioned could supply 20 milligrams a day. Supplements greatly exceeding the RDA can be helpful in B-6 dependency states such as certain anemias (very rare), alcoholism, and isoniazid treatment for tuberculosis. Depression and abnormal tryptophan metabolism in oral contraceptive users can sometimes be corrected by about 50 milligrams a day.

Doses up to 150 milligrams have been used with variable results in the treatment of skin problems, premenstrual syndrome, neuromuscular and neurological disease, and nausea and vomiting in pregnancy. Large doses have also been used in recurring oxalate kidney stones and loss of muscle tone due to levodopa therapy in Parkinson's disease. (The latter use may reduce the drug's effectiveness.) Supplements have been advocated for the prevention of atherosclerosis and coronary artery disease in people with low dietary intakes, but supporting evidence is weak.

Hazards. Vitamin B-6 is apparently safe in amounts several times the RDA, but the very large doses recommended by some orthomolecular and megavitamin advocates are hazardous. Doses over 200 milligrams per day taken for months or years can cause severe, crippling nerve damage. Even smaller doses might be harmful to a fetus, so pregnant women should not take supplements exceeding the RDA without consulting a physician.

VITAMIN B-12 (COBALAMINE)

Like folacin (below), cobalamine is a coenzyme in the synthesis of nucleic acids and DNA. It is also involved in the production of myelin (a protective coating of the nerves), protein synthesis, and other processes. Deficiency causes anemia due to inadequate red blood cell production, as well as myelin destruction followed by numbness and tingling in the hands and feet, poor muscle coordination, mental slowness, depression, confusion, and poor memory, and sometimes full-blown psychosis with delusions and hallucinations.

Sources. The only natural source of vitamin B-12 is synthesis by microorganisms, including those in the digestive tracts of most animals. All animal products (meat, fish, eggs, dairy products) are good sources. Plant foods are devoid of cobalamine unless bacteria-containing root nodules in legumes are included. In some poorer countries grains and vegetables are contaminated with enough insect parts and dirt to prevent deficiency in strict vegetarians. Vitamin B-12 has even been reported in some rain water, probably due to dust particles in the clouds.

Who Needs Supplements? The dietary requirement for vitamin B-12 is extremely small, partly because it is recycled (excreted in the bile and reabsorbed from the intestine) many times. And, unlike the other water-soluble vitamins, an excess is not all flushed right out, but is stored (mostly in the liver) so efficiently that after all dietary sources are withdrawn, it takes two to ten years before symptoms are seen. However, by the time symptoms occur it may be too late to reverse the damage to the nervous system.

Evidence indicates that .5 microgram (a half of a millionth of a gram) per day will sustain normal functions in a healthy person. The RDA is set at 2 micrograms to allow a safety margin. The average intake is higher still, about 6 micrograms a day; thus, deficiency due to dietary lack is very rare. However, there have been a few cases of breast-fed infants of strictly vegetarian mothers who developed B-12 deficiency anemia even though the mothers were fine. Therefore, strict vegetarians who use no milk or other animal products, especially pregnant and lactating women, should take supplements. People lacking intrinsic factor (a substance required for B-12 absorption) usually receive monthly injections of the vitamin for life.

Others who often require supplements include those with malabsorption disorders, gastrectomy, hyperthyroidism, and liver disease. Chronic alcoholics sometimes develop low levels.

Cobalamine is advocated by some as an appetite stimulant and a remedy in various neurological disoders. Studies point to the placebo effect at work rather than any nutritional or pharmacological benefit.

Hazards. Simultaneous ingestion of large doses (100 micrograms) of vitamin B-12 with large doses of vitamin C has been reported to cause nosebleeds, ear bleeding, dry mouth, and decreased ejaculate volume (see **Vitamin C,** below). These may signify serious metabolic abnormalities.

FOLACIN

Folacin (folic acid and related compounds) is a coenzyme in the synthesis of nucleic acids that become components of DNA. It is therefore essential for normal growth, reproduction, blood production, and replacement of all tissue with a high turnover rate, like that of the digestive tract.

Deficiency causes macrocytic anemia, in which red blood cells are few in number and larger than normal due to failure of the young cells to mature in the bone marrow. Early symptoms of deficiency include gastrointestinal disturbances, such as diarrhea and a smooth red tongue. Although folacin deficiency does not damage the nerve myelin, it often causes irritability, forgetfulness, hostility, and paranoid behavior; these symptoms usually improve dramatically within twenty-four hours of folacin therapy.

Sources. As indicated by the name, foliage is an excellent source of folacin. Other good sources include asparagus, broccoli, citrus fruits, nuts, seeds, beans, whole grains, wheat germ, and liver. The richest source is brewer's yeast. A tablespoon can provide almost half the RDA. Heating destroys up to two-thirds of the folacin in food.

Poor sources include most meats, eggs, root vegetables, most fruit, refined grains, and processed milk (especially dried milk). A diet heavy in these foods with very little from the above group can cause deficiency, especially in pregnant and lactating women.

Who Needs Supplements? The requirement is less than once believed, and the RDA is now set at .2 milligrams. Deficiencies are most common in those with malabsorption syndromes, infants with low birth weight, alcohol abusers, pregnant women, and those with various diseases.

Hazards. Large doses of folacin are rapidly excreted. Single doses hundreds of times the RDA are apparently without harmful effects, but prolonged use could lead to precipitation of folacin crystals in the kidneys which may damage them. There is no benefit from such large doses, and they can mask vitamin B-12 deficiency by lessening the anemia while allowing the irreversible nerve damage of B-12 deficiency to continue. Strict vegetarians should not take folacin without also taking vitamin B-12.

CHOLINE

Not exactly a vitamin for humans, choline is a constituent of phospholipids (like lecithin) which aid in the transport and metabolism of fats. It is also part of acetyl choline, an important neurotransmitter, and plays a role in the synthesis of some hormones. Dietary choline is required for normal growth in some animals, but clear-cut deficiency has not been produced in humans because other substances, such as betaine and the amino acid methionine, can do choline's job to some extent.

Sources. Good sources are whole grains, legumes, wheat germ, brewer's yeast, vegetables, and milk. Fruits have little choline. A mixed diet of natural foods provides about .5 to 1 gram of choline a day.

Who Needs Supplements? Choline supplements, usually lecithin, have been tested in age-related memory loss, tardive diskinesia (a neurological disorder often associated with certain antipsychotic drugs) and other neurological disorders, with some successes and some failures reported. There is no clear evidence that anyone benefits from choline supplements.

BIOTIN

This water soluble B-vitamin is required in the synthesis of fatty acids, in the production of energy from carbohydrates, and in the synthesis of DNA, glycogen, and some amino acids. Deficiency causes depression, lassitude, muscle pains, loss of appetite, nausea, anemia, dermatitis, grayish pallor, elevated blood cholesterol, and electrocardiogram abnormalities.

Sources. Biotin is abundant in natural foods with other B-vitamins. It is stable to heat, processing, and storage. Large amounts are also produced by intestinal bacteria.

Who Needs Supplements? The average intake of biotin in the U.S. is about 2 milligrams per day. At least twice this much is made in the intestines. Because intestinal synthesis of biotin is sufficient to meet the human requirement and because it is widespread in food, deficiency is almost unheard of and difficult to produce in volunteers. However, a deficiency can be induced in about one month by eating eight or more raw egg whites a day and by eating only highly refined foods. Raw egg whites contain the protein avidin, which blocks biotin absorption.

A diet high in natural foods can easily supply several milligrams a day. Even the most potent supplements supply less than 1 milligram, so they are usually a waste of money.

PANTOTHENIC ACID

This water-soluble B-vitamin is essential for the production of coenzyme A, one of the most important substances in the body, essential for the synthesis and metabolism of proteins, fats, carbohydrates, and several hormones. Deficiency causes fatigue, headache, insomnia, nausea, personality changes, impaired coordination, numbness and tingling of the hands and feet, and loss of antibody production. Experimental deficiency has been induced with a highly refined diet (supplemented with other vitamins) plus the use of a chemical antagonist to pantothenic acid, without which it would take many months to produce deficiency. Such well-defined deficiency does not occur naturally; a very poor diet causes other deficiencies that confuse the picture. (This is true to some extent with most nutrients.)

Sources. Pantothenic acid exists in all living cells and is therefore present in all natural foods. Its very name means *from everywhere.* Freezing and canning destroy up to half of it and cooking at moderate temperatures up to about 30 percent.

Who Needs Supplements? No RDA has been set, but 5 milligrams per day seems to be a borderline amount. Fifty milligrams can be easily obtained from a diet of natural foods. People who eat a lot of refined foods or drink a lot of alcohol, and those under severe stress due to injury, surgery, or illness, may benefit from supplements. Beans, brewer's yeast, and wheat germ are especially rich sources and are preferable to pantothenic acid pills because they contain several B-vitamins and other nutrients.

This vitamin is often touted as a remedy for graying hair. However, while deficiency causes graying in some animals, large doses do not prevent or reverse graying of hair in humans.

Bioflavinoids, such as rutin and hesperidin, are widely distributed in natural foods, especially those containing vitamin C. They are not considered vitamins because no deficiency state has been induced or discovered in humans or animals. However, they may potentiate vitamin C, allowing a smaller dose to effectively protect people from scurvy, although this is debatable.

Para-Aminobenzoic Acid (PABA), although an important growth factor for lower animals, is not a required nutrient, not a vitamin. It is an excellent sunscreen when applied to the skin, but not when taken internally. Large doses can cause adverse changes in the liver, heart, and kidneys, and a drop in white blood cell count. The marketing of PABA supplements is highly questionable since they provide no benefit and can be hazardous.

Inositol, or myoinositol, is a sugarlike substance very widespread in natural foods. It is a constituent of certain phospholipids, but the human body makes it and it is no longer considered a vitamin. Inositol pills are sold, but they are quite expensive and there is no known benefit from taking them.

VITAMIN C (ASCORBIC ACID)

Ascorbic acid is an essential cofactor in the synthesis of collagen, a protein important in the formation of connective tissue, skin, tendons, and bone. It helps maintain blood vessel strength and is involved in the formation of hemoglobin. Vitamin C is also an antioxidant, like vitamins E and A, helping protect essential oils from oxidation.

Nitrates in food are suspected of forming carcinogenic nitrosamines in the stomach. Vitamin C, whether taken in the food or added, tends to inhibit this reaction. Increased consumption of fresh produce may be partly responsible for the decline of stomach cancer in the United States over the last several decades.

Vitamin C deficiency causes (roughly in order of appearance) fatigue, rough skin with many small hemorrhages under the surface, hemorrhages in the eye, coiled hair, swollen and bleeding gums, pain in the joints, loss of dental fillings, dental caries, a tender mouth, and hair loss. Susceptibility to infections and bacterial toxins increases. Children fail to grow properly.

Sources. Fruits and vegetables are by far the most important sources of vitamin C. Fresh and fresh-frozen produce have higher concentrations than cooked or canned, but even these are left with significant amounts intact. Prolonged storage and drying decrease the vitamin C content.

Some of the richest sources, approximately in order of vitamin C concentration, are: black currants, chili peppers, sweet peppers, broccoli, Brussels sprouts, collards, guavas, kale, parsley, cabbage, cauliflower, oranges, lemons, limes, passion fruit, strawberries, papayas, mangoes, spinach, watercress, asparagus, lima beans, swiss chard, grapefruit, okra, bananas, tangerines, potatoes, tomatoes, peas, melons, pineapple, squash, and corn.

To minimize losses, use produce promptly or store in the refrigerator. After preparation (cooking or cutting up), serve right away. Don't overcook or reheat. Use as little water as possible in cooking; steaming is preferable to boiling. Never add baking soda, and don't thaw frozen produce before cooking.

Who Needs Supplements? It has been determined that the minimum amount of ascorbic acid required to prevent scurvy in most people is approximately 5 to 10 milligrams per day. To provide a margin of safety, the recommended allowance in some countries is 20 to 30 milligrams. To provide a greater safety margin, the RDA is 60 milligrams, about the amount in an average orange or medium mixed salad. The RDA for smokers is 100 milligrams.

There is no question that certain factors increase the need for vitamin C by increasing its excretion or decreasing its absorption. These include certain diseases, severe physical or mental stress, cigarette smoking, aspirin, alcohol, and probably amphetamine, cocaine, and marijuana use. The effect of such factors is grossly exaggerated by vitamin peddlers, who would have everyone take megadoses. All of the factors together would no more than double or triple the vitamin C requirement.

Vitamin C for Colds? Large doses of ascorbic acid have some antihistamine effect, and may be slightly useful in colds and allergic reactions, especially hay fever. Huge doses (several grams a day) on a regular basis are recommended by some for the prevention and treatment of influenza and the common cold. Many studies have been done and the results generally do not support the mega-C advocates. However, some relief may be obtained because of the antihistamine effect.

Hazards. Chewable vitamin C, even in moderate doses, may cause severe dental erosion and should be avoided. (These products perhaps should be removed from the market.) Most people cannot take megadoses of vitamin C for long because they cannot bear the loose bowels and intestinal cramps that so often occur.

At least 10 percent of American blacks, Sephardic Jews, and some people of Mediterranean and Middle Eastern ancestry are deficient in an important red-blood-cell enzyme, glucose 6-phosphate dehydrogenase (G6-PD), and are highly susceptible to drug-induced hemolytic anemia (red cell destruction). Megadoses of vitamin C act as a powerful chemical reducing agent and can cause potentially fatal anemia in these people.

Excessive vitamin C can cause excessive absorption of iron and consequent iron poisoning, especially if iron intake is also high. At least one young man has died of heart failure apparently due to this effect.

People with sickle-cell disease are likewise vulnerable because the vitamin C converts their oxidized hemoglobin to reduced hemoglobin, which takes the sickle shape, clogs capillaries, and causes severe illness. Without treatment, they may die.

Diabetics must be careful with vitamin C. Megadoses can cause the Testape test for urine sugar to be falsely negative, and the Clinitest to be falsely positive. This could lead to underdose or overdose of insulin, and consequent diabetic crisis or insulin shock.

The strong reducing action of mega-C can also distort the occult blood test for colon cancer. Because of the large number of people who take megadoses, this is becoming an important problem in older people and those deemed at risk for the disease.

Ascorbic acid is normally converted to oxalic acid, which is broken down and excreted in the urine. Some people's bodies can't break down oxalic acid fast enough, and prolonged use of megadoses of vitamin C may increase their susceptibility to oxalate kidney stone formation.

Vitamin C deficiency can impair immunity, but extra amounts do not confer extra benefits; they may, in fact, impair the bactericidal power of leucocytes.

Perhaps the strongest argument against the use of megadoses of ascorbic acid is an increased rate of catabolism and excretion of the vitamin, leaving the person more vulnerable than ever to deficiency symptoms should the intake be reduced to natural levels. In essence, the requirement is increased. If you take two or more grams for as little as two weeks and then stop you may experience bleeding gums, loosened teeth, and aching muscles in the following weeks. Such symptoms don't normally occur until several months after total withdrawal of all vitamin C. Cases of infantile scurvy in spite of an intake of at least 60 milligrams per day have been attributed to excessive doses taken by mothers during pregnancy.

One other very disturbing effect of mega-C has been reported. A thirty-five-year-old chemist took 1 gram of vitamin C and 100 micrograms of vitamin B-12 every day. After only one week he experienced nosebleed, spontaneous bleeding from the external ear, dry mouth, and decreased ejaculate volume. Several repetitions of the experiment by him and others confirmed the effect. This illustrates the complex, and sometimes dangerous, interactions of megadoses of nutrients.

How Much Is Safe? No one knows for sure. It depends largely on an individual's blood chemistry and use of other supplements. Probably no one is immune to the development of increased tolerance from taking large doses. Several large servings (five to ten) of vitamin C-rich foods could provide about a gram (1,000 milligrams) a day. This probably wouldn't cause adverse effects because the vitamin C would gradually enter the blood throughout the day rather than in one huge dose. But it is far more than most bodies could use, and most would be excreted unused.

Dr. Linus Pauling suggests up to 9 grams on a regular basis, since this amount could theoretically be obtained from foods alone. But to get this amount from food, you would have to eat nothing but chili peppers, sweet peppers, and black currants—not exactly a natural diet.

If you already eat lots of vitamin C-rich foods, supplements would just increase destruction rate and make you more susceptible to deficiency should your intake suddenly drop. If you are not eating such foods and want some protection from your smoking, aspirin use, emotional stress, and so on, 300 milligrams per day (thirty times the minimum to prevent scurvy) would surely be all your body could use on a regular basis. It should be considered an upper limit of regular supplementation in almost all cases. If more is used, say for its antihistamine effect, two or three days should be the limit. Large amounts should be spread throughout the day, not taken all at once. This decreases the likelihood of adverse reactions occurring.

VITAMIN D (CHOLECALCIFEROL)

Vitamin D is necessary for the absorption of calcium from the intestine and for normal bone metabolism. Without it, bone mineralization is impaired and rickets (in children) or osteomalacia (in adults) occurs. It has been known for almost a hundred years that sunshine is a specific cure for rickets, although vitamin D was not discovered until the 1920s.

Sources. The precursor of vitamin D, dehydrocholesterol, is present in the lubricating oily material in and on the skin of animals and humans. When ultraviolet radiation from the sun falls on the skin, one of the four rings of the molecule is broken, forming the three-ringed cholecalciferol, or vitamin D, which is absorbed into the blood.

Vitamin D occurs naturally in fatty fish (such as tuna, sardines, and herring), eggs, liver, butter, and other animal-produced foods. A large number of packaged foods are vitamin D fortified, especially milk, breakfast cereals, and margarines.

One hundred International Units (IU) per day prevents rickets and ensures normal mineralization and growth in practically all children, but the RDA is set at 400 IU for all ages to allow a large safety margin. This amount can be synthesized on the skin by exposure of only the arms to moderate intensity sunshine for about twenty minutes. Clouds decrease the effectiveness only a little, unless they are very thick and the sky quite dark, because ultraviolet rays penetrate the clouds; on the other hand, they are blocked by glass and reduced by air pollution.

Who Needs Supplements? Vitamin D is one of the most potent vitamins; the RDA of 400 IU is only 10 *micrograms,* a barely visible speck. It is also toxic, oil soluble, and cumulative, so excessive intake must be avoided. Those who don't get a daily dose of sunlight or vitamin D foods should consider a supplement. A good example would be a vegetarian who doesn't eat fortified foods and gets little sun exposure. Vitamin D deficiency is a very common factor in hip fractures in elderly people who don't get out much and get little of the vitamin in their diet. Some experts recommend up to twice the RDA for the susceptible elderly.

Hazards. Some vitamin promoters advocate doses many times the RDA and contend that they are harmless. They are apparently not familiar with several reports of the devastating consequences that excessive vitamin D can have. For example, infants given excessive doses have developed generalized hardening of the arteries; severe mental retardation;

a peculiar facial structure with large ears, a high narrow palate, and irregular, carious teeth; kidney damage; recurrent infection; loss of appetite; and failure to grow. Discontinuing the vitamin D leads to dramatic improvement if it is not too late.

In Great Britain in the 1950s there was a rash of such cases associated with excessive fortification of dried milk and other foods provided by the government with vitamin D. Several hundred children were affected, many of whom died. The intake in these cases was generally only 1,000 to 2,500 IU, much less than the ten-fold increase over the RDA said by some to be safe. In 1957, the British Ministry of Health recommended a 70 percent reduction of vitamin D in fortified milk and cereals.

Adults are by no means exempt from these problems. Combined with moderately high calcium intake, excessive vitamin D can cause calcium deposites in vital organs. The kidneys are especially vulnerable to damage. Animal studies also indicate dangerous increases in cholesterol and triglyceride levels.

The widespread fortification of foods in sunny climates for consumption by sun-loving whites is highly questionable. Consider, for example, a white person of northern European ancestry who tans poorly, lives in a sunny area, surfs, eats fortified breakfast cereal with fortified milk (in addition to drinking half a gallon a day), and takes a multivitamin with D in it and antacids with calcium carbonate. This amounts to twenty or more times the vitamin D RDA in a sensitive person with a very high calcium intake, and it spells *danger*. The sun exposure alone would unquestionably be more than adequate. All the rest probably increases, rather than decreases, the risk to health.

VITAMIN E (TOCOPHEROL)

In 1922 it was learned that rats fed mostly rancid lard with adequate amounts of the known vitamins could not bear offspring. Adding the fat-soluble substance tocopherol, from lettuce or wheat germ, restored fertility. It was dubbed vitamin E. Deficiency also harms muscles and the nervous and circulatory systems. It has been established that vitamin E is an antioxidant, that it protects vitamin A and unsaturated fats from oxidation, and that it prevents cell membrane damage from naturally occurring peroxides. In healthy humans deficiencies are very rare. In cases of sprue, cystic fibrosis, and other malabsorption problems, deficiencies may cause impaired red blood cell survival, elevated platelet count, skin lesions, and other changes.

Sources. Vegetables, seeds, grains, and their oils are the best sources of tocopherol. Fruits, meats, beans, eggs, and dairy products contribute significant amounts, as do most margarines, salad oils, and shortenings.

Who Needs Supplements? There is no question that most premature infants and people with malabsorption problems should have supplements, but beyond that, controversy rages. The Food and Nutrition Board says 10 milligrams is plenty and that adequate amounts are found in a varied diet. Although increasing vegetable oil consumption increases the requirement, the oil almost always provides that extra vitamin E.

Vitamin industry representatives and a few physicians advocate up to 800 milligrams, about eighty times the RDA, on a regular basis to prevent and cure a long list of ailments including heart disease, varicose veins, phlebitis and other circulatory disorders, cancer, menopausal symptoms, leg cramps, shingles, arthritis, and diabetes. It is also used in efforts to promote wound (especially burn) healing, fertility, and libido functioning. So far all the dramatic claims of cures have been anecdotal, not scientific. Several scientific studies have failed to detect any real benefits, nor is there any evidence that vitamin E supplements can improve atheletic performance or stamina.

Hazards. Vitamin E, like vitamins A and D, is oil-soluble, and an excess is not readily excreted. This alone is grounds for caution. Excessive vitamin E has been shown to reduce blood thyroid levels in some people. This may account for some of the reported side effects of megadoses: headaches, severe fatigue, nausea, blurred vision, dizziness, inflammation of the mouth, chapped lips, muscle weakness, low blood sugar, increased bleeding tendencies, inhibited wound healing, increased blood fats (especially in women), increased cholesterol levels, and gastrointestinal disturbances. The elevated levels of fat and cholesterol could promote heart disease, which is ironic in view of the claims that vitamin E can prevent atherosclerosis. Some people who suffer fatigue and weakness from large doses (800 IU per day) excrete large amounts of creatinine, a protein that indicates possible skeletal muscle damage.

VITAMIN K

Vitamin K is necessary for the synthesis of prothrombin and other blood clotting factors in the liver. A deficiency causes poor clotting and hemorrhage. At least half the requirement is met by production by intestinal bacteria; the rest comes from leafy greens.

Who Needs Supplements? It is difficult to produce a deficiency by dietary restriction alone. However, combined with antibiotics, which destroy intestinal bacteria, poor diet can lead to a deficiency and poor blood clotting. Newborn infants, especially if premature, are sometimes deficient before their digestive tracts are fully mature. Breast milk has low levels of vitamin K, so supplementation may be advisable for the first few months. Chronic fat malabsorption, which occurs in certain uncommon ailments, can lead to deficiency, and liver disease sometimes increases the requirement.

Hazards. The natural forms of vitamin K, K-1 (phylloquinone), and K-2 (menaquinone) are apparently completely safe, even in very large doses. However, the synthetic K-3 and its various derivatives can be toxic even in moderate doses.

Minerals

Nutrient minerals are those basic chemical elements that are required in the diet for normal growth, reproduction, and health. They are often classified as "major" or "trace" minerals, depending on the amounts required. Although requirements for calcium and phosphorous are many thousands of times greater than those for iodine, chromium, and other trace minerals, the minerals in the middle range are difficult to classify. Moreover, the distinction may imply that the major minerals are more important than the others which is not true. Therefore, we will simply discuss the minerals in alphabetical order, with chloride discussed under sodium chloride and "other trace minerals" discussed last.

CALCIUM

Calcium is required for normal bone development, blood clotting, muscle tone, nerve transmission, and heart muscle function. The mineral also appears to provide some protection against hypertension and colon cancer. If insufficient amounts are ingested, the blood level is maintained (by parathyroid hormone) at the cost of bone calcium. Poor growth and poor bones and teeth result.

Sources. The richest sources are milk, hard cheese, dark green leafy vegetables, and soft-boned fish. Other good sources include legumes, broccoli, string beans, artichokes, almonds, sesame seeds, soft cheeses, tofu made with calcium, and figs. Fair sources include cottage cheese, nuts, whole grains, carrots, eggs, oranges, dates, and prunes. Most meats, fruits, and vegetables are poor sources.

Who Needs Supplements? One and a third cups of milk provide about 400 milligrams which, along with another 400 milligrams from vegetables and other sources, supply the RDA for most children and adults. However, those age eleven to twenty-four should get 1200 milligrams, as should pregnant and lactating women.

A handy rule of thumb in calculating your calcium intake is the "rule of 300s." You can get about 300 milligrams of calcium from each of the following: a cup of milk; a cup of yogurt; one and a half ounces of cheese; two and a half ounces of canned sardines or salmon (with bones); and several average servings of all lesser food sources combined—beans, grains, vegetables. Any combination of four of these supplies 1200 milligrams of calcium. Women should get one major source of calcium at each meal. If their diet is good the lesser sources will provide the rest of the requirement.

If these guidelines cannot be followed, supplements may be in order. Food sources are much preferable, though, and pills should not be taken for "insurance" if the diet is adequate because excess calcium can affect the absorption of other minerals. The safest supplements are pure calcium carbonate, while those made from powdered oyster shell, bone meal, and dolomite often contain lead, cadmium, and mercury, and they should be avoided. Calcium from supplements is better absorbed if taken with a meal or snack. Prolonged excessive calcium intake can cause calcification of soft tissues and kidney stone formation, especially if vitamin D is also taken. Most people should avoid total calcium intake of more than 2 grams per day including food sources, supplements, and calcium-containing antacids.

COPPER

Copper is involved in the formation and functions of blood, bones, nerves, reproductive organs, and various enzymes. Deficiency can cause anemia, skeletal defects, degeneration of the nervous system, elevated cholesterol levels, and possibly cardiovascular disease.

Sources of copper include various meats, nuts, seeds, peas, grains, beans, and many whole, unprocessed foods. Dairy products are a poor source.

Supplements of up to 5 milligrams a day, preferably in a multimineral formula, should be taken by anyone who eats poorly.

FLUORIDE

Fluoride is incorporated into the teeth and greatly increases resistance to tooth decay. It is also incorporated into bones and may be essential for normal growth and development.

Sources of fluoride include almost all foods, especially seafood, and drinking water, but the amounts present may be less than necessary to prevent dental decay.

Supplements are advisable for people whose drinking water is deficient; fluoridation has proved to be a safe and very effective way of reducing the incidence of dental caries. (See **Dental and Gum Disease** in Section Two for more on this.)

IODINE

Iodine is a component of the metabolism-regulating hormone thyroxin. When iodine is lacking, the thyroid gland enlarges, sometimes to a volume greater than the whole head. In spite of simple and inexpensive means of prevention, endemic goiter is possibly the most common single deficiency disease in the world, with more than two hundred million people affected. Most of them are in developing nations, isolated villages of Europe, northern India, and South and Central America.

Sources. The best sources of iodine used to be seafoods, including seaweed, which the Chinese have used to treat goiters for five thousand years. The ancient Egyptians and Incas also used this remedy. The biggest source of dietary iodine in the United States now is dairy products. Farmers feed cows lots of iodine in the belief (unproved) that this prevents foot rot. Moreover, many iodine-containing chemicals are used as antiseptics to clean and sanitize milking machines, storage vats, transport tankers, and other equipment.

The use of iodine chemicals in cleaning food processing equipment has also led to high levels in grain products, sugars, and sugar products such as candies, jams, and puddings. Other important sources include iodized salt and fast foods.

Iodine deficiency was once a problem in the midwestern United States where the soil and the foods grown in it had little of the mineral. This led to the widespread use of iodized salt to prevent goiters. But now most Americans get far more iodine than they need, typically five to ten times the RDA, which is 150 micrograms for adults. These high levels are safe for most people, but pose certain hazards for some, especially those with thyroid problems. Extremely high intakes, fifty or more times the RDA, are common among seaweed gatherers in Japan and cause many of them to develop goiters.

Who Needs Supplements? Strict vegetarians who do not eat dairy products, processed grain, or sugar products, and whose vegetables and fruits are grown in noncoastal areas, should use iodized salt or take supplements. One gram of the salt provides about half the RDA.

IRON

Iron is an essential component of the metabolic enzymes in every cell of the body. Most of it is present in the blood cells as hemoglobin. Deficiency, especially when combined with chronic blood loss such as with hemorrhoids and heavy menstrual bleeding, causes anemia, the lack of sufficient red blood cells or hemoglobin. It leads to fatigue, weakness, pallor, shortness of breath, lack of appetite, and a general slowing of vital functions. Mild deficiency in children has been linked to clumsiness, low IQ scores, inattentiveness, and restlessness.

Sources. Good sources include lean meats, fish, eggs, legumes, nuts, some fruits, whole grains, and leafy greens. Most whole, natural foods provide significant amounts of iron. Cow's milk is a poor source; human milk is generally much better. A varied diet of whole natural foods easily supplies the required amounts. For example, 2,500 calories worth of potatoes, broccoli, whole grains, carrots, and other mediocre iron sources supplies the generous RDA (15 milligrams) for women of child-bearing age. The requirement for men is less, and so is even more easily met.

Who Needs Supplements? The body uses iron very economically, absorbing it much more efficiently when stores are low and storing large amounts of reserves, that last for months, when the intake is large. Therefore, deficiency develops only after a long period of unusually high need, as during pregnancy and growth, and after severe blood loss, as in active ulcers, hemorrhoids, and heavy menstrual flow. Borderline intake in young girls for months or years prior to the onset of menses may result in deficiency when blood loss begins. Repeated pregnancies are especially costly to women's iron stores. In these situations, supplementation is usually advisable. IUD users often have heavy menstrual flow and often need supplements. However, supplements should not be taken without proper blood studies because iron can be very upsetting to the stomach and an excess can be hazardous.

Sources of iron, such as ferrous sulfate, fumarate, and gluconate, are all well absorbed. If one causes gastrointestinal distress, another can be tried.

Hazards. There is no advantage to taking supplemental iron unless anemia is present or stores are very low. Prolonged intake of 250 milligrams per day can cause serious problems due to iron build up. While 60 milligrams per day is a common therapeutic dose, even this amount, if not needed, can decrease absorption of zinc and possibly other trace minerals, and can be toxic if vitamin C intake is high.

MAGNESIUM

Magnesium is an essential cofactor in the metabolism of carbohydrates, protein synthesis, normal calcium and potassium metabolism, and other important biochemical processes. It is involved in the regulation of body temperature and in nerve and muscle function.

Symptoms of deficiency include loss of appetite, nausea, apathy, tremors, convulsions, and coma. Even mild deficiency may cause cardiac arrhythmias.

Sources. The best sources are whole grains, nuts, beans, peanuts, leafy greens, wheat germ, and brewer's yeast. Hard water and most fruits and vegetables have fair amounts, which can add up to a lot. For example, a mixed fruit salad would contain about 200 milligrams per 1,000 calories, or 500 milligrams per 2,500 calories. The RDA is 250 to 400 milligrams. Clearly, a diet with generous amounts of natural foods easily provides the requirement. Diets heavy in refined foods may present a problem; for example, brown rice has about 250 milligrams per 100 grams, but white rice has only 25 milligrams.

Who Needs Supplements? People most likely to need supplements are alcoholics, malnourished infants, pregnant or lactating women with poor diets, those taking high doses of diuretics for long periods, people who fast frequently, those on highly refined diets, and heavy exercisers with mediocre diets. The best supplement is pure magnesium oxide; dolomite often contains toxic heavy metals and should be avoided. Excessive magnesium frequently causes diarrhea, which should not be surprising since one of the most popular and heavily advertised laxatives, Milk of Magnesia, is a slurry of magnesium hydroxide. Excessive magnesium can also affect the absorption of other minerals, so no more than the RDA should be taken.

PHOSPHOROUS

Phosphorous combines with calcium to mineralize bones and teeth. Small amounts are also essential to almost every reaction in the body. Deficiency causes stunted growth and weak bones and teeth.

Sources. Phosphorous is widely distributed, especially in protein-rich foods like meat, fish, and milk, but also in whole grains, vegetables, and fruits.

Who Needs Supplements? Because of its widespread availability, deficiency is almost unheard of except in cases of very poor diet and heavy, prolonged use of aluminum-containing antacids. Strict vegetarians who avoid dairy and other animal products (vegans) might also have borderline intakes. Isolated phosphorous supplementation is almost never necessary or desirable. Some believe that excessive phosphorous from a diet heavy in meat and soda pop may induce a relative calcium deficiency, but the evidence is weak.

POTASSIUM

Potassium is the major intracellular element, and deficiency results in muscle weakness or even paralysis. Potassium is widely distributed in both plant and animal foods. The best **sources** are fruits and vegetables and their juices.

Who Needs Supplements? Potassium is lost in fasting, severe protein deficiency, injury, diuretic use, and diarrhea. Endurance athletes should be especially careful to get adequate amounts. However, potassium supplements, like potassium chloride, can be hazardous; an excess may cause death by depression of heart function. Those who need large amounts should eat fruit and vegetables and drink their juices.

SODIUM AND CHLORIDE

These essential nutrients are important in the electrolyte and water balances in cells, nerves, muscles, and the body as a whole. Chloride is also a component of gastric acid (hydrochloric acid). Depletion causes muscle cramping, loss of appetite, and, progressively, apathy, convulsions, coma, and death.

Sources. Sodium chloride (table salt) is widely distributed in foods, so depletion is very rare except from prolonged vomiting, diarrhea, or diuretic use, and heavy sweating.

Who Needs Supplements? Moderate to heavy work in hot conditions can increase the sodium requirement by several grams a day, but salt should be added to food, not taken as tablets. It can also be added to water, but no more than a half teaspoon (2 grams) per liter. If little sweating occurs, little sodium is required, and there is usually no need to salt foods, most of which already have some sodium. Excessive salt intake is believed to be a major factor in hypertension in sensitive people, perhaps in one-third of all cases.

ZINC

Zinc is an essential coenzyme in a long list of reactions in the body such as the synthesis of RNA, DNA, and proteins. Deficiency causes dwarfism, failure of sex glands to mature, anemia, abnormal hair and nail growth, decreased pancreatic enzymes, decreased hormone synthesis, decreased alcohol tolerance, poor wound healing, and impaired immunity.

Sources. Zinc is very widely distributed in plant and animal tissues. All natural foods have some, but fruits and green vegetables tend to have less than whole grains, legumes, and nuts. These latter sources, however, have high levels of phytates, which tend to bind much of the zinc and prevent its absorption. The richest sources of available zinc are wheat germ, fish, and meats. Nuts are generally better than beans and grains. Sprouting grains and seeds reduce the phytate activity and increase zinc availability. Making bread with yeast and allowing it to rise eliminates much of the phytate activity and greatly increases zinc availability.

Who Needs Supplements? The RDA is about 10 to 20 milligrams. Slow-growing children, especially if they eat poorly or are strict vegetarians, and those with sickle-cell anemia often benefit from daily supplements of about 1 milligram per kilogram body weight (about .5 milligrams per pound). Zinc directly promotes growth and may also improve the appetite.

While up to 150 milligrams per day have been used for treating deficiency, alcoholism, acne, and ulcers, such doses should not be taken by normal healthy persons for prolonged periods because excessive zinc may cause nausea, vomiting, low blood copper, and anemia. It might also promote atherosclerosis by interfering with copper function, increasing LDL-cholesterol, and decreasing HDL-cholesterol. It may inhibit immune responses. Large doses taken by pregnant women may induce premature birth.

Zinc for Colds? In recent years zinc has been promoted as a cold remedy. Proponents say that sucking on zinc tablets at the first sign of a cold can nip it in the bud by inhibiting the viral infection. One of our associates tried this once. It did not work, but even if it had it could not be recommended: Zinc tastes so horrible that sucking on it for even ten minutes is worse torture than a week-long cold. This is one potential fad that will never catch on.

OTHER TRACE MINERALS

Recent research reveals that tiny amounts of the unlikeliest elements are essential nutrients without which reproduction, growth, and health are not possible. Who would have guessed, for example, that we have a dietary requirement for tin, chromium, or nickel? Others proved or strongly suspected to be essential include manganese, boron, molybdenum, vanadium, and silicon. Selenium deficiency may damage heart muscle, promote cancer, and weaken the immune system. Even cadmium may have a biological function, though it is toxic in large amounts, as are the others.

Sources. As with so many other essential nutrients, these elements are very widely distributed and present in hundreds of natural foods but are largely removed by refining. For example, by milling wheat 40 to 90 percent of the chromium, manganese, zinc, molybdenum, and copper are removed. Other trace nutrients are also lost. "Enriched" bread is a consumer fraud since it contains added amounts of only a few of the many nutrients removed by processing. Besides trace minerals, amino acids, fiber, vitamin E, and other components are lost and not replaced. This is yet another reason to eat more natural and fewer refined foods.

Since the presence of trace elements varies a great deal and is dependent on soil content, a variety of foods from different areas should be eaten. Dependence on locally grown foods, as advocated by macrobiotics, can contribute to deficiencies, as dramatically illustrated by the high incidence of goiter in many areas of the world where the iodine content of the soil is poor, and high cancer incidence where selenium levels are low.

Who Needs Supplements? Many trace element preparations are on the market and people wonder if they should take them. If one has a highly refined diet, trace mineral supplements might be of value, but it would make a lot more sense to simply eat a variety of natural foods. Taking high doses of trace elements can be dangerous. For example, as little as two weeks of high-potency selenium can cause hair loss, fatigue, vomiting, and other symptoms of toxicity.

What About Hair Analysis? Some commercial labs claim they can determine your trace mineral needs by analyzing your hair. Such claims are false. Many variables affect hair mineral content, and no clear association of hair levels with tissue levels or nutritional needs has been established. Hair analysis may reveal high levels of lead, mercury, and other toxic heavy metals, but we wouldn't trust a lab that makes claims about detecting deficiencies to do a proper job on heavy metal detection.

Food Poisoning and Parasites

We have known for a long time that foods can be infested and contaminated with organisms and toxins that cause illnesses (usually nausea, vomiting, and diarrhea) that can sometimes become very severe and occasionally fatal. While even our most ancient ancestors had to contend with visible molds, which they probably recognized as a source of illness, most of the offending organisms and toxins have been identified only in recent decades. The most important ones are bacteria and bacterial toxins, mold toxins, protozoa, viruses, and worms. Hundreds of thousands of Americans are stricken by such organisms each year.

Bacteria and Bacterial Toxins

There are many bacteria that contaminate foods and, either by infection or poisoning, make us sick. For example, more than 1700 kinds of *Salmonella* bacteria thrive in raw meats, poultry, fish, eggs, and milk and multiply rapidly at room temperature. Within twelve to forty-eight hours after the foods are eaten symptoms begin. The nausea, vomiting, diarrhea, abdominal cramps, headache, and fever can last for a week. The infection may be lethal in infants, the elderly, and the infirm.

Staphylococcus bacteria poison foods if they are left too long at room temperature. Cream-filled pastries, meats, poultry, eggs, tuna, and all the products and dishes made from them are especially vulnerable. Seemingly minor staph infections of the skin of food handlers can be the source of the bacteria. Typical symptoms of poisoning are similar to those caused by *Salmonella* toxins. They usually begin within one to eight hours of eating and last a day or two. The toxins are rarely lethal.

Shigella, Campylobacter, Clostridium, and *Yersinia* are bacteria that have similar sources and produce illnesses similar to those above. **Shigellosis** is especially troublesome and difficult to get rid of in day-care centers, where good hygiene must always be strived for. *Yersinia,* often from raw milk, can produce symptoms that mimic appendicitis so closely that unnecessary surgery may be done.

Vibrio cholerae bacteria cause **cholera.** The symptoms range from mild to very severe diarrhea, which can lead to dehydration and death. The most common sources are fish and shellfish, especially raw oysters taken from waters contaminated by human sewage.

Prevention of Illness from Bacteria in Food. All food must be handled, cooked, and stored properly. Be aware that bacteria are lurking on your skin, nails, and hair, and that they can multiply and produce toxins in foods. All raw animal products will rapidly breed bacteria when left at room temperature. Be careful to wash cutting boards, plates, knives, and other utensils used with raw poultry or meat before using them again. Do not touch your face, hair, or body while handling food. Don't handle any animals and then food without first washing your hands. Don't drink raw milk; even "certified" raw milk has been associated with serious illness and death. Even cooked foods can breed dangerous bacteria; they generally must be refrigerated within an hour or two of cooking. Foods should be refrigerated at 40° F or below.

Undercooked and raw eggs and dishes containing them should be avoided. There is a growing problem with eggs being contaminated during formation in chickens' ovaries, so that no matter how carefully they are handled, stored, and inspected, they can cause illness. Therefore, all eggs should be thoroughly cooked: boiled for seven minutes, poached for five minutes, or fried for three minutes on each side. Eating eggs with runny yolks is risky. Ice cream, Caesar salad dressing, hollandaise sauce, eggnog, and mayonnaise containing raw eggs should *not* be homemade. Commercial products are safe because the eggs used in them have been pasteurized.

Botulism is caused by a toxin produced by *Clostridium botulinum* bacteria. These bacteria are widespread but they produce the toxin only in an oxygen-free environment of low acidity (high pH). Low-acid foods, such as beans, olives, beef, mushrooms, and spinach, that are canned without adequate cooking are ideal for *botulinum* toxin production. The most common source of botulism is home-canned foods. Honey also may have large amounts of *botulinum* spores, which are harmless to adults but can cause botulism in infants. Honey should not be fed to infants (see **Infant Nutrition**).

Botulism is rare but important because it is potentially lethal and will occur whenever we get careless about canned foods. Neurotoxic symptoms of botulism start within eight to thirty-six hours after eating and include double vision, difficulty in swallowing and talking, and progressive paralysis of the respiratory system. The latter leads to death if the person is not treated. *Botulinum* antitoxins are effective if given in time. If the above symptoms appear, get medical help immediately.

Prevention of Botulism. Do your home canning with the utmost care, and never cut corners; above all, don't reduce pressure cooking time. Don't eat food from cans (commercial or home-prepared) that are swollen, leaking, or broken.

Will French Convenience Foods Cause Botulism Outbreaks? A new type of convenience food, already very popular in Europe and making inroads in the United States, is considered by the Food and Drug Administration (FDA) a potential bacterial monster (however, the FDA cannot take action until the products actually hurt someone). The French invention is called *sous-vide* (under vacuum) refrigerated foods. These fresh, lightly cooked, tasty dishes, vacuum-sealed in plastic pouches and spared the temperature extremes of freezing and canning, are ready to be dropped into boiling water. The problem is that the oxygen-free environment in the pouches provides a breeding ground for some very dangerous bacteria, including those responsible for botulism and listeriosis, another potentially lethal form of food poisoning.

The *sous-vide* process kills the harmless microorganisms whose foul odor might have warned of spoilage, but does not kill dangerous bacteria that produce no odor: The food could look and smell fine but be poisonous. Therefore, the chain of refrigeration from factory to boiling water must not be broken. Some experts fear slip-ups during shipping and storage could lead to massive outbreaks of deadly food poisoning. However, the products have an excellent record in Europe, and some American restaurants have been using vacuumed-packed refrigerated foods for a decade without any reported problems. Because the foods taste better than frozen and canned foods, their popularity is sure to grow. One possible safety measure would be color indicators on the labels to indicate if the refrigeration chain has been broken. If you buy these foods get them from the store to your refrigerator as fast as you can and follow cooking instructions carefully.

Traveler's diarrhea, frequently contracted by American tourists in parts of Latin America, the Middle East, Africa, and Asia, is most often caused by food- and water-borne strains of *Escherichia coli* bacteria that attach themselves to the intestinal lining and produce toxins provoking diarrhea. To prevent traveler's diarrhea avoid fruits, vegetables, and other raw foods that may have been handled or rinsed with bad water, which is common in Mexico and some other countries. Stick to cooked foods and fruits that you peel yourself. Avoid raw dairy products. Avoid water and ice if it has not been chlorinated or otherwise treated. Brush your teeth using boiled or bottled water or mouth rinse.

Prevention of Traveler's Diarrhea. Although commonly prescribed by doctors, some experts believe that taking antibiotics for prevention is not recommended because the risk of adverse side effects and emergence of resistant bacteria outweigh the benefits. However, bismuth subsalicylate (like Pepto-Bismol) is an effective preventive for about 75 percent of those who try it. The necessary dose is quite large, about a quarter cup or two tablets, four times a day. Tablets are often more convenient for travelers. The regimen is expensive, about five dollars a day; it should be started the day before departure and continued for two days after returning. It should *not* be taken for more than three weeks. Bismuth subsalicylate should not be taken by people who are allergic to aspirin, or by those who are taking large doses of aspirin or any prescription drug without consulting a physician. Moreover, it can be constipating, and therefore may aggravate hemorrhoids. Some experts believe the cost and risks of using bismuth subsalicylate to prevent traveler's diarrhea outweigh its benefits, and they recommend against it.

Mycotoxins

Several types of molds establish themselves on a variety of foods, especially grains, beans, peanuts, and their products. Some of them produce toxins that can cause liver and kidney disease. *Aspergillus flavus,* which is found on corn and grain, for example, is one of the most potent carcinogens known and is responsible for thousands of cases of liver cancer worldwide each year.

Prevention of Mold Poisoning. Don't eat foods with visible mold. Don't eat moldly or shriveled peanuts. Store grains and other susceptible foods in closed containers in a cool, dry place.

Protozoa

Some varieties of these single-cell organisms can infect the human intestinal tract, cause sickness, and be spread through the feces. For example, **giardiasis** is caused by the flagellate *Giardia lamblia* and **amebiasis** is caused by the ameba *Entamoeba histolytica.* Symptoms of these infections include diarrhea, abdominal pain, gas, anemia, and weight loss. Several effective drugs can usually clear up the infections.

Prevention of Protozoal Infection. Avoid raw fruits and vegetables in areas where protozoa are endemic. Food handlers must keep their hands clean at all times, especially if food is to be served raw. Sewage must be properly disposed of and local sanitation laws must be obeyed to avoid contamination of drinking water supplies. When hiking and camping don't drink water from streams or lakes, no matter how clean it appears, without boiling it for a few seconds.

Viruses

Several varieties of enteroviruses, rotaviruses, parvoviruses, and others exist in human digestive tracts and are expelled in feces, which may then contaminate food and water. Symptoms of infection include severe diarrhea, nausea, and vomiting and usually last less than a week but they may last longer and respiratory symptoms may develop.

The most important food-borne virus is **hepatitis A.** Primary food sources include shellfish from waters contaminated with human sewage, and foods, usually raw, handled by those carrying and shedding the virus, whether or not they have symptoms of infection. (Hepatitis is discussed in detail in Section Two.)

Prevention of Diseases from Viruses in Food. Patients and known carriers of hepatitis viruses should not handle food to be eaten or utensils to be used by others. Food handlers at all levels must make sure their hands are absolutely clean. It is especially important to wash the hands thoroughly after using the toilet. Shellfish from contaminated waters should be avoided and local sewage disposal laws should be obeyed to avoid contaminating water supplies.

Worms

The worms that make foods hazardous to eat are not the visible insect larvae on our lettuce and in our apples that we mistakenly call worms: Those little beasties are specialized for crop devastation and cannot directly harm humans or animals even if swallowed alive. The worms we are concerned about here are usually microscopic eggs or larvae of real worms, not insects. They occur in the tissues and wastes of cattle, hogs, fish, and other animals, and may grow to prodigious size once the adult form is settled in a host.

Trichinella spiralis is a tiny roundworm that infects swine, rats, bears, walruses, and other wild animals. Young larvae settle in skeletal muscle fibers, grow into the adolescent spiral form, and develop protective shells. They stay largely unchanged for years. If the flesh is eaten, their shells protect them from stomach acid. They mature and mate in the intestines, die, and are evacuated, while their larvae bore through the intestinal wall and ride the blood to the muscles.

The severity of symptoms of this worm infection, known as **trichinosis** or **trichinellosis,** depends on the number ingested and the individual's immunity. During the intestinal phase there is rarely more than mild diarrhea, but after the muscles have been invaded symptoms may include muscle pain, fever, nausea and vomiting, headache, facial swelling, and difficult breathing. In severe cases death may occur in about a month, but drug treatment is usually successful. Severe illness and death are not common, but experts suspect that a quarter million or so mild cases go unreported each year.

Prevention of Trichinellosis. Don't eat raw or undercooked meat of swine, wild boar, bear, walrus, or other game, as cool spots in the meat can leave surviving worms. Microwave oven cooking is especially troublesome in this regard. For microwave cooking of pork and other potential sources of *trichinella,* the U.S. Department of Agriculture recommends that evenly shaped cuts of five pounds or less be cooked at a medium setting (300 to 350 watts), with frequent rotation, to 170°F throughout, then allowed to sit at least ten minutes under aluminum foil. Swine should not be fed garbage because it sometimes contains raw, *trichinella*-infected meat.

Tapeworms, most commonly *Taenia saginata* from infected beef, but also *T. solium* from infected pork, develop into adults in the human intestine. Symptoms include diarrhea, frequent hunger pangs (the large worms expropriate what you have eaten for themselves), and chronic indigestion. Their eggs, which can also be consumed in vegetables contaminated with animal feces, hatch, and the larvae (of *T. solium* but not *T. saginata*) penetrate to the blood and are carried to soft tissues. In the brain they can grow to large masses and cause death.

Prevention of Tapeworm Infection. Take the same precautions as for preventing trichinellosis, but cook beef to 160° F.

Fish worms, that is, various roundworms, tapeworms, and flukes consumed in some raw or undercooked fish, can infect humans and cause serious illness. For example, several related roundworms called anisakines exist as larvae in the flesh of many fish. If eaten by humans they anchor themselves to the gastrointestinal tract and cause ulcers, pain, bleeding, and nausea. They sometimes wander up the throat and may be coughed up. They can spread throughout the body, settle in other tissues, and form granulomas, tumorlike masses sometimes misdiagnosed as cancerous. Horrible as this may sound, such infections are rarely life threatening, which is fortunate because there is no cure.

A dangerous fish tapeworm is *Diphyllobothrium latum*, which can grow to 60 feet long in the human digestive tract and cause pernicious anemia. In recent years it has frequently been associated with raw, undercooked, pickled, and salted salmon, especially in Japan and on the west coast of the United States. Fortunately, effective drug treatment is available.

Prevention of Infection with Fish Worms. Freeze fish to -4° F for three days, or fry at 140° F for five minutes, or bake or broil until the meat flakes easily. Smoking and salting the fish also work. Don't worry unduly about sushi bars. The chefs are usually well trained in choosing fish unlikely to be infected and in removing larvae should they be present. You are more likely to be infected by eating home-prepared sushi or sashimi, or simply lightly cooked fish, than by eating at a sushi bar.

Ascaris worms are large roundworms that can grow as thick as a pencil and cause severe symptoms in infected humans. The eggs are found on fruits and vegetables grown in contaminated soil or sewage sludge. When swallowed they hatch in the gut and the larvae travel to various tissues. Intestinal blockage and an asthmalike condition may develop. The infection is especially severe in children, sometimes lethal in infants. Several effective drug treatments are available.

Prevention of Ascaris Infection. Rinse unpeeled fruits with water and rinse or scrub vegetables before eating them raw.

Toxins In Fish

Ciguatoxin is a poison sometimes present in a variety of coral-reef fish such as barracuda, grouper, red snapper, surgeonfish, and sea bass. It is derived from dinoflagellates, algae eaten by herbivorous fish and stored harmlessly (to them) in their bodies. Carnivorous fish that eat such contaminated fish can accumulate large amounts, thus larger predators are the most likely to be toxic. Since the poison is heat stable, cooking the fish doesn't help. Symptoms may occur any time within about twenty-four hours of eating the fish. They include vomiting, diarrhea, muscle pain, chills, itching, flushing, burning tongue, numbness, tingling, and a strange reversal of temperature sensation of objects held in the hand—hot feels cold, and vice versa. The last four may linger for months or even years. Coma and death occasionally occur. Treatment is with intravenous mannitol (see **Mannitol,** under **Food Additives,** below). There is no way to test for the toxin in people, but a new test can detect it rapidly in fish. If the price is right it may become widely used.

Scombroid poisoning occurs after ingesting the dark meat of fish that have not been promptly refrigerated after being caught. Bacterial decomposition of the flesh gives rise to the toxins. Symptoms resemble an acute allergic reaction: facial flushing, sweating, burning of the mouth and throat, dizziness, diarrhea, nausea, abdominal cramps, heart palpitations, headache, and hives. In severe cases rapid heartbeat, blurred vision, and breathing difficulties may occur. The symptoms usually last about four hours, but they may persist for a day or two. Treatment is with antihistamines and cimetidine, a histamine blocker used to treat ulcers. Because the symptoms are so similar to an allergic reaction, patients are sometimes told to never eat fish again, which is most unfortunate.

The fish most commonly affected are tuna, albacore, mackerel, bonito, mahi-mahi (dolphin), and bluefish. Taste, aroma, and texture do not reveal the presence of toxins. Once contaminated no method of preparation, including cooking, freezing, salting, drying, or smoking, can destroy the toxin. **Prevention** requires proper handling and prompt refrigeration of fish. Use of a gaff (an iron hook) should be avoided if possible, and handling of the fish should be minimized. Fish should not be rinsed in sea water during cleaning because it contains microbes capable of causing the toxin production.

Tetrodotoxin is an extremely potent nerve toxin present in several species of fish, the best known being the blowfish or puffer fish. It is estimated to be 500 times as potent as cyanide and 160,000 times as potent as cocaine. Ingestion causes paralysis and death within minutes. In Japan *fugu,* as the blowfish are called, is a delicacy that commands premium prices. The flesh is usually eaten as sashimi, that is, raw. Shiny little slices are beautifully arranged on platters in the shape of a bird, fish, or geometrical design. Only specially trained and licensed chefs are allowed to prepare *fugu;* they know how to remove the highly toxic livers, ovaries, and other organs. Nevertheless, about a hundred fatal poisonings occur each year. Many of these deaths are due to a kind of Russian roulette played by *fugu* lovers. In very low doses, such as might be ingested from eating *fugu* sashimi, tetrodotoxin causes a mild numbing and tingling of the tongue and lips, flushing of the skin, a feeling of warmth, and euphoria. Overzealous aficionados sometimes talk a chef into (illegally) preparing a dish with a little liver or intestine so they can get a bigger thrill from the meal. It's a very dangerous game.

Food Additives

The complex chemical names on food labels sometimes cause people to wonder whether they are being slowly poisoned. Food additives are nothing new, of course. Since prehistoric times, smoke, salt, spices, herbs, plant dyes, thickeners made from seaweed, and flavor enhancers extracted from fish have been added to food. But recent application of modern chemistry and technology to food production has given rise to an enormous proliferation of semiartificial foods made from refined starch, sugar, and fat, plus thickeners, emulsifiers, moisturizers, flavors, stabilizers, colorings, preservatives, and other additives—several thousand in all.

In most cases the additives are harmless in themselves, but a long list of them in a foodstuff indicates a lot of processing, often with nutritional losses at each step, in spite of so-called enrichment. Highly processed foods tend to be high in fat, sugar, and salt and low in fiber, vitamins, and minerals. This is generally of more significance to the consumer than any toxicity of additives. However, a few additives do present problems. They are discussed below.

These are perfectly safe: acetic acid, agar, alginate, alpha tocopherol (vitamin E), amylases, ascorbic acid (vitamin C), ascorbyl palmitate (fat-soluble vitamin C), beta-carotene (pro-vitamin A), calcium proprionate, carrageenan, casein (avoid if you are allergic to milk), carboxymethylcellulose and microcrystalline cellulose, citric acid, natural colors, cysteine (an amino acid), dextrin, dextrose (glucose), dioctyl sodium sulfosuccinate, EDTA, ergosterol (pro-vitamin D), ferrous gluconate (iron), fumaric acid, furcelleran, glycerin (glycerol), iodides and iodates, isopropyl citrate, lactic acid, lecithin, malic acid, oxysterin, pectin, polysorbates, silicates, silicones (methyl silicone and others), sodium propionate, stannous chloride, and stearyl citrate.

The following additives are viewed with some concern:

Antioxidants—BHA, BHT, Propyl Gallate. These substances protect fats and oils from oxidation (rancidity) and are very common ingredients in processed foods. How well they work, their necessity, and their safety are controversial subjects. In the body BHA and BHT spare (protect) vitamin E to some extent. In food they all spare vitamin E and unsaturated oils, and under certain conditions they appear to protect animals from some cancers.

Animal tests have failed to consistently show toxicity at high levels of consumption, but there are reports of liver damage in rats given very large amounts. These are synthetic chemicals; they do accumulate in body fat (and Americans have particularly high levels); and some experts think they have not been adequately tested for carcinogenicity, fetus-deforming effects, and liver damage.

Because of evidence of toxicity in animal studies, Japan has banned BHA. Eventually the United States and other countries may also ban one or more of these substances. Your best bet is to avoid them unless you can't get fresh-tasting cereals, oils, and nut butters without them. Stale oils may be more hazardous to your health than these preservatives.

Aspartame is a synthetic combination of two amino acids that are naturally present in many foods. It is almost two hundred times as strong as sucrose but loses its sweetness when heated, so it is not useful in cooking. It is added primarily to soft drinks, breakfast cereals, and various low-calorie sweets.

Aspartame is metabolized down to the amino acids aspartic acid and phenylalanine. The latter cannot be metabolized by those with the genetic disorder phenylketonuria (PKU), so they *must* avoid aspartame. Some critics believe that even those without PKU may experience changes in mood, sleep, and appetite if they consume large amounts of aspartame because the phenylalanine can affect the levels of some brain neurotransmitters. However, aspartame is probably the most tested food additive ever used and arguments against it are weak. Until there is hard evidence of harm to people the sweetener will stay.

Artificial colors are derived from chemically treated coal tar. Thousands of tons are added to all kinds of processed foods every year. Although they have been used for over a hundred years, the list of allowable colors keeps shrinking as hazards are discovered. Some people develop allergic reactions to some colorings. These chemicals are completely worthless nutritionally and serve only to deceive the consumer, or enhance the enjoyment of highly processed foods, depending on your point of view.

Artificial Flavors. Thousands of these are used, some of which are entirely synthetic but most of which are synthetic replicas of natural compounds. These are very leniently regulated and little tested. They are probably as harmless as the substances they imitate, but their presence indicates that there is little or none of the natural foods that would normally supply the flavor.

Caffeine is naturally present in the kola nut that was used to make the first kola (or cola) drinks. This is apparently the reason the U.S. Code of Federal Regulations has long required that caffeine be present in any beverages called colas or pepper drinks, unless specified as caffeine-free. Many noncolas also have added caffeine, supposedly as a flavoring (albeit a bitter one) but perhaps also simply as a stimulant drug that subconsciously enhances the appeal of the products. (The effects and hazards of caffeine are discussed in Section Four.)

Fat substitutes are likely to be approved soon. The primary contenders for this multibillion-dollar market are NutraSweet's Simplesse and Procter and Gamble's Olestra, two very different products. Simplesse is made from milk and egg proteins that have been subjected to a patented heating and blending process that makes them smooth and creamy like fat. It contains about one-sixth the calories of fat. Since heat denatures it, Simplesse can only be used in cold-processed foods such as mayonnaise, whipped cream, frozen dairy products, and the like. One potential problem is that people who already eat lots of protein and add large amounts of Simplesse to their diets might end up with far too much protein in their diets. This carries a theoretical risk of excessive calcium excretion and thus osteoporosis, as well as premature aging of the kidneys.

Olestra is a sucrose polyester, that has properties similar to fat but passes through the digestive tract without being digested or absorbed. Because it might interfere with the absorption of fat-soluble vitamins, Procter and Gamble proposes to mix Olestra with fats and oils for use in cold products as well as for cooking. Olestra is unlike any natural food, so it requires more extensive testing than Simplesse. Some toxic effects have been reported in test animals given high doses, but their significance for humans is unclear. On the positive side, Olestra seems to lower LDL-cholesterol (the worst kind). In any case, if fat substitutes catch on the way artificial sweeteners have, fat consumption will not necessarily go down: American consumption of artificial sweeteners nearly tripled in the last twenty years; at the same time per capita sugar consumption increased almost 15 percent.

Flavor enhancers like monosodium glutamate (MSG), disodium guanylate (GMP) and disodium inosinate (IMP) all occur naturally in many protein-containing foods ("GMP" and "IMP" come from alternative chemical names). They are generally safe, but large amounts of MSG, often used in Chinese cooking, should be avoided by those who are sensitive to it. MSG is believed to be at least partly responsible for Chinese restaurant syndrome, which consists of headaches, numbness in the limbs, burning sensations, weakness, dizziness, nausea, and tightness in the chest. Symptoms last three or four hours after the meal. Pregnant women and infants should ingest a minimum of MSG to decrease the chances of this sensitivity developing. If you are sensitive to MSG request that it be left out of your food when eating out. Also, read labels and avoid products with hydrolyzed vegetable protein, as well as those with MSG. These products contain glutamic acid, which can form MSG when cooked. If you are on a strict low-sodium diet you should avoid MSG.

Feeling unwell after eating Chinese restaurant food seems to be fairly common, but it is not always caused by sensitivity to MSG. Chinese food often contains very large amounts of sodium from salt, soy sauce, and flavor enhancers, primarily MSG. Up to 5 grams of sodium may be ingested in one meal, perhaps ten times one's daily requirement (which varies enormously with sweating). This may cause symptoms for up to about four hours of severe thirst, bloating, and headache.

Glycyrrhizin, extracted from licorice root, is fifty times as sweet as sucrose and is widely used to flavor processed foods. It is safe in small amounts, but as little as two ounces of licorice candy a day may cause edema, hypertension, headaches, and other circulatory problems in some people. Licorice candy labels should warn against excessive consumption for those who have high blood pressure.

Lactose is the slightly sweet milk sugar and is safe except for people with lactase deficiency (lactose intolerance), in whom it can cause intestinal bloating, cramping, gas, and diarrhea (see **Double Sugars,** under **Carbohydrates,** above).

Licorice Flavoring. (See **Glycyrrhizin,** above.)

 Mannitol is a naturally occurring sugar used in "sugarless" chewing gum and low-calorie desserts. It is poorly digested by bacteria and therefore cannot promote tooth decay. It is also poorly absorbed by humans. Large amounts may have a laxative effect and may cause diarrhea, especially in children.

Monoglycerides and **diglycerides** are fats naturally present in many foods as well as throughout the body. They are used as texturizers and stabilizers in some foods. While harmless in themselves, they are empty calories that displace more nutritious components when large amounts are added to foods.

Nitrates and **nitrites** are naturally occurring essential plant nutrients used to form plant proteins. Substantial amounts occur naturally in many vegetables. They also occur in water leached from the soil. Fertilizers are a major source of nitrates in the soil, food, and water. For many centuries nitrates and nitrites have been added to meats, especially canned and cured products, to give them a pink color—they are normally a gray-brown. In large amounts they can impair hemoglobin function and accidental overdose is sometimes fatal.

These additives also inhibit *botulinum* growth, so they aid in the prevention of botulism. But critics charge that some foods they are added to do not harbor the deadly bacteria and therefore their use is purely cosmetic. Since these additives are strongly suspected of forming carcinogenic nitrosamines in the digestive tract, cosmetic use should not be allowed. (This reaction can apparently be inhibited by vitamin C eaten at the same time as the nitrate-containing foods.)

Saccharin has been used as a calorie-free sweetener for about a hundred years. It is extremely sweet but has a slightly bitter aftertaste that is often masked by the addition of the amino acid glycine. It is absorbed into the blood and excreted unchanged in the urine. Animal studies indicate it might be a very weak carcinogen or cocarcinogen, but extensive study of human users has not revealed a cancer hazard. It has *not* been shown to help in weight loss or control of diabetes.

Sodium benzoate occurs naturally in many fruits and vegetables, and may even be a natural metabolite in the human body. It has been used almost since the turn of the century as a preservative. It effectively inhibits the growth of microbes in acidic foods. It is generally safe, but a few people are allergic to it.

Sodium erythorbate is sprayed on cured meats like hot dogs, bologna, and pastrami to keep them pink. It has no important advantages over its chemical relative, sodium ascorbate (a form of vitamin C) and, though there is no evidence of a hazard, some critics believe it has not been sufficiently tested for health hazards.

Sorbic acid (or **potassium sorbate**) is a fatlike substance very effective in preventing the growth of molds and fungi. It is metabolized like any natural fat, and many studies indicate it is safe. However, reports that it may combine with nitrates in the digestive tract to form potential carcinogens are stimulating a closer look.

Sorbitol is a close relative of glucose and almost as sweet. It is slowly absorbed and converted to glucose, and is considered better for diabetics than sugar because of the slow absorption. It is also safer for teeth than sucrose because it does not stick to them. Many human and animal studies indicate that it is safe, although it tends to have a laxative effect and often causes gas, bloating, cramps, and diarrhea. Children seem to be especially susceptible, sometimes to very small amounts, but many adults are also affected. Unexplained chronic abdominal complaints should prompt consideration of sorbitol intake and possible intolerance.

Sulfites and **bisulfites** (of sodium and potassium) have been used since the time of the ancient Egyptians; the Romans preserved wine with them. They are also widely used in beer, soft drinks, bottled and canned fruits, vegetables, and soups. Until recently the largest amounts were used in restaurant salads. Vegetables could be cut ahead of time for quick serving during peak hours or left in the salad bar for several hours. The FDA has banned restaurant use however, and required labeling in packaged foods. Bisulfite destroys thiamin and so is banned from foods with large amounts of the vitamin.

These compounds are rapidly converted to innocuous sulfate, and are apparently safe for most people, but they can cause serious reactions in some, especially those with asthma. Reactions include nausea, diarrhea, hives, itching, anaphylactic shock (which has led to death in some cases), acute asthma attacks, and loss of consciousness. Up to one million of the ten million asthmatics in the United States may be sulfite-sensitive. All asthmatics should be alert for this sensitivity and do their best to avoid foods with the preservatives. Furthermore, nearly one-third of all people sensitive to sulfites are not asthmatics and have no known allergies, so the problem is one of concern to the general population.

Sulfur dioxide is a gas used in beverages, dried fruits, and other foods. It is easily metabolized and excreted and appears to be safe for most people, but the large amounts present in some wines can provoke severe reactions in sensitive persons.

Tartrazine is a yellow coloring used in hundreds of foods and drugs. In sensitive people it can cause hives, asthma, and other allergic reactions.

Xylitol is a sweetener naturally present in many plants including plums, strawberries, raspberries, and some vegetables. The main sources for commercial use are corncobs and birchwood chips. Xylitol has the same taste, appearance, and caloric value as sucrose, but it does not stick to the teeth, feed bacteria, or promote acid formation and tooth decay; this is naturally considered an advantage for chewing gum and some candies. However, it is rarely used now and may eventually be banned because animal studies indicate it might cause or promote tumors.

Air, Water, and Food Pollution

The fouling of our air, water, and food supplies has become an enormous problem and a threat to good health. The growth of population and industry and the rise of chemical agriculture have led to the proliferation of hazardous chemicals throughout the thin film covering the earth known as the biosphere. Hundreds of volumes have been written on the complex problems, the answers to which generally require group and community action more than lifestyle changes. Individual awareness is important, however, as a prerequisite to effective political action and is necessary to avoid some of the worst hazards in the environment. The following is a brief survey of some of the more important pollution problems.

Air Pollutants

The major gaseous pollutants are carbon monoxide, nitrogen oxides, hydrocarbons, and sulfur oxides. Liquid and solid particles from smoke, dust, and the like can also pollute the air. All of the gases and many of the particles, including asbestos, lead, nickel, selenium, and sulfuric acid droplets, are health hazards. In high concentrations most of them are very toxic and potentially lethal. In the lower concentrations found in polluted air they cause, promote, or aggravate chronic respiratory and circulatory problems and various cancers.

Nature, of course, contributes substantially to air pollution. For example, most of the atmosphere's nitrogen oxide is produced naturally by bacteria; carbon monoxide is produced by volcanoes and electrical storms; and dust, including naturally occurring asbestos, is kicked up by the wind. However, nature is rarely responsible for the dangerously high concentrations found in urban areas. It is well known that motor vehicles, industrial processes, and the burning of solid wastes are the major sources of air pollution severe enough to be a threat to health.

Laws regulating emissions from these sources generally prevent catastrophe, but in some areas special precautions may be in order. This is especially true on days of temperature inversion, when a lack of wind and other factors combine to trap large masses of polluted air in a populated basin or valley.

INDIVIDUAL REMEDIES

If possible, live away from polluted areas. If not, reduce your activity level on smog alert days, don't jog or bicycle during peak traffic hours or on the busiest roads, and try to avoid long, slow drives in bumper-to-bumper traffic, especially through tunnels. Exercise when you can to help clear particulate matter from your respiratory system. Remember that some air pollutants increase the harm done by cigarette smoke, which is a major indoor pollutant especially to the smoker but also to those who share his or her air.

If you live in a rural area and use a wood-burning stove, remember that its smoke can be a major air pollutant if too many such stoves are used in an area which has little wind. Moreover, unless the stoves are installed and used properly, and ventilation is adequate, their use can cause carbon dioxide, carbon monoxide, and other gases to accumulate to potentially dangerous levels inside the home.

Water Pollutants

Water pollution in the United States is caused by agricultural pesticides draining into waterways and seeping into water tables and wells; toxic industrial wastes dumped into streams and rivers or buried where they seep into water supplies; and run-off from mining operations, barnyards, and feed lots. While we have not experienced an epidemic of health problems associated with impure drinking water, there are certainly reasons for concern and action.

For example, tap water in some areas has high levels of chloroform and related carcinogens that are formed when chlorine (added to kill bacteria) reacts with decaying vegetable matter. Preliminary studies suggest that people who drink such water for many years are more susceptible to bladder and colon cancers. In some communities, farming activities have contaminated the water tables and well water with a wide variety of pesticides. Some water is polluted by dirty air even before it falls as rain—acid rain, that is. Water flowing through pipes, especially if it is acidic, can corrode the metals and take lead, cadmium, and copper to your tap.

Another reason for concern is that, in spite of the growing number of major pollutants and ways they can get into our water, the Environmental Protection Agency (EPA) demands that only a handful of chemicals be checked for by the water utilities, who frequently ignore even these meagre requirements. Moreover, millions of wells, both private and public, have never been tested for any pollutants.

INDIVIDUAL REMEDIES

If we cannot solve the problem of water pollution as a nation by cleaning up dump sites and ending the polluting of waterways and water tables, individuals and families will have to fend for themselves. Millions have already lost faith in their local water supplies and have taken remedial steps. **Ask your water utility or your local public health department** what is added to the water, what is or might be present as a pollutant, and how the levels compare to EPA safety guidelines.

If you are not satisfied with the information or if you still have questions, call some chemistry labs and get cost estimates for a thorough analysis of your water. Depending on where you live, how old your plumbing is, and other variables, some logical things to check for are lead, cadmium, chloroform and other trihalomethanes, dieldrin and other pesticides, copper, hydrocarbons and bacteria. If you decide that you and your family should not drink your tap water you have two alternatives, both fairly expensive but probably worth the cost in many cases.

Bottled water is a fast-growing industry, partly because of concern about water safety. However, there are hundreds of brands on the market, they come from many and varied sources, and there is no guarantee that they are pure and safe. Tests have shown that some bottled water has more chloroform and other pollutants than tap water, some have less, and most have about the same amount. In fact, seltzers and club sodas are almost all simply carbonated tap water and naturally have all the pollutants common to the water they are made of. Some bottled spring waters, especially mineral waters, have small but significant levels of arsenic, barium, and other potential toxins. Other bottled waters have been shown to be completely free of pollutants. If you have any doubts write to the bottler(s) and ask for proof of purity.

Home water filters have become a billion-dollar-a-year business. There are many brands on the market and they work in a number of different ways. The most effective systems use activated carbon, made by heating coal or wood to a very high temperature. This etches channels and craters in the carbon, and when water is forced through, the pollutants get trapped in the tiny pockets.

When comparing models of water filters, most of which fit under the sink, check the initial cost (usually $200 to $500), the filter replacement cost ($50 to $150 per year), and the efficiency of the systems. Look for 99 percent removal of trihalomethanes and halogenated organics, and at least 35 percent removal of nonpurgeable total organic carbon (NPTOC). Fortunately, most Americans have clean tap water and don't need filters.

Food Pollution

Our foods are almost never pure and completely free of potentially harmful contaminants. Even if we grow them ourselves without using chemicals they may pick up lead from the soil or drifting pesticide spray from the neighbors' farms and gardens. The potential for contamination is multiplied when the food is grown on large farms and transported long distances. Insecticides are among the most troublesome of the pollutants because they are so widespread and because heavy exposure can cause or promote serious illnesses, including cancer.

There is no evidence yet that pesticide residues in foods have become a major public health problem, and the hazards to the consumer have been greatly exaggerated by some. Most people are exposed to far more potentially carcinogenic chemicals in the form of natural pesticides that occur in most plants than in the form of synthetic pesticides that contaminate their food. The health hazards of pesticides are mostly to the workers who make and apply them, and to wildlife. Nevertheless, there are steps worth taking to minimize your intake of hazardous chemicals with your food.

INDIVIDUAL REMEDIES

Wash your fruits and vegetables with diluted soapy water or soak them in diluted vinegar (¼ cup per gallon of water). Even if they have to be peeled, washing may be advisable. For example, oranges are sometimes coated with a strong-smelling white crystalline fungicide, which is used to suppress molds during transport. If you peel the orange without washing it first, you inevitably smear the chemical all over the orange and end up swallowing it.

Peel or scrub root vegetables. The soil they were grown in likely contains pesticides and heavy metals. Little nutrients are lost by peeling carrots and the like.

Be wary of produce from Mexico and Central America, where pesticides banned in the United States are sometimes heavily used and government controls are not very tight. The FDA monitors imported foods for pesticide residues, but it can only sample a small percentage of imported food. When other factors are equal, buying American is usually better, though it is not always easy to tell where produce comes from. We're not saying don't buy foreign produce; but be extra thorough in cleaning it if you suspect it was imported.

Grow your own fruits and vegetables and use an absolute minimum of pesticides. Learn how to control pests without using chemicals; read books and ask local gardening and farming experts. If you do have to use pesticides, at least you can be sure to use them in accordance with safety requirements and with the law. If you live in an urban area with very polluted air, especially near heavy traffic, have your garden soil analyzed for lead, most of which comes from vehicle exhaust.

The problem of lead is especially important for children, who can suffer long-term neurological problems, including learning deficits, from excessive exposure. The major sources of lead contamination, in addition to gasoline fumes, are industrial emissions, leaded paint, food grown in soil with lead or exposed to lead-polluted air, and contaminated soil. Tin cans were once a significant source of lead in our food, but techniques have greatly improved and the cans now impart very little or no lead to the food. Children in high-risk areas (with paint chips and dust in the soil) can be protected by keeping the homes as free of dust and paint chips as possible, keeping their hands clean, and discouraging them from eating nonfoods.

Finally, you can reduce the impact of pesticides, heavy metals, and other pollutants on your health by eating well. Low levels of essential nutrients slow down the metabolism and excretion of the pollutants, while a healthy diet helps to get rid of them.

Staying Fit for Health and Pleasure

Born to Move

Humans are commonly thought to differ from animals primarily in the areas of tool-making, language, laughter, and other manifestations of intelligence and mental capacity, but human physical feats are just as impressive. There are, of course, swifter and stronger animals, and those that can fly and do other things humans need mechanical aids to accomplish. But what animal could keep up with a physically fit human as he or she runs ten miles, swims three more, scampers up and then down a fifty-foot tree, throws five rocks a hundred yards with great accuracy, and then does a short ballet or gymnastics demonstration?

We are clearly as gifted physically as we are mentally, which is not surprising since the human mind and body evolved together. The intelligence to understand what is needed for food and shelter would be worthless without the physical strength, stamina, dexterity, and courage to go get them.

Since the rise of agriculture, and especially since the industrial revolution, most of us no longer need much physical strength and stamina to put food on the table, and so we tend to be much more sedentary than our hunting and gathering ancestors. But our biology has not changed in this short time. We are still born to move. Children naturally enjoy roaming and romping, skipping, jumping, running, and climbing. Unfortunately, American kids seem to be losing this natural exuberance at a younger age as they spend more time watching television than running around. This makes them more susceptible to obesity and a variety of health problems as adults, including atherosclerosis and heart disease, diabetes, osteoarthritis, hypertension, constipation, hemorrhoids, and mental depression.

Degrees of Fitness

Consider two extremes: a triathlon finisher, who swims a couple miles, bicycles about a hundred, then runs twenty-six, all in less than ten hours; and a flabby sedentary office worker who would strain to walk a fast mile. There are visible and invisible differences between them associated with the tremendous differences in performance. Unfit muscles lose fibers and become marbled with fat, like the prime steaks (muscles) from grain-fed, penned-up cattle. The office worker may have fifty pounds of fat, while the triathloner at the same weight may have only five pounds of fat.

Fitness, of course, is a matter of degree, not an all-or-nothing state. Most people fall somewhere along the spectrum between the sedentary office worker and the triathloner, with the vast majority closer to the office worker. Methods of estimating one's place on the spectrum are outlined below.

The only way to improve fitness is to exercise, but not all exercise is equally beneficial. In dynamic exercise such as walking, running, swimming, and pedaling there is rhythmic contraction and relaxation of the flexor and extensor muscle groups that promotes blood flow through the arteries as well as the return of venous blood to the heart. At the right pace such activities can be continued for long periods. On the other hand, in isometric exercises, in which muscles are held in contraction for prolonged periods, the sustained contraction limits blood flow by compressing the small arteries and fails to help pump venous blood back to the heart. Moreover, the acute increase of blood pressure associated with isometrics can be hazardous to people with heart disease or high blood pressure.

How Exercise Improves Health

Body fat can be reduced and obesity controlled. Aerobic exercise stimulates the production of fat-burning enzymes in the muscles. After fifteen to twenty minutes of steady exercise, even a simple brisk walk, the muscles start to burn fat. In addition, regular exercise increases your muscle mass, which requires more maintenance energy than fat tissue. Theoretically, at least, as your muscle mass increases due to exercise you should burn more calories even at rest. (The significance of this effect is a subject of dispute.)

The heart's strength and efficiency are increased. The heart, like any muscle, responds to exercise by growing stronger. An unfit person's heart is small and thin-walled, and pumps only small amounts of blood with each contraction. With proper exercise it can increase in muscle mass, chamber volume, and efficiency. Being more efficient, the heart can pump more blood with each beat, so it beats less rapidly for a given level of activity.

The resting pulse of a highly trained athlete may be as low as 35 beats a minute, compared to 70 to 100 for an unfit person. If a sedentary person starts exercising at about 75 percent capacity for twenty minutes every other day, his or her resting and exercise heart rates will decrease about one beat per minute for each week of the program. With prolonged, intensive training, the maximum heart output per minute can be doubled to as much as 40 liters per minute.

Heart muscle circulation is improved. Oxygen-carrying blood is supplied to the heart muscle by two arteries arising from the aorta (which carries oxygenated blood out of the largest heart chamber, the left ventricle). These coronary arteries branch into smaller and smaller arteries that form a network that can shunt blood to any area of the heart muscle. During heavy exercise these channels open wide.

Animal studies and clinical observations show that regular aerobic exercise increases this network of tiny arteries, as well as the size of the coronary arteries. Should one of these arteries get plugged (a coronary occlusion), a well-developed network can provide adequate blood to the whole heart until the blockage is cleared. Without this detour system, a region of heart muscle could go without blood long enough to damage it and cause a heart attack.

Blood lipids are improved. Exercise tends to decrease the undesirable LDL form and increase the desirable HDL form of cholesterol, thereby reducing the formation of fatty plaques in the arteries.

Clot formation is made less likely by exercise, which enhances fibrinolysis, the body's mechanism for dissolving dangerous blood clots that cause stroke or heart attack.

High blood pressure can often be reduced to safe levels, especially if aerobic exercise is accompanied by proper diet. However, blood pressure may actually be increased dangerously in those with hypertention, so careful monitoring is essential.

Glucose tolerance, which is poor in diabetes, **can be improved.** Type 2 diabetes, the more common type, can often be kept under control without drugs with good nutrition and regular exercise.

Exercise promotes muscle and bone development by increasing blood levels of anabolic hormones like growth hormone and testosterone. The risk of osteoporosis developing is decreased by regular exercise. Increased levels of testosterone also tend to increase libido in men and women. However, overexercise may decrease bone strength and libido, like any strain or overexertion.

Psychological benefits of exercise include reduced muscle tension and anxiety, and increased self-confidence and emotional stability. Many people exercise simply because it makes them feel good for hours after. Some psychiatrists prescribe running to their depressed and anxious patients and the results are often very good, with great improvements in mood and functioning. Some people also experience improved concentration, memory, creativity, and mental speed and stamina. These beneficial effects are apparently due to increased levels of brain hormones (called endorphins) and to improved cerebral blood circulation resulting from general cardiovascular improvement.

Stress resistance is a general benefit of fitness. A person who is fit and strong with muscles full of fat-burning enzymes is more capable of withstanding a sudden illness, injury, surgery, and possibly even a heavy emotional stress like grief than a physically weak and unfit person. The fit body is less susceptible to wasting, but if wasting does occur it can continue far longer before causing a crisis. In emergencies requiring prolonged swimming, running, or walking for safety or for help, the fit person has a clear advantage. In short, the reserve of strength and stamina can speed recovery and tip the balance in favor of life in many critical situations.

Added fun is a major benefit of being fit rather than fat. Whether hiking in the hills, strolling on a beach, or snorkling on a coral reef, the fit person can go much further and longer and see and do more with much less effort than the unfit person.

A decreased rate of aging seems to be the net effect, the sum of the above individual effects of regular exercise. The degenerative changes common to many body tissues and functions can be slowed by exercise. Sedentary people experience a reduction of maximum oxygen consumption, probably the most reliable indicator of fitness and life expectancy available, of about 1 percent per year. Proper exercise can bring this under control and effectively decrease the rate of aging. Regular exercise maintained over a lifetime holds much more potential as a "fountain of youth" than any drugs or nutritional supplements available or even on the drawing boards.

Apparent Effects of Aging That Can Be Modified by Exercise

Increased blood pressure
Decreased cardiac output
Increased tendency to clot formation and thrombotic disease
Increased blood fat and cholesterol
Fatty degeneration of the arteries
Reduced maximum oxygen consumption
Protein wastage; loss of lean body tissue
Calcium wastage; bone weakening
Insensitivity to insulin; poor glucose tolerance
Lower levels of dopamine, norepinephrine, other neurotransmitters
Sleep disturbances
Tendency to depression
Decreased immune function
Lower testosterone levels

Decreased risk of cancer of the reproductive system and breast seems to be a long-term, perhaps lifetime, benefit for female athletes. Sedentary women have double the risk of these cancers compared to women who were athletes in their late teens and early twenties.

How Much Exercise is Best?

Guidelines are needed to assure an adequate workout without overdoing it. One approach is to simply walk, run, swim, dance, or bicycle at a steady pace as fast as you can without becoming breathless when you talk. Another rule of thumb is that you should feel good after the exercise, not exhausted. These guidelines are probably adequate for most people, but some prefer a more precise approach.

The 75 Percent Rule. One widely used rule of thumb is to exercise at a level that makes your heart beat at about 75 percent of its maximum rate, the very fastest it could be driven to beat. (Some say 80 percent, but we'll play it safe.) Up to the age of 20 the maximum rate is about 200 beats per minute. This decreases according to the formula, maximum heart rate = 220 − age. So the proper training rate to aim for is given by the formula:

$$\text{training rate} = .75 \times (220 - \text{age})$$

For example, a forty-year-old person should aim for a training rate of 135 beats per minute. If the person is not fit, brisk walking might be all it takes to get to the training rate. If he or she is fit, it would take jogging or running.

The Five- and Ten-minute Rules. If five minutes after you stop exercising your pulse is above 120 beats per minute, you went too hard or too long. If ten minutes after you stop exercising your breathing rate is more than 16 per minute, you went too hard or too long.

To Measure Your Pulse. Using the fingertips rather than the thumb (to avoid counting your thumb pulse), count the beats in ten seconds and multiply by six to get your beats per minute rate. The pulse can be felt on the inside of the wrist, on the side of the neck, or just in front of the ear in the temple area. It may be necessary to stop the exercise, but with practice the pulse can be measured while walking or jogging. A battery-operated, digital pulse gauge simplifies matters greatly, but before relying on one test its accuracy against a good watch.

How Often and How Long Should You Exercise?

The benefits of aerobic exercise begin to be significant with regular workouts of about fifteen consecutive minutes every other day. Two eight- or ten-minute workouts are of less benefit than a nonstop fifteen-minute session. The duration and frequency can be steadily increased as fitness improves.

The amount of exercise required for maximum protection from heart disease is a controversial issue, although twenty nonstop minutes of aerobic exercise every other day clearly improves fitness and reduces the risk of cardiovascular disease. Some experts believe that more exercise than this improves the situation only a little, but there is evidence that improvement increases at the higher levels (up to about thirty minutes every day and possibly more). However, as exercise increases, so does the risk of harm from overexercise. To be sure of substantial benefits while avoiding the point of diminishing returns, twenty minutes of aerobic exercise every day is a practical level for most people. Thirty minutes every other day is another effective option worth considering.

Why Overexercise Is Harmful

It is important not to exceed your capacity for exercise, or you will do more harm than good. Exercising at a level that makes the heart beat at or near its maximum capacity forces the muscles into more anaerobic metabolism, quickly using up the available glucose and increasing the breakdown of muscle tissue. There is always some degree of muscle breakdown during prolonged exercise. Normally the lost tissue is more than replaced over the next twenty-four hours, but if exercise resumes before full recovery, there will be a net loss of muscle tissue rather than a gain.

Overexercise can result in a significant loss of muscle mass and fat-burning capacity, especially if repeated for many days. The older a person is, the more likely this is to occur because tissue repair tends to slow down with age. People who consistently overexercise in a compulsive effort to get in shape end up feeling sore and tired and in worse condition than before they started.

Overexercise can precipitate a heart attack, even in apparently healthy people. Do not ignore symptoms such as tightness or pain in the chest, dizziness, light-headedness, stomach pain, or breathing trouble. This cannot be overemphasized. Failure to heed symptoms with rest and a check-up have cost even experienced runners their lives. For example, the popular fitness writer Jim Fixx, who had a family history of early heart disease, apparently ignored early warning symptoms in the days before his much-publicized fatal heart attack while jogging in July of 1984.

One forty-nine-year-old runner began having chest pains eight kilometers into a race, but kept going. He had a massive heart attack six kilometers later. Another runner, said by his wife to be obsessed with training, put these words on his T-shirt: "You haven't really run a good marathon until you drop dead at the finish line—Pheidippides." He did just that a week later. Another man had trouble breathing after running a marathon, yet raced his wife in a final dash home, where he dropped dead. The majority of such cases are caused by coronary atherosclerosis, a major blockage in coronary arteries by cholesterol-laden plaques. In athletes under thirty most such cases are caused by structural abnormalities of the heart. Screening young athletes for congenital abnormalities might help prevent some of these deaths.

Careful contemplation of these examples might save your life. Serious endurance athletes over thirty should pay special heed. Those with risk factors like high cholesterol level, hypertension, or a family history of early heart disease, should consult a physician about a stress test to determine risk.

Decreased immunity is a definite risk for marathoners and other serious endurance athletes who push themselves to their limits. For a week or so after a marathon, runners seem to have a much higher incidence of colds and flu. The cause may be the hormone cortisol, which suppresses immune function and is greatly increased during severe physical stress. The effect lasts a half day or so after a race. During this time and perhaps for a couple more days racers should practice germ avoidance by limiting social contacts, keeping away from people with respiratory infections (especially runny-nosed toddlers), and avoiding crowds. Moderate runners who don't overly stress themselves don't seem to be affected, and may even have slightly increased immunity.

No Pain, No Gain? This little aphorism, which implies that exercise must make you feel miserable or it is not beneficial, is absolutely false. On the contrary, exercise that causes pain and exercising while experiencing pain can lead to severe injuries. It's true that in intensive body-building programs the muscles one is trying to build should burn after they are worked, but in moderate to intensive aerobic training programs there is no reason to experience pain in order to gain.

Infertility Due to Heavy Exercise. Serious training for prolonged periods can cause temporary infertility in both men and women. When body fat is reduced to extremely low levels the activity of the hypothalamus (the part of the brain that controls the pituitary gland and hormone output) is altered. Women may stop ovulating and having periods, and men's sperm count often declines. The effect is completely reversible by gaining fat, and is not often considered a serious hazard. Some women even consider such infertility a natural form of birth control and a bonus for being superfit.

Bone Damage and Increased Risk of Osteoporosis. The price of this natural birth control may be very high. Women who exercise to the point of amenorrhea (suppression of menstruation) can loose bone mass at a frightening rate—up to 4 percent during each year of amenorrhea—and experience more stress fractures. Their bone loss approaches that of postmenopausal women. Most important, if amenorrhea lasts three years or more the demineralization may not be reversible and early osteoporosis could become a real possibility. To prevent amenorrhea due to heavy exercise, the level of exercise should be increased very gradually. If amenorrhea does occur and you refuse to decrease your exercise level, at least be sure to get adequate calories, including some from fat if necessary, and adequate calcium. And consult a physician about estrogen supplements and monitoring for bone injuries and bone thinning.

Exercise and Illness. Some people are so enthusiastic about their exercise routines that they will not skip them for anything, not even illness. This is a serious mistake. In illness, even a cold or flu, tissue repair is greatly slowed and exercise causes substantial muscle breakdown. Even the heart muscle can be inflammed and damaged; fatal rhythm disturbances may occur. Rest is essential when one is sick.

Proper exercise can be very beneficial for persons with hypertension or diabetes, but a vigorous exercise program should not be started without consulting a physician to discuss the intensity, frequency, and possible adjustments in drug therapy. Those susceptible to exercise-associated asthma attacks should discuss the problem with their physicians; there is usually no reason to discontinue activities, but some adjustments may be in order.

How Fit Are You?

There are several ways of estimating your level of cardiovascular fitness. Direct measurement of maximum oxygen consumption is the most precise, but others are also useful. None of the fitness measurements, which are based on averages of real performances, should be taken too seriously in themselves. The important thing is to make steady progress in your performance; the tests are useful guides for measuring your progress.

The Maximum Oxygen Consumption Test, also known as aerobic power, is the most precise measure of fitness. The subject walks or runs on a treadmill while his or her oxygen consumption is monitored. The maximum rate, adjusted for weight, is a clear indicator of the efficiency of the heart and lungs in getting oxygen to the working muscles as well as the capacity of the muscles to use it. Aerobic power can increase with training for about eighteen months of optimum effort; then it levels off at a plateau probably determined by each person's genes. Further training cannot take a person beyond his or her genetic capacity for aerobic power.

The Resting Pulse Test. A fast pulse at rest may be a sign of a weak heart. As fitness increases, the heart becomes more efficient (pumps more with each beat) and the resting rate decreases. In very fit athletes it can go as low as 35 beats per minute. More common (and not far from unhealthy) is about 70 for men and 80 for women; 75 and 85, respectively, are clear signs of lack of fitness in apparently healthy persons. Keep in mind, though, that caffeine and other drugs, as well as anxiety and excitement, can speed up the heart.

The Pulse Reduction Test. After prolonged exercise, the heart slows to its resting rate in two stages. The first drop is the largest and most significant, and usually occurs within the first minute. The second reduction occurs several minutes to an hour later. The significance of its rate is not clear. The first reduction is used to determine one's level of fitness. A commonly used formula to gauge recovery rate is:

recovery rate = exercise pulse − one-minute pulse

The recovery rate is the measure of how fast the pulse slows down after exercise. The exercise pulse is obtained while standing still or walking slowly immediately after exercise. Count the beats in the first ten seconds after the exercise and multiply by six. This is the exercise pulse. Repeat after one minute for the one-minute pulse.

A recovery rate of less than 20 is considered a sign of poor fitness; 30 is about average. More than 40 is excellent; more than 60 is super.

The Five-Minute and Twelve-Minute Tests. Dr. Kenneth Cooper, the popular fitness advocate, and other physiologists have developed standardized tests and methods of estimating fitness levels. Years of data collected from thousands of subjects of all ages have led to detailed tables for twelve-minute tests for running/walking, swimming, and cycling. The point is to cover as much ground as you can in twelve minutes without exceeding about 80 percent of your maximum heart rate unless you are very fit. Other researchers have come up with a five-minute test, but this would seem an inferior measure of aerobic capacity, which implies stamina. There will probably be other tests. Most people need consider only the following simple facts:

Assuming the test is for at least five minutes, and preferably more (up to about fifteen minutes among healthy, nonhandicapped men under sixty), the range of performance is about 140 to 270 yards per minute. The range for women is about 120 to 220. If you can cover 200 yards a minute (say, 1,000 yards in five minutes), your fitness level is fair if you are a man under fifty, good if you are older. A good performance by a younger man would be at least 220 yards per minute. For a woman, 200 yards per minute is good if she is in her twenties and excellent if she is in her fifties.

The goal should be to improve fitness until performance is in the "good" range and keep it constant or increasing from year to year. This gets harder as the decades go by and inevitably cardiovascular fitness and performance decline. But in the process of trying, healthy years can be added to your life.

The Best Fitness Activities

Dynamic exercise that is rhythmic, steady, moderate in intensity, and prolonged has the most aerobic value and the most potential for improving fitness and health. Isometric exercises, as we noted earlier, tend to inhibit efficient circulation and oxygen consumption. They have little value in improving cardiovascular fitness. They are also hazardous to those with atherosclerosis, heart disease, or high blood pressure because they tend to greatly increase blood pressure.

In choosing a dynamic exercise, the most important consideration is surely pleasure. An activity that one enjoys will be performed more frequently and consistently than one that is a chore. Even if it has half the aerobic value of others, in the long run it will be more beneficial. Ideally, one should enjoy several different types of exercise, and switch frequently so different muscles are developed and none is worked beyond its capacity for self-repair. This is especially true for those over fifty who exercise every day since their tissue regeneration is slower than when they were younger. Switching exercises can also minimize stress injuries and prevent boredom with a single routine. Swimmers and cyclers should jog, jump rope, or dance periodically; a little of these more jarring exercises will help keep the bones strong.

The following activities are listed approximately in order of their aerobic value and effectiveness in improving cardiovascular fitness. However, the most important factors in choosing are practicality, enjoyment, and likelihood of producing injury.

Cross-country skiing is generally considered to be the very best aerobic exercise. It provides all the benefits of running without the jarring stresses on various tissues. The large leg muscles are used more than in swimming, and very high levels of oxygen consumption can be reached by the fit cross-country skier. Unfortunately, the sport is not accessible or affordable for most people, though it is much cheaper than downhill skiing. Some exercise devices mimic cross-country skiing very well and are excellent for skiers and nonskiers.

 Jumping rope is quite strenuous and difficult to do for long periods. It is especially hard on the feet, Achilles tendons, and knees. The stress should be minimized by the use of a soft carpet and tennis, basketball, or running shoes, and by alternating from foot to foot rather than jumping with both feet. Bouncing on a mini-trampoline is not hard on the joints, but it may not be strenuous enough to provide a good workout for those already in good shape.

Running in place and jumping jacks (the scissorslike jumping calisthenics most of us learn in P.E. classes) are convenient for almost everyone but, like jumping rope, they can be rough on the feet, joints, and tendons. Stress can be minimized by using a soft carpet and good shoes.

Jogging and running are excellent aerobic exercises, but they can be quite stressful and lead to injuries. During running the feet, knees, and lower back absorb the shock of about 150 foot strikes a minute, each one transmitting a force of about four times the runner's weight to the heel, ankle, knee, hip, and lower back. It is not surprising that people who run a lot often suffer injuries. The most common injuries are of the knee, shin, Achilles tendon, forefoot, hip, thigh, heel, ankle, arch, and groin, in that order. Injury can be avoided by careful choice of shoes, running surfaces, and running habits.

Polluted air is another hazard to the jogger. Running near traffic can increase the carbon monoxide in the blood to the same amount as smoking one to twenty cigarettes a day, depending on the length of the run and the density of pollution. This suggests that smokers should absolutely not run in polluted air. For healthy nonsmokers, though, the benefits of exercise probably outweigh the risks except in the heaviest pollution. For urban joggers the best advice is probably to run in the morning and avoid the busiest roads. Warm and windless days tend to be worse. Pregnant women and people with heart trouble should be especially careful.

Women and Jogging. There has been some concern that the stress of the repeated impact of jogging could weaken the connective tissue supporting the uterus and drive it down so that it causes pressure on, and protrusion into, the vagina. These fears are unwarranted; surveys of thousands of female runners indicate the problem does not exist. However, women who already have a prolapsed uterus (usually caused by giving birth several times) should be aware that running as well as lifting heavy weights and other stressful activities can aggravate the condition. They should be alert for a feeling of pressure on the vagina or leakage of urine when exercising. Running on soft grass with good shoes or on sand lessens the risk.

Jogging can cause breast sagging and pain. This problem can usually be prevented by wearing a sports bra that prevents lateral and spiraling motions of the breasts. The bra should not bind, but should be rigid enough to limit bouncing. It should have wide nonelastic straps, cotton cups, padded seams, and covered metal fasteners.

Women who regularly run or engage in other strenuous exercise and lose too much fat may develop symptoms of estrogen deficiency. Aside from this and the fact that men appear to be more susceptible to heart attack and sudden death during and shortly after exercise than women, the main hazards of running are the same for both sexes, namely, stress injuries to muscles, bones, joints, and connective tissues.

Hiking and hill climbing are excellent fitness activities, especially with a small pack on the back. Try to maintain a steady, brisk pace for at least a mile between breaks.

Aerobic dancing is a fitness program originally designed for people who found jogging inconvenient or boring. An aerobic dance session resembles a rehearsal for an amateur dance show. Accompanied by Broadway, rock, and disco music, the participants follow the leader in kneelifts, kickjumps, ballet reaches, and rhythmic running, hopping, jumping, stretching, and skipping. A session should include at least ten minutes of stretching and warming up exercises, fifteen to thirty minutes of nonstop aerobic movements (at a pace determined by one's fitness and the 75 percent rule), and five minutes of cooling down activities like walking and stretching. It is important to go at your own pace and not try to keep up with the leader or fastest person in the group.

These programs can be very effective in improving fitness and shedding fat; even some professional sports teams have taken them up as an integral part of their training. However, the workouts in some commerical aerobic dance programs and some television shows are not intensive enough to provide significant benefits. Remember that, to be of real value, a workout should get your heartbeat up to 75 percent of its maximum rate for at least fifteen minutes. Moreover, whether they are intensive enough or not, they are stressful and can cause foot, leg, and back injuries, so good shoes and a resilient surface are necessary.

Disco, jazz, ballet, and other dancing can be good aerobic exercise if the movement is nonstop for fifteen minutes or so, and if it does not take place in a smoke-filled room.

 Rowing and paddling are good aerobic activities, but not quite as beneficial as those that use the leg muscles more. People who enjoy these activities can reach high levels of fitness with a little supplementary running, bicycling, or dancing.

Walking should be brisk, nonstop for at least twenty minutes a session, and engaged in nearly every day. It will not take you to your maximum potential level of fitness, but it is much less likely to cause injuries than any other exercise that improves fitness, and it is the most practical for most people. For these reasons it is perhaps the most important exercise in a public health sense, one that should be strongly promoted by health agencies and educators.

Bicycling is in some ways the best exercise of all, although the peak oxygen load is not as great as with running or cross-country skiing. It is also much less stressful than running and other sports. Cycling has been increasing in popularity because we can fit it into our daily lives, saving energy and lessening parking problems as we cycle to work, school, and shopping. But to be of significant benefit you must ride hard enough to increase your heart rate for at least fifteen minutes nonstop, which is often difficult in urban areas.

A human on a bicycle is the most efficient living locomotion system known, capable of moving a pound of flesh a given distance on less energy than a salmon, horse, pigeon, or bee. A large slice of bread can take you about five miles. This efficiency is a disadvantage in terms of fitness value. The main problem with bicycling is that it is simply too dangerous in many areas. If you live in such an area you might consider a stationary cycle for your home. If you do ride a bike, wear a helmet.

Swimming is an excellent aerobic activity, and a regular program can develop a high level of fitness. However, the maximum oxygen capacity generally does not get as high as with running because the large upper leg muscles are not used as much. There also seems to be a tendency to retain upper body fat in regular swimmers. This is apparently an adaptation for warmth and bouyancy and does not interfere with fitness.

Ice and roller skating are aerobically valuable in theory, but all too often the skating area is too small, crowded, and dangerous to allow a high-speed, prolonged workout.

Tennis, racquetball, basketball, and ping pong can be very tiring, but they consist largely of bursts of action, and are not as aerobically valuable as steady, smooth, continuous movements. It has been estimated that jogging at the proper rate for fifteen minutes is worth an hour or more of these sports, but this depends on how vigorously and quickly the games are played.

Baseball, football, and volleyball are even less effective since they consist mostly of standing around between short bursts of mostly anaerobic movements. However, a brisk game of two-on-two volleyball can be valuable, especially if played on sand between players good enough to keep long volleys going. Baseball and football players keep in shape with jogging, sprinting, and other exercises during practice, not by playing their games.

Can Work Be Good Exercise? Some people think they get enough exercise because they do a lot of housework, gardening, carpentery, or other strenuous work. However, such work is usually done in short bursts rather than in sustained output at a proper training rate and, strenuous though it may be, has little aerobic value. The muscular construction worker is often unfit because he feels too tired to exercise after work. However, some workers, such as pedestrian letter carriers and longshoremen with the more active jobs, do gain substantial aerobic benefit from their work. And even some domestic chores, such as lawn mowing, raking, and mopping, can be good workouts if they raise the heart rate to the training level for at least twenty minutes.

Exercise and Nutrition

Many dubious claims are made about commercial products that supposedly fill the extra need that physically active people allegedly have for this and that nutrient. Does a moderate fitness program or accelerated training for a marathon change a person's nutritional requirements? Yes and no. Consider the following details.

Water is the nutrient most affected by exercise. Dehydration can cause muscle cramps, headache, and fatigue and progress to heatstroke, collapse, and, if the condition is severe and untreated, even death. Ample amounts of water should be drunk before, during, and after prolonged exercise, especially in hot weather. In general, enough water should be taken to keep the urine clear or slightly yellow (this will usually be more than is dictated by thirst), at least one cup for each fifteen minutes of exercise. Bright yellow urine is a sign of inadequate fluid intake unless it is caused by a recent large dose of B vitamins or brewer's yeast.

Some people advise against taking ice-cold drinks during and after exercise. They believe the cold may set off reflexes that result in spasms of the coronary arteries, heart arrythmias, and heart attack. There is no good evidence for this belief and we are unaware of any reported cases. The biggest hazard seems to be a wave of nausea or a brief headache.

Salt lost from sweating needs to be replaced, but salt tablets should generally not be taken even if it is hot and you sweat a lot. This is because too much salt can upset the electrolyte balance and promote heatstroke. It is better to drink lightly salted water (a quarter teaspoon per quart) and moderately salt your food if you have a craving for it. People with hypertension who want to exercise regularly should discuss their need to take or avoid salt with their physicians.

Calorie intake generally must be increased if exercise is increased. The exception is in the case of an obese person who wants to combine moderate exercise with moderate calorie restriction. Those who are not fat and maintain a constant calorie intake while involved in an accelerating exercise program risk losing lean tissue, especially muscle mass, and thereby becoming less fit and less strong.

Women especially are likely to be harmed by heavy exercise and inadequate calorie intake. Continued over several months the combination can lead to estrogen deficiency symptoms, including anovulation, amenorrhea, and insidious bone thinning. No special diet or supplements are required to prevent the problems, just an increased intake of all the good foods one presumably eats.

Protein requirement is not increased by moderate exercise, but heavy exercise can result in excessive protein breakdown and nitrogen loss, in which case extra protein might be of value. High-level training that significantly adds to muscle mass may slightly increase the protein requirement, but the added food intake that comes naturally usually takes care of it. There is no need to gorge on high-protein foods, nor are protein supplements (powders, pills, liquids) necessary or desirable. However, vegetarians, especially vegans (vegetarians who avoid dairy and other animal products), would be prudent to eat more high-protein foods like tofu, nuts, and seeds.

The idea of pushing protein in order to increase muscle mass is untenable. The small amount of extra protein that may be needed because of an accelerated fitness or weight lifting program can be easily provided by the extra amounts of foods one would naturally eat. Excessive protein, especially from concentrated supplements, can cause excessive calcium excretion, poor zinc absorption, and possibly even kidney damage.

Potassium must be replenished daily to prevent weakness, fatigue, irritability, and other signs of deficiency. Problems are especially likely for those taking diuretics or suffering from diarrhea. The best sources of potassium are fruits and vegetables and their juices. Those with hypertension who want to exercise regularly should discuss their potassium needs with their physicians.

Iron is sometimes in low supply in athletes, especially marathoners and female athletes. Prolonged exercise tends to increase the excretion of iron in sweat, urine, and feces. Anemia itself, the lack of adequate hemoglobin in the blood, is not very common, but low blood stores of iron, determined by blood ferritin levels, can cause some of the same problems as anemia, including reduced performance, fatigue, headache, and muscle cramping. Once the condition occurs, iron supplements and careful monitoring of blood ferritin will be necessary. It can usually be prevented with a good diet, but supplements may be in order for those who train at the marathon level. Because excess iron can accumulate in the liver and muscles, where it is toxic, doses larger than the RDA (10 milligrams for men, 15 for women) should not be taken without consulting a physician.

Magnesium is excreted in the stool in large amounts by heavy exercisers; deficiency can cause cramps and chronic fatigue. Good sources are nuts, seeds, leafy greens, whole grains, and magnesium oxide tablets. We would advise against dolomite supplements unless the manufacturer can guarantee it to be lead-free.

Vitamin requirements are not increased by exercise beyond the increase which naturally accompanies increased food consumption with training. There is no evidence that massive doses of any nutrient can improve athletic performance or stamina. There is no need for anyone to take commercial vitamin preparations supposedly formulated for athletes and other active people. Vitamin E in particular has been heavily promoted as an athletic performance booster. A very thorough study done at Tulane University put such claims to the test. Forty-eight members of the swimming team were put into two groups matched for age, sex, and swimming ability. For six months one group was given 900 IU of vitamin E, while the other group got an identical-looking pill with none. No one, not even the coaches or research assistants, knew who was getting which pill until the study was completed. As it turned out, there was no detectable difference in performance, endurance, or improvement between the two groups. Several other studies have come to similar conclusions. Such studies are not reported in "health food" magazines, which is not surprising since the purpose of these publications is to sell supplements, not to tell the truth about them.

Carbohydrate loading is a popular method of increasing stamina for extreme endurance competition. While fit people burn fat very effectively for energy, it is desirable to have large reserves of glucose (stored as glycogen in the muscles and liver) available for anaerobic metabolism in the final stretch. Training increases muscle glycogen storage capacity, which promotes stamina and sprint capacity for the end of the race.

The idea in carbo loading, as it is commonly called, is to pack the muscle cells with as much glycogen as possible just before the race. One method that seems to work is to exercise to full capacity and eat your normal diet for a week before the race; then exercise lightly for three days on the same diet; then exercise lightly for three days on a very-high-carbohydrate diet; then rest and splurge on carbos on the last day. It's best to eat lots of whole grains, potatoes, beans, fruits, and vegetables, and not fill up on sugary foods. Contrary to common belief, athletic performance is not improved by a high-sugar snack just before exercise. In fact, the sugar may prevent optimum performance and promote early fatigue. Interestingly, carbo loading can cause substantial weight gain due to water retained with the glycogen. This presents no problems; it is quickly lost in the competition. All this aside, the very fit person burns about 80 percent fat during a marathon and probably does not benefit from carbohydrate loading.

Prevention and Treatment of Common Sports Injuries

While exercise can be beneficial, there are also certain hazards, some of them serious, but with awareness and care the risks can be minimized. Most injuries and health problems associated with exercise have the same general cause: the overstressing of muscles, tendons, ligaments, bones, or other tissues. It is important to know your body's limits and warning signals and not push yourself too hard; the following principles should also be kept in mind.

1. **Drink plenty of water.** Before, during, and after prolonged exercise (more than fifteen minutes), drink enough water to keep the urine clear

or light yellow. Otherwise there is a risk of dehydration and heatstroke, especially in hot weather.

2. **Do not eat a heavy meal** within a couple hours of starting heavy or prolonged exercise. After eating, blood concentrates in the digestive organs, and so not enough is available to keep the skeletal muscles and heart going at a fast clip for long. Exercising hard soon after (or before) eating can lead to indigestion, stomach cramps, and side stitches. In extreme cases, especially if coronary artery disease is present, eating and exercising too close together can contribute to a heart attack. On the other hand, you don't want to go into prolonged exercise on the verge of hunger, so plan ahead.

3. **Warming up** slowly before exercising hard is very important in avoiding stress injuries, especially muscle cramps, pains, and strains. Proper warmup involves the use of the muscles in the same way as in the "main event," but at a slower pace and with less stress. Joggers should walk for several minutes, then jog slowly before hitting their stride. Sprinters should walk and jog first. Exercises that do not use the same muscles as the main event are of little value for warming up.

4. **Stretching** muscles and tendons is appropriate before most activities in order to prevent a variety of stress injuries, especially tendon rupture. Stretching should always be done slowly and gently, particularly in the morning when muscles are cooler and more susceptible to injury. However, some experts doubt that stretching is terribly important and feel that many tend to overdo it.

5. **Cooling down** properly after heavy exercise is one of the most important and least appreciated rules of fitness training. After a hard run or other workout, you should slowly walk or otherwise keep moving for a few minutes and not just stand still. You also should not jump into a hot bath or shower because the demands on your heart will continue for a while. Being still or applying heat suddenly will cause the blood to pool in the large muscles, like those in the legs.

Moreover, the enormous increase in norepinephrine and epinephrine (blood vessel constrictors) associated with exercise continues for several minutes after the exercise stops. These hormones can induce dangerous arrhythmias, especially when standing still. Those with known or suspected cardiovascular problems should be especially alert to these dangers.

Exercises That Help Prevent Injuries

The following simple exercises strengthen and stretch muscles and thereby help prevent sprains and strains. Try them all, then choose those you like best or need the most and do them regularly and carefully.

Each exercise should last two to five minutes, but serious athletes may benefit from longer stationary stretches, especially of the calf and hamstring.

If you do these in the morning upon arising, be extra careful and start slowly. Your muscles are at their coldest and stiffest and are easily injured. It is good to at least walk around a little and perhaps take a hot shower before working out.

These exercises should be done to the point of mild stretching discomfort or muscle fatigue, not pain or exhaustion.

Groin stretch

With soles of the feet together, lower your head and trunk while pressing down on your legs with your elbows.

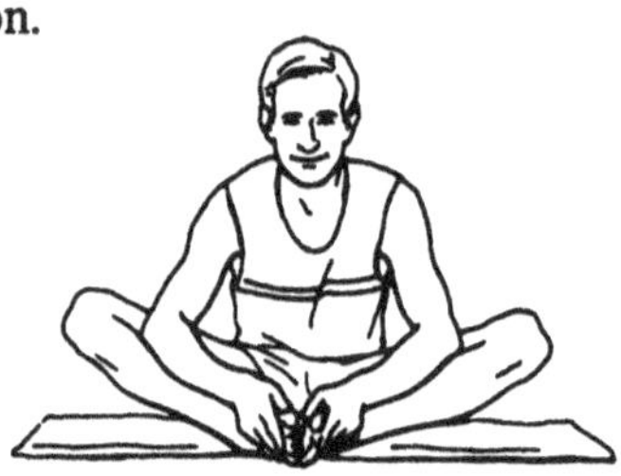

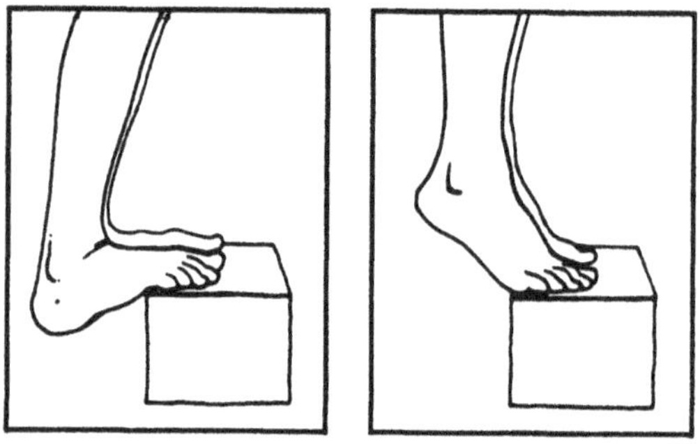

Calf stretch and strengthener

Let your heels drop over the edge of a block or step. Stay in the low position for stretching. Go up and down for strengthening.

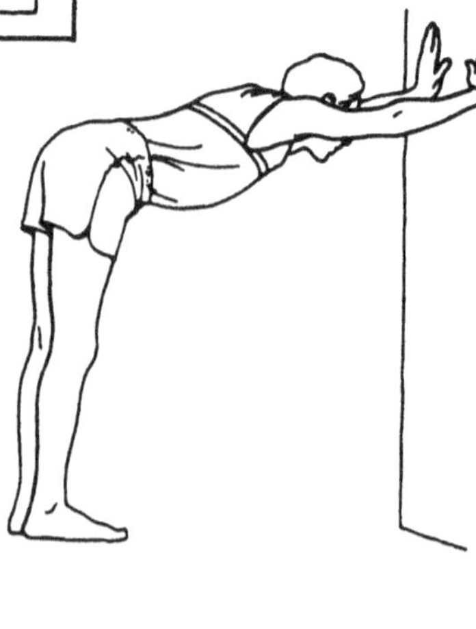

Back-leg stretch

Keep your hands on the wall and your feet flat on the ground while slowly moving away from the wall.

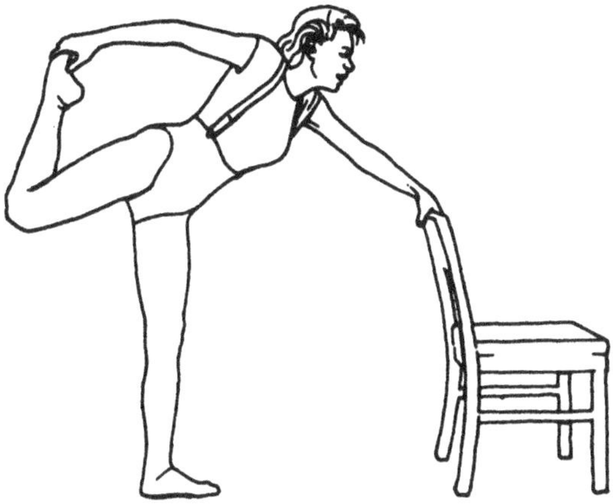

Quadriceps stretch

Support yourself with one hand and grab a foot with the other. Pull the foot up to increase the stretch.

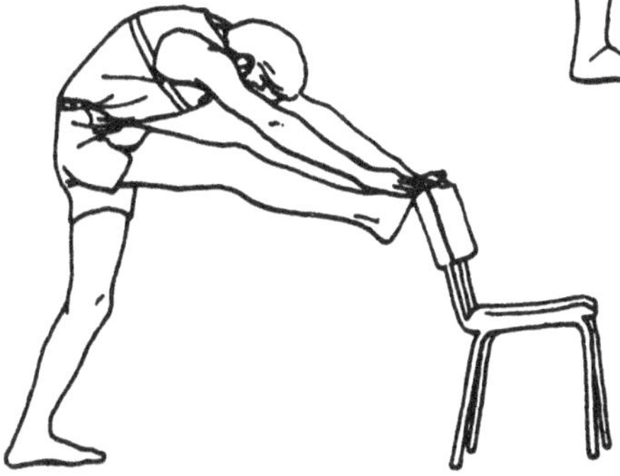

Hamstring stretch

Put one foot up on the back of a chair or a railing and grasp your toes. Straighten the knee and bend the body forward.

Hamstring stretch

Lie on your back. Bring one leg up and grasp the toes with your hands. Slowly straighten your leg as much as possible and pull your head up toward the knee.

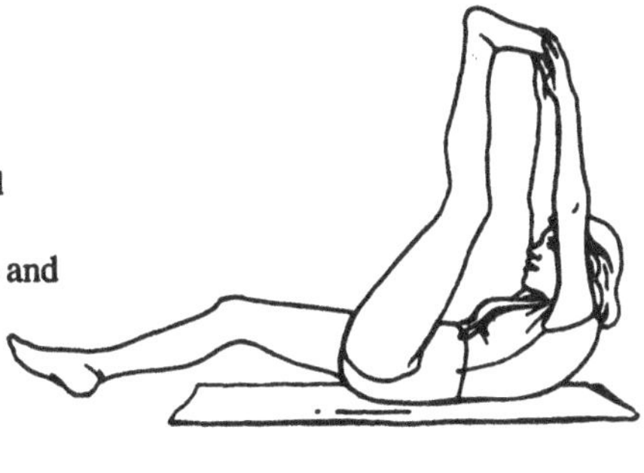

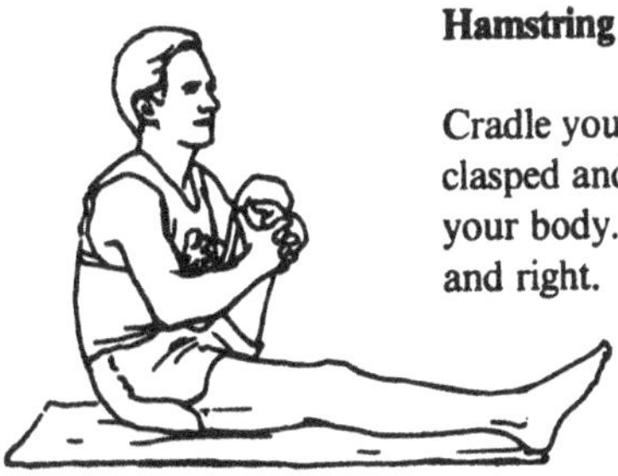

Hamstring stretch

Cradle your leg with your hands clasped and gently pull it toward your body. Gently twist to left and right.

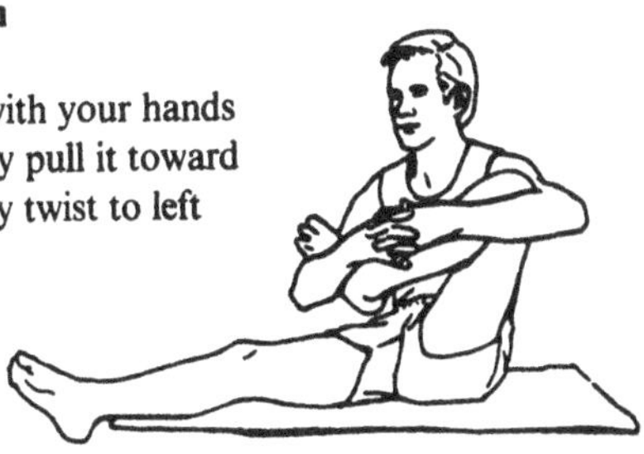

Side leg lifts

Lie on one side with both legs straight. Lift the upper leg about 45 degrees; lower. Repeat several times. Do both sides.

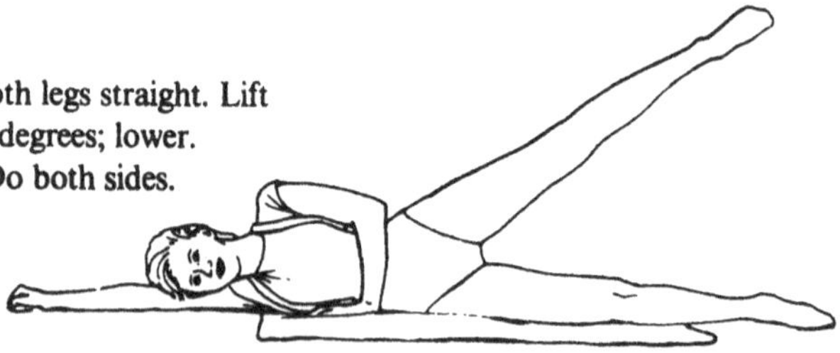

Rocking sit-ups with knees bent

Use adequate padding to protect your spinal column. This type of sit-up is less likely to cause stress injury of abdominal and back muscles than standard sit-ups with legs held down.

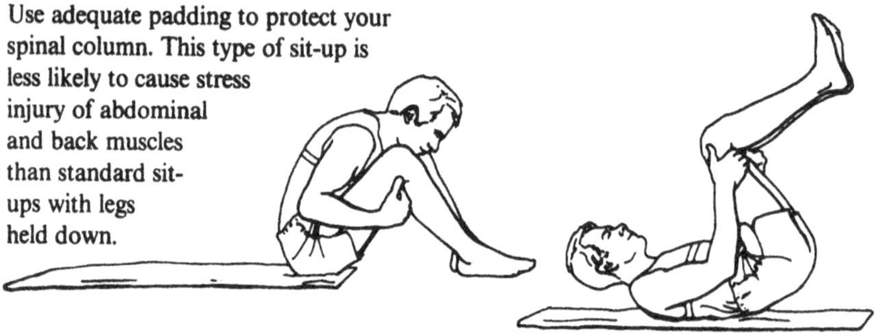

Bicycling on your back

Move your legs in a circling fashion, as if cycling. This is an excellent toner of the abdominal muscles.

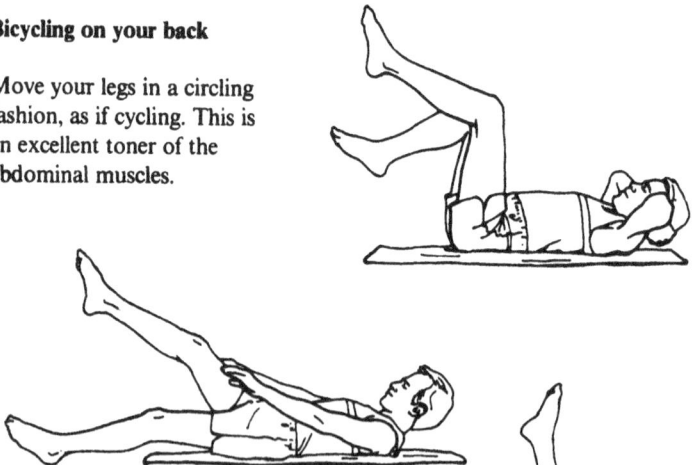

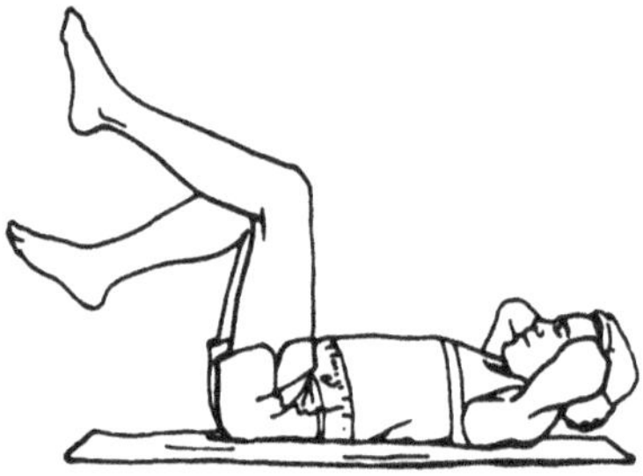

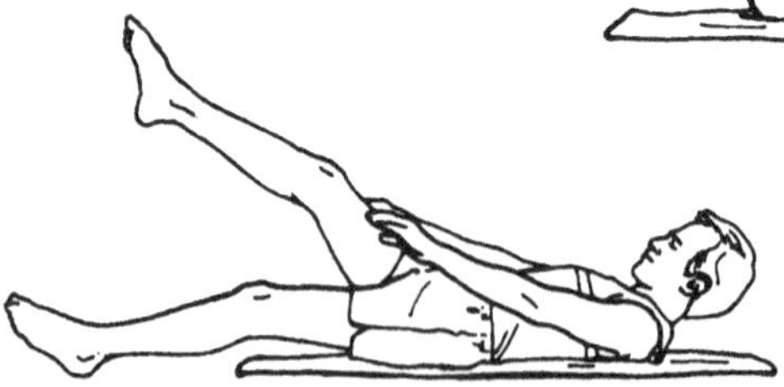

Single leg lift

Start flat on your back. Now lift one leg while bringing your head up. Lower your leg and head. Now lift the other leg, and so on. Inactive leg can be straight or bent.

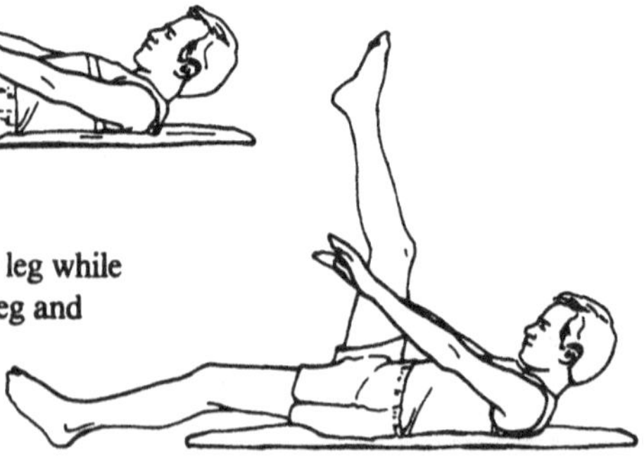

The poor person's weight gym

A stout piece of surgical tubing, an inch or two in diameter and five or six feet long, can be used for a variety of strengthening exercises. You may want to work with two at a time. Be sure to fasten the ends securely, or you'll risk a painful whack.

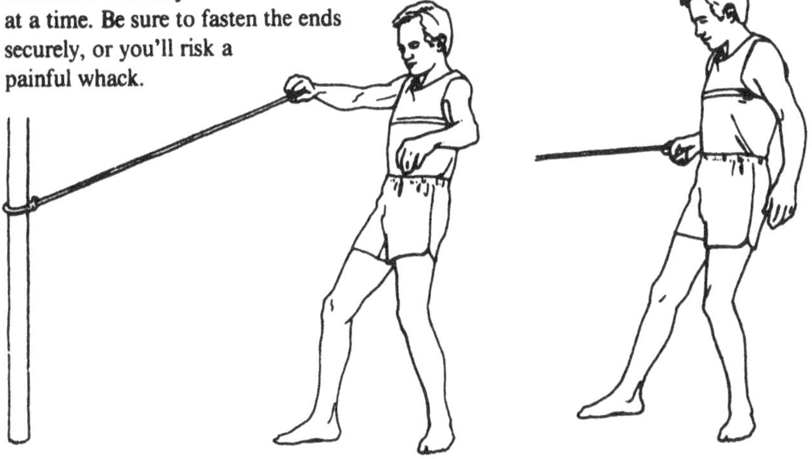

Full arm flex

Stand still and pull tubing forward using only your arm, not your body. Let back slowly. Do both arms.

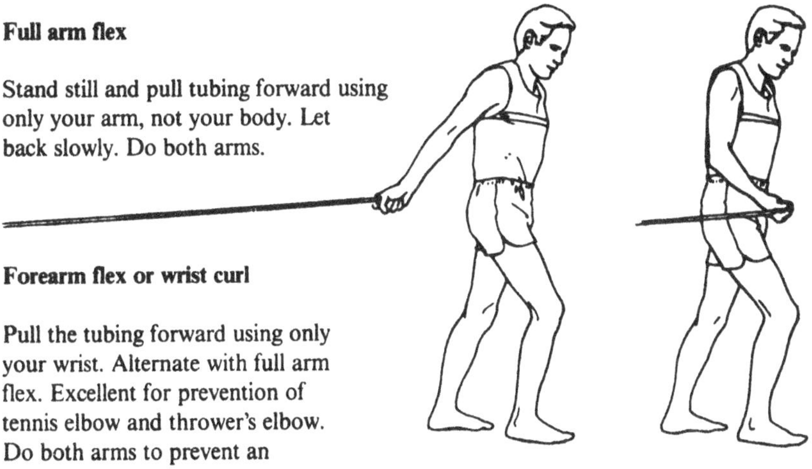

Forearm flex or wrist curl

Pull the tubing forward using only your wrist. Alternate with full arm flex. Excellent for prevention of tennis elbow and thrower's elbow. Do both arms to prevent an imbalance of development.

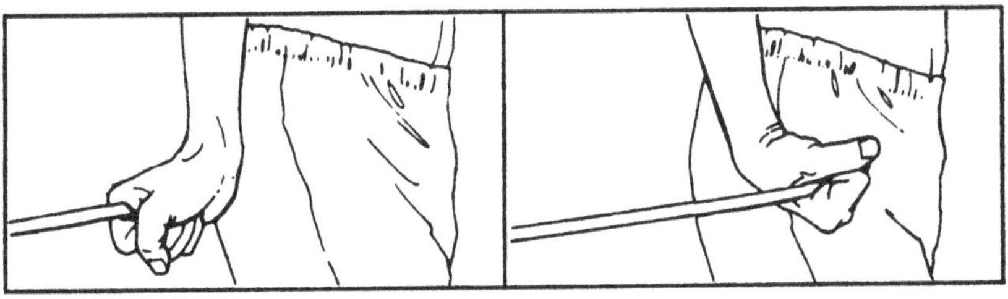

100 Treatment of Stress Injuries

Many stress injuries common in sports, particularly strains and sprains, have traditionally been treated with rest (often with immobilization), ice, compression, and elevation, commonly referred to as RICE. The point of all four steps is to reduce movement, blood flow, inflammation, and pain. There are some arguments against immobilization; sometimes controlled movement along with cooling is preferable in order to prevent stiffness and weakness that complicate the injury. Pain is usually a good guide to how much movement is safe.

Coaches, trainers, and physicians often use ethyl chloride spray for cooling injured tissue. It will not relieve pain or allow movement in severe sprains (with ligament rupture or fractures), so it is safe. The spray is applied directly over the painful area, which is carefully flexed and moved until the pain is reduced or gone. It is believed to work by relieving the muscle spasms that usually accompany strains and sprains; this allows movement and reduces swelling.

Ice is cheaper, more likely to be available to most people, and probably just as effective as ethyl chloride. An ice cube in a plastic bag wrapped in cloth can be applied to the painful area for ten to twenty minutes several times a day. It should reduce pain, swelling, and muscle spasms.

Summing up, there is agreement on the value of cooling, whether by ice or ethyl chloride, and on elevation of the injured area to prevent the pooling of blood and increased inflammation and pain. The only question concerns movement, which is apparently harmless and probably beneficial in nonsevere injuries if done carefully. However, *in no case should injured tissue be stretched.* Rest is surely necessary, even if some movement does help. So, we are left with cooling, careful movement, elevation, and rest, or CMER, for stress injuries that can benefit from home treatment. In more severe injuries a physician should be consulted: for any obvious or apparent fracture; if a limb is crooked, cold, numb, or blue; if a joint is deformed or moving abnormally; or if you are limping.

Heart Attack

Everyone, no matter how fit, is more likely to have a heart attack while active than while doing nothing. The risk is especially great for those who rarely exercise though it can be decreased by regular exercise. Other risk factors also increase the danger of exercise overloading the heart muscle and precipitating a heart attack: simply being a man over forty (though women are not immune), smoking, high cholesterol levels, high blood pressure, obesity, diabetes and a family history of heart disease or sudden death. The risk can be minimized in the following ways:

Drink adequate amounts of water and warm up and cool down properly as described above.

After warming up, **exercise at a moderate pace;** the 75 percent rule is a good guideline. In particular you should be careful if you are just starting an exercise program or otherwise greatly increasing your activity level. Start out slowly and gradually increase the length and intensity of your workouts. If you are under a physician's care for hypertension, angina, asthma, or any other chronic condition, discuss any large change in your activity level with your doctor.

No matter how healthy you think you are or how careful you think you have been, always be alert for signs of trouble such as chest pains, nausea, dizziness, and difficulty breathing. If any of them occur, stop exercising and sit down. If it continues, call a physician.

Do You Need a Stress Test? In order to detect early silent heart disease, some people should have a stress test, an examination of the heart's function during exercise. The most common stress test is treadmill electrocardiography in which an ECG is taken while the person walks or jogs on a treadmill. More sensitive tests using radioactive tracers and computer imaging are done when the stress ECG gives ambiguous results.

A stress test is generally advisable before a major increase in activity for all those with risk factors for coronary artery disease, including most men over forty or as young as thirty-five with two or more risk factors, and all women past menopause. Some physicians advocate that all exercisers past these milestones have a treadmill ECG every year or two. This may be excessive for those with no risk factors except age, but it does make sense for others. This whole area is controversial, clouded by lawsuits and threats of lawsuits, so the trend is for physicians to recommend more stress tests to decrease their malpractice lawsuit threat. The problem is that a large number of false positives have the effect of putting people through more expensive tests.

Heat Stress and Heatstroke

Exercising in the heat, especially with inadequate water intake, can lead to fatigue, syncope (fainting), muscle cramps, heat exhaustion (sometimes with headache, dizziness, profuse sweating, and vomiting), and heatstroke. All of these problems except heatstroke can be dealt with by rest in a cool environment and drinking plenty of water. Slight elevation of the feet helps in syncope. Heatstroke, which is characterized by extreme fatigue, collapse, hyperventilation, fast heart rate, confusion, headache, and hot, dry skin, requires immediate cooling and hospitalization.

Heat stress can be prevented by avoiding overexercise, particularly in hot weather, and drinking plenty of water before, during, and after a workout. Young athletes are still sometimes subjected to water restriction by their coaches in the erroneous belief that this improves stamina. This practice should not be tolerated by youngsters or their parents. Also, acclimation is very important. If you move to a warmer climate or if it suddenly gets much hotter than you are used to, give yourself a couple weeks to acclimate before exercising at your normal level. When active in hot weather, it's best to wear light-colored, light-weight, cotton clothing.

Heat stress can happen to anyone, but among the most susceptible are children, the obese, the very thin, the elderly, diabetics, heart patients, and those taking diuretics, aspirin, antihistamines, stimulants, antidepressants, atropine, and phenothiazines. In these cases all the preventive measures are very important. For example, as you get older you should be generally more careful about exercising in extreme temperatures and drinking enough water. Child athletes also deserve extra care because their heat regulating systems are not yet efficient.

Impingement Syndrome

Also known as swimmer's shoulder, bursitis, and rotator cuff tendonitis, impingement syndrome occurs when the shoulder is repeatedly raised over the head as in swimming, throwing, or playing volleyball. The upper-arm bone (humerus) impinges upon the top-of-the-shoulder joint bone (acromion) in such a way that the tendons, bursa, and other soft tissue are squeezed, causing inflammation and pain.

Aspirin and ice are usually sufficient, but other remedies, like ultrasound or cortisone, may be necessary in severe cases. The activity that caused the problem should be minimized; if it must be continued, aspirin before and ice after should help. A coach in the problem sport may be able to improve your technique or style so that less stress is put on the soft tissues. A physiatrist familiar with the problem may be able to prescribe helpful exercises.

Knee Injuries

The knee is a common site of injury because it is an unstable joint where two weight-bearing long bones are held together only by ligaments and tendons. There is no ball and socket to fit the bones together, and the ligaments allow movement in only one plane. When the knee is severely stressed by a blow, a fall, overuse, or excessive lateral force, injuries of various degrees can occur to one or more of the ligaments, tendons, bones, cartilages, muscles, or bursi in or near the knee. These stresses can occur in various sports.

Knee injuries that are not properly treated can lead to a lifetime of problems (commonly known as "trick knee") in which the knee locks, collapses, clicks, pops, or otherwise annoys and incapacitates you. The nature of the "tricks" depends on the exact location and extent of the injuries.

Sprains (ligament tears) are the most common knee injuries. Depending on the direction and force of the blow or the nature of the stress, different ligaments suffer varying degrees of damage.

Runner's knee, also known as chrondromalacia patellae, is a disfunctional kneecap, characterized by pain during exercise and while climbing or descending stairs. Pain also occurs if the kneecap is pressed or the quadriceps contracted.

Jumper's knee is very painful tendonitis of the patellar tendon just above the kneecap. It is caused by overstressing the tendon which attaches the thigh extensors (the quadriceps) to the kneecap by repeated vertical jumping as is common in basketball and volleyball.

PREVENTION

Always warm up slowly and train patiently and properly for your sport with attention to the areas of major stress. For example, if you play volleyball and spike a lot, you should strengthen your quadricep muscles with appropriate exercises such as straight leg lifts while lying on your back (raise one leg at a time to avoid back stress). Beware the deep knee bend, or full squat. It is sometimes recommended for strengthening the quadriceps and developing flexibility, especially in dancing and gymnastics, but it can produce cartilage tears and wearing of the kneecap. In short, it tends to age the knee joint.

TREATMENT

Many knee injuries can be treated with CMER and, when pain and inflammation have subsided, proper exercise. But if you have severe, persistant, or recurring knee pain you should see a physician. Special exercises, surgery, or other treatment could save you years of knee troubles. The proper exercises to help speed rehabilitation depend on the exact nature of the injury. For example, stair climbing is helpful in some injuries, but can aggravate others like runner's knee. It is important that the injury be properly evaluated so a rational exercise program can be applied. Professional physical therapy is important in most cases.

Muscle Cramps

Muscle cramps, whether constant or intermittent, can be painful and incapacitating. The causes include muscle fatigue due to increased lactate in muscles, excessive loss of body fluids or minerals, strain injury, and blood supply obstruction by prolonged isometric exercise.

PREVENTION

Warm up carefully before exercising hard, and avoid overworking any muscles. Eat plenty of fruits, vegetables, and grains to get adequate minerals. Drink water before and during exercise. Salt tablets should not be taken, but eating salty foods is okay if you do not have hypertension. Do not use rubberized exercise suits or heavy clothes; they promote excessive water and mineral loss.

TREATMENT

Relax the affected muscle, the whole body, and the mind, and gradually stretch the muscle. It often helps to flex the muscles opposing the ones in spasm. For example, if a calf muscle is cramping, flex your foot towards your shin.

Muscle Strain

A muscle strain (or pull) is a tearing of a muscle or its tendon or both. The injury can range from a few torn muscle or tendon fibers to a complete rupture. Runners often pull hamstring muscles (leg flexors in the rear thigh) and swimmers pull shoulder muscles. Strains are caused by excessive tension on a muscle-tendon complex caused by trying to do more than one's strength allows.

PREVENTION

Always warm up properly by beginning slowly and gently before working out hard. Increase your training level gradually and do not work out hard too often. Each vigorous exercise session causes some damage to the muscle, which must heal before being stressed again. Muscles should be balanced in strength with their opposing muscles. For example, hamstring pulls are common in running sports because the quadriceps (the knee extensors in the front thigh) are usually much stronger than the hamstring; during running they exert tremendous tension on the hamstrings and may stretch them to the point of tearing.

TREATMENT

If the injury is severe, with nearly complete loss of function, consult a physician right away. Surgery may be required. Milder cases can be treated with CMER for two or three days followed by mild stretching and range-of-motion exercises. The muscle and tendon must be thoroughly rehabilitated before full resumption of activity, or re-injury is certain.

Plantar Fascitis

A fascia is a sheet of strong connective tissue that surrounds and supports a muscle, tendon, or other organ. Most of the body's organs are covered by fasciae, which are subject to injury from stress or trauma. Probably the most common fascia injury is plantar fascitis, a stress-induced tear of the plantar fascia that covers the muscles of the bottom of the foot. The plantar fascia can withstand only so much pressure or stretching. When the pressure is great enough to flatten the arch or spread the toes, the fascia may tear. A sharp pain in the bottom of the foot may occur at the moment of injury or it may develop slowly over hours or days. It will then be most painful while taking the first steps in the morning and with each step in running, which can cause further tearing if done too vigorously.

PREVENTION

Wear the proper shoes for your feet and for the surface you are running on. A shoe with inadequate arch support and too much flexibility can transmit too much pressure to the fascia. A shoe that is too stiff in the sole requires too much force to bend; when the foot strike is hard, the fascia may give before the sole of the shoe does. People with flat feet, which tend to pronate (turn inward) excessively when they walk or run, may need extra arch support or even orthotics, shoe inserts that must be specially made for each individual.

TREATMENT

The affected foot must be rested to allow healing. Switch to a nonrunning sport for awhile, or run gently and not to the point of pain. Inflammation is rarely severe, but ice may help relieve pain. Cortisone and other drugs should *not* be used to allow continued training because this could lead to further injury. Taping and friction massage may help, but the proper methods should be demonstrated by an expert. Sometimes foot imbalances are responsible and must be corrected with in-shoe orthoses. In rare cases surgery is necessary.

Shin Splints

This term refers to a spectrum of pain syndromes in the overstressed shin muscles and tendons that pull the foot up. Trauma-induced inflammation and spasms may squeeze shut the veins and cause the injured muscles to become engorged, swollen, and hard. Depending on the extent of the injury and the care taken not to aggravate it, it should clear up within one to three weeks. The problem is most common in joggers, basketball and soccer players, and other runners.

PREVENTION

Warm up by walking, stretching, and slow jogging before vigorous workouts. Train patiently. Work your way up gradually, and heed pain and fatigue as warning signs that you may be overstressing your legs. Minimize your activities on hard surfaces, and wear good shoes that will cushion the repeated shocks involved in running, aerobic dancing, and jumping rope. People with low arches may need arch supports or orthotics.

Strengthen and stretch your shin muscles with ankle and toe exercises, and stretch your calf muscles and Achilles tendons. Try to pick up marbles and other objects with your toes. Vary your speed to strengthen all the tissues of the lower legs. (Always running at the same speed is believed to contribute to shin stress.) Knee-high socks or leg warmers may help by improving blood supply and waste removal during exercise.

TREATMENT

Rest, move gently, and use ice massage (see **Treatment of Stress Injuries,** above) until the pain and hardness are gone. If this takes more than three weeks or so, you should see a sports physician or orthopedic surgeon. If the pain occurs while just walking, you should see a physician right away to check for stress fractures.

Sprains

A sprain is an overstretching, tear, or complete rupture of a ligament. Swelling, pain, and dysfunction are proportional to the degree of injury. Ligaments hold bones together and stabilize joints. While they are very strong, they are not designed to withstand the strong lateral forces that occur in many sports requiring sudden changes of direction. A sprained ankle is one of the most common athletic injuries and usually involves the foot turning inward under the ankle. Sprains also occur in the knees, elbows, fingers, and other joints.

PREVENTION

Strengthen the muscles of the lower legs and feet to decrease the stress on the ankle ligaments. Always warm up slowly before running hard. When walking, jogging, running, or hiking, watch out for ruts and holes. If you are susceptible to ankle sprains because of pronated (flat) feet or other reasons, you may need arch supports or high-top shoes. Other joints can be protected by preventing blows of various kinds.

TREATMENT

If you suddenly develop a pain in a joint, stop exercising. If the pain persists, apply CMER. A mild sprain will heal in a few days, but severe pain should be evaluated by a physician who will check for torn ligaments and broken bones. Crutches, immobilization, and even surgery may be necessary. As a sprain heals, the exercise of the joint should be gradually increased. With an ankle sprain, for example, activity can increase from bending the joint up and down to walking and standing on the toes, to slow jogging, and then short and long runs.

Stitches (Side Pains)

A stitch is a sharp pain in the left or right side of the upper abdomen that usually occurs during running. The weekend athlete is more likely to experience stitches, but even highly trained people can get them. There are two common causes: cramping of the diaphragm or the muscles of the rib cage when they are forced to produce deep, rapid breathing (this is often due to pushing too hard and running while out of shape), and accumulation of gas in the colon. Exercise increases peristalsis, which pushes gas toward the rectum. If it does not escape, pressure can build up to the point of cramping.

PREVENTION

Run within the limits of your fitness level; do not push too hard. Do not eat just before working out, as this takes blood from the breathing muscles and makes them more likely to cramp. Eat more high-fiber food that is less likely to form hard stools that block gas in the colon. Be alert for signs of milk intolerance: Some people otherwise unaffected get gas and cramps from it upon exercising.

TREATMENT

Sometimes the pain will stop if you push your fingers deep into the affected area while you keep running, but usually you must slow down or stop and rest for a few minutes. If the pain continues, lift the arm of the affected side high and stretch that side, or bend forward at the waist and stretch both arms over your head. Also, try deep breathing while at rest. Stitches go away by themselves and do not require medical help, but if pain occurs in the chest, shoulders, neck, or arms, stop exercising and see a physician.

Stress Fractures

Stress fractures are shallow cracks found most commonly in bones of the feet, legs, and hands. Running, basketball, football, baseball, skiing, and skating are some of the sports that often lead to stress fractures. Sharp pain from walking or pressing the bone with a finger is an indication of a possible stress fracture.

PREVENTION

As is the case with most sports injuries, stress fractures can usually be prevented by using proper equipment (like good shoes and an appropriate running surface), and by being aware of the stresses and alert to your body's warning signals.

TREATMENT

A cast is rarely required (and carries the risk of atrophying the muscles), but rest is important. The activity that caused the fracture should be suspended, but fitness can be maintained without extending the crack by switching to another type of sport like swimming or bicycling.

Tendonitis

Tendonitis is inflammation of a tendon with swelling and pain. The pain tends to be worse in the morning and subsides as the tendon is used. This encourages abuse, however, which may aggravate the problem. Tendonitis commonly occurs in the Achilles tendon in runners, in the elbows in tennis players, and in the shoulders in swimmers and throwers. It is caused by overstressing the tendons with exercise when the muscles are tight.

PREVENTION

Strengthen your muscles so they will take stress off the tendons. Always warm up properly before working out. Exercise within your limits and heed your body's signals. If you can avoid muscle tightness you can generally prevent tendonitis. If you are prone to tendonitis in a certain area or if you plan on increasing your exercise level and the stress on certain tendons, then you should regularly do tendon-stretching exercises for several minutes before heavy workouts. For example, to stretch your Achilles tendons, stand with your heels on a board inclined toward a wall and your back against the wall for up to twenty minutes. Gradually increase the incline. Or lean against a wall with your heels on the floor, and move your feet farther and farther from the wall.

TREATMENT

Apply an ice massage for the first two days or so, and do gentle stretching and movement. Stretch slowly and pause; jerky stretching could cause further irritation and injury. Resting the affected area is important to avoid further injury. For example, running with Achilles tendonitis could rupture the tendon, a serious injury that could lay you up for months. Cortisone injections can relieve pain due to tendonitis, but they can be risky because they mask the pain and allow continued activity, and may directly weaken the tendon.

Tendon Rupture

A tendon rupture is a complete tear in a tendon or, more commonly, the rupture of a tendon's attachment to a bone or muscle. There is often an audible pop and very severe pain. The area becomes swollen, painful, and black and blue. The most common site by far is the Achilles tendon, in which case the heel cannot be lifted. The cause of a tendon rupture is usually a forceful contraction of a muscle in such sports as sprinting, skiing, handball, or tennis. A rupture is more likely if the attached muscle is tight, fatigued, or weak.

PREVENTION

Strengthen your calf muscles so they will take some stress off the tendons. A good exercise is to walk with an exaggerated tiptoe bounce. Or stand on a curb or book with your heels hanging over. Lower your heels and then push up on your tiptoes. Repeat until fatigued. Always stretch and warm up slowly before working up a sweat or making sudden strenuous movements. A rupture in an Achilles tendon is usually preceded by a partial tear or by Achilles tendonitis. These painful conditions are clear warnings to rest or risk the more serious danger of rupture.

TREATMENT

Immobilize the injured tissue, apply ice or ethyl chloride, and call a physician right away. Partially torn tendons reattach and heal by themselves, but complete ruptures usually require surgery and immobilization, especially if the tendon recoils too far or tears a piece of bone off.

Tennis Elbow

In this condition there is pain in the elbow and the forearms that is aggravated by any action involving gripping or rotating the wrist. In severe cases simple acts like shaking hands, turning a doorknob, or brushing one's teeth can be agonizing. The pain is due to injury and inflammation of the wrist-moving tendons and muscles at the elbow. The term is often applied to similar injuries to other elbow tissues because the causes, symptoms, therapy, and preventive measures are much the same.

The cause of tennis elbow is almost always overuse of a poorly conditioned forearm and hand, such as in sporadically playing tennis vigorously with little other arm exercise. Chopping wood, swinging a hammer, beating a rug, paddling a canoe, throwing a ball or javelin, and many other activities can also precipitate the condition. The tendons and their points of attachment to the bones are subjected to enormous stresses time and again. Strong, properly conditioned forearm muscles can help absorb the shock, but in weaker arms the tendons and their bone attachments are easily irritated by the stress.

PREVENTION

If you play tennis or similarly stress your forearm, always warm up slowly and don't overdo it. Heed symptoms of fatigue and tightness. Develop stronger forearms with exercises like wrist curls or by swinging a weighted racket. Improve your stroke with more shoulder and body action and less wrist action. Hit backhands with two hands at least until your forearm is strong. Improve your racket: In general, more string tension and a larger handle diameter put more stress on the muscles and tendons. You may want to try a racket with a slightly bent handle. It puts less stress on the muscles and tendons of the forearm and reduces the risk of elbow injuries. Aluminum rackets absorb less shock and transfer more up the arm than wood rackets.

TREATMENT

In the acute situation, right after the injury and for two or three days following, immobilization and intermittent cold packs are recommended. If the pain is very severe, consult a physician; injection of a long-acting local anesthetic or cortisone usually brings relief. The arm should be immobilized to avoid aggravating the injury. Movement can be gradually increased as the pain decreases. Excessive immobilization and rest can lead to atrophy, slow healing, and rapid re-injury. Friction massage properly done can be useful (a physiatrist should be consulted for this). If simple treatment does not bring relief and the condition persists for some weeks, surgery may be required to remove granulation from the areas of inflammation.

112 Thrower's Elbow

Almost everything we said about tennis elbow applies to thrower's elbow, but the affected site is the medial epicondyle rather than the lateral epicondyle—the point of attachment of the forearm's flexor muscles on the inside of the elbow, rather than the extensor muscle attachment at the outer elbow that is affected in tennis elbow. Thrower's elbow is generally more serious than tennis elbow because of the nearness of the ulnar nerve ("funny bone"), involvement of which can cause severe pain and disability.

Throwing too hard or with improper warmup is the most common cause. But just as throwing can precipitate tennis elbow, so playing tennis can cause thrower's elbow. The causes, treatment, and prevention are essentially the same, but thrower's elbow is more likely to require surgery due to ulnar nerve involvement.

PREVENTION

Prevention can be accomplished by properly warming up before throwing hard, and strengthening the forearm with wrist curls and other arm exercises.

Sports and Drugs

Many drugs are used in professional and amateur athletics in the belief that they will provide a shortcut in training or an edge in competition. In spite of laws forbidding this and studies showing the drugs to be mostly ineffective and dangerous, doping for sports remains popular. We will discuss the drugs most commonly used and their effects on athletes.

When athletes consider taking a drug because others say it helps, they should keep in mind the tremendous power of the placebo effect; even the most sophisticated people can be fooled by their hopes and expectations. And if they are still convinced that a certain drug will do wonders, they should ask themselves whether the long-term costs are worth the short-term gains: Should the purpose of athletics be to help you live a healthy, happy life, or to win some medals and money regardless of the cost to your health and sanity?

Amphetamine and its relatives such as methylphenidate (Ritalin) are potent stimulants and mood elevators, and are among the most commonly abused drugs in sports. They produce self-confidence, aggressiveness, and delusions of outstanding performance. They tend to mask pain and reduce the perception of fatigue, increasing the risk of injury and heatstroke, a very serious hazard for amphetamine users in strenuous competition. Deaths have occurred. Moreover, the user takes longer to recover from workouts and competition, and is prone to depression and lethargy unless he or she takes more of the drugs, all of which are addicting.

Anabolic steroids. (See **Testosterone analogues,** below.)

Androgens. (See **Testosterone analogues,** below.)

Antibiotics do not go well with very heavy exercise because the stress can provoke a reaction to the drug, like diarrhea or vomiting, or difficulty in breathing, that otherwise might not occur. Moreover, if you have an infection worthy of antibiotics it could be serious enough to cause a reaction to heavy exercise, which increases susceptibility to bacterial toxins.

Blood packing is also called blood doping, but this is a poor term since no drugs are used. It involves removing a couple pints of your blood, training for a few months to bring the red cell level back up to the normal 45 percent (40 in women), and transfusing the removed red cells back before the competition. This is done to elevate the number of red cells and increase the oxygen-carrying capacity of the blood in order to improve performance in endurance events.

The concentration of red cells increases to about 50 to 52 percent (45 in women) and it apparently helps, but not much. The result is similar to training at several thousand feet elevation for several months before competing at sea level. There is a slight risk of the thickened blood slowing circulation and even clogging capillaries. The practice is illegal in most competition, but practically impossible to detect.

Caffeine and its relatives, found in coffee, tea, colas, and various non-prescription drugs, are among the more innocuous drugs used by athletes to get a lift for working out or competing. For most people they are harmless in moderation, but some people will experience a racing heart or palpitations. They should cut out the caffeine or theophylline and consult their physicians. However, for athletes susceptible to exercise-induced asthma, theophylline, taken an hour or so before exercising, is an effective and safe treatment. It is also approved for use in competition, as are cromalyn sodium and albuterol. Very large doses of caffeine are banned, but the illegal amounts are enough to make most people feel sick anyway.

Cocaine was one of the big scandal drugs of the eighties, with hundreds of proved and suspected users in professional and amateur sports. Its effects and hazards are nearly identical to those of amphetamines (see above).

Cortisone and its relatives can do wonders when injected into areas with stubborn, painful, incapacitating inflammation. But it can mask pain and even directly weaken some tissues, so its use must be coupled with rest. Using cortisone to allow use of slightly injured tissue carries a risk of severe injury.

Ephedrine is a stimulant related to adrenalin with effects similar to those of amphetamine but usually without the mood elevation. Heatstroke is a potentially lethal hazard.

Erythropoietin is a prescription drug given to some AIDS patients to stimulate the bone marrow to produce more red blood cells, thus increasing the oxygen-carrying capacity of the blood. The effect is similar to blood packing, but is potentially more dangerous, as it could thicken the blood enough to clog an artery and cause a stroke or heart attack.

Human growth hormone has effects similar to those of testosterone derivatives (below) and is in much demand by athletes because the extra amounts cannot be detected in the blood or urine. The hazards include abnormal glucose metabolism (similar to diabetes), abnormal growth of some tissues, and severe reactions to pig and cow hormones passed off as human growth hormone. Moreover, the demand for the drug (some athletes pay hundreds of dollars a month for it) has driven the price out of sight for many dwarf children who could be helped by it. In this respect, the use of this hormone is perhaps the most reprehensible of all the efforts athletes make to gain an edge with chemicals.

Psychedelics such as LSD, peyote, mescaline, and psilocybin mushrooms are sometimes used in long-distance running and other events that test one's stamina. However, the effects are too unpredictable so such use is not very common.

Oxygen is not usually considered a drug, but as it is used by athletes during competition it is a drug of sorts, though only a placebo. The lift that football and basketball players and others get from inhaling pure oxygen during time-outs is all in their heads. They would probably reduce their blood lactate levels faster if they walked around rather than sat and breathed oxygen (lactate builds up during exertion and causes muscle pain and fatigue). Walking helps remove the lactate from the muscles. Athletes become conditioned to the oxygen in college and feel they can't play as well without it, but it's a foolish practice because by sharing oxygen masks teams pass around viruses and bacteria. This modern superstition has no place in our educational institutions.

Speed. (See **Amphetamines, Caffeine, Cocaine, Ephedrine,** above.)

"Steroids" are a group of hormones and other biochemicals with a particular chemical similarity. Cortisone, other adrenal hormones, and sex hormones are examples of steroids. Since these have very different and sometimes opposing functions, it is better to specify the substance in question rather than speaking of "steroids" in general.

Testosterone analogues, or anabolic steroids, are the focus of much recent scandal and controversy. Testosterone is responsible for the rapid increase in muscle mass in boys at puberty. Now, many weight lifters, body builders, and football players take large doses of synthetic analogues of the male sex hormone to help build up their muscles. They get them from doctors, health club owners, drug companies, pharmacists, and other athletes. It appears that the vast majority of athletes in some sports, especially body building, spend hundreds of dollars a month on the injections and pills.

There does seem to be an increase in the size of muscle fibers with the use of these drugs, but this appears to be due to the retention of fluid in the tissues. There is *no* evidence that in trained athletes and other normal people there is an increase in strength. The dubious benefit should be weighed against a host of side effects. Here are the most important ones reported or suspected so far:

- atrophy of the testicles with decreased libido and sperm count;
- chemical hepatitis and possibly liver cancer;
- neurological and behavioral symptoms such as increased aggressiveness, psychotic behavior ("roid rage"), sleep disturbances, headaches, fainting, and dizziness;
- greatly decreased HDL-cholesterol (the "good" type) and an increased risk of atherosclerosis and heart disease (especially given the high-fat diets many body builders are on);

- gynecomastia, the growth of the nipples and surrounding tissue, which often requires cosmetic surgery;
- male pattern baldness;
- masculinization of females, mostly irreversible, with increased facial and body hair, baldness, acne, and leathery skin;
- abnormal sexual maturation and stunted growth in adolescents, perhaps the greatest danger of these drugs.

Section Two

COMMON DISEASES: A PREVENTIVE APPROACH

Common Diseases

- AIDS
- Allergies
- Asthma
- Atherosclerosis
- Backaches (Low Back Pain)
- Birth Defects and Sickness in the Newborn
- Cancers
- Chickenpox and Shingles
- Colds
- Dementia and Alzheimer's Disease
- Dental and Gum Disease
- Diabetes
- Eating Disorders
- Epilepsy
- Female Disorders
- Gallstones
- Hearing Loss and Ear Infections
- Heart Disease
- Hepatitis
- Hypertension
- Influenza (Flu)
- Kidney Disorders
- Malaria
- Measles (Rubeola)
- Mumps
- Obesity
- Osteoporosis
- Pneumonia
- Rabies
- Rubella
- Sexually Transmitted Diseases (STDs)
- Stomach Acid Related Disorders
- Stroke
- Tick-Borne Diseases
- Tuberculosis
- Vision Loss

AIDS

Acquired immune deficiency syndrome (AIDS) is a highly lethal disease first recognized in male homosexuals in 1979. It has stricken over 100,000 Americans in the years since. By 1991 there will likely be more than 300,000 cases in the United States and tens of millions worldwide. Despite improvements in treatment, 80 percent of victims die within three years of diagnosis.

AIDS is caused by infection with the human immunodeficiency virus (HIV), also called the AIDS virus. Most infection is caused by a form of the virus called HIV-1, but a second form, HIV-2, has been reported in West Africa, which raises the alarming prospect of still more forms. The virus produces illness in two ways: by direct injury to tissues and by destruction of the immune system's T cells.

In some cases, a few weeks after infection a flulike illness occurs with fever, sweating, headache, bodyache, diarrhea, sore throat, rash, and enlarged lymph nodes. At this stage blood tests for HIV are negative. After this acute illness the person may feel well until later effects of the virus emerge. In most cases there is no initial illness, just the insidious onset of enlarged lymph nodes and sometimes fever, fatigue, and weight loss. Full blown AIDS follows in subsequent months and years.

More specifically, AIDS patients come down with severe cases of Pneumocystis carinii pneumonia (PCP), thrush (an oral fungus infection), virulent herpes that attacks internal organs, atypical tuberculosis, toxoplasmosis, protozoa, and other infections that intact immune systems usually handle with ease. They are also prone to such cancers as Hodgkin's disease and other lymphomas, and Kaposi's sarcoma. The latter was, until recently, a mild skin cancer that affected mostly the elderly but is now aggressive and lethal in young AIDS patients.

120 Direct effects of the virus include injury to the brain and nerves, leading to intellectual deterioration (known as AIDS dementia), as well as weakness, loss of coordination, and incontinence. Ninety percent of AIDS patients suffer some degree of brain or nerve involvement.

Who Gets AIDS?

The AIDS virus is passed from person to person through sexual contact, by injection of infected blood and blood products, and from infected mothers to their unborn children. Consequently, almost all cases in North America fall within one of six categories. About 90 percent are homosexual men or intravenous drug abusers. The rest are patients who received infected blood by transfusion (mostly before blood testing for HIV became routine), those who had heterosexual contact with infected partners, infants born to infected mothers, and hemophiliacs who inject blood clotting products that are sometimes contaminated with the virus.

The greatest risk is from injection with contaminated blood products, including accidental jabs with a bloody needle. Next most dangerous is passive anal sex with an infected partner. With genital sex the risk of male to female transmission is much greater than female to male. Female to female sexual transmission has been reported, but appears to be very rare. In all cases the risk is greater if a genital lesion from a sexually transmitted disease is present.

In parts of Africa and in Haiti AIDS is just as common in women as in men, and the disease runs rampant. Heterosexual transmission is, for unknown reasons, much more common in these areas, and this helps account for the high incidence. But another possible factor deserves serious consideration: In areas where AIDS is endemic blood rituals and tatooing are very common, AIDS is not understood, and precautions are rarely taken. The careless splashing around of blood during these rituals and the shared use of cutting and tatooing instruments may be a significant factor in the spread of AIDS in some cultures.

The AIDS virus is not transmitted by casual contact such as shaking hands, sharing meals, using toilets or showers, or working together. Children don't spread the virus to schoolmates and playmates. Nurses and family members don't get it caring for patients. Mosquitoes and other insects do not spread the virus. Nor can you get the virus by donating blood since only new needles are used for this purpose. Receiving a blood transfusion carries a tiny risk, about one in 40,000 to 100,000. With improved blood screening methods this small risk is sure to decrease.

- **Don't share needles** to inject illicit drugs.
- **Don't use crack**—ever. This form of cocaine is so addicting that even the best and brightest, whether from inner cities or neat suburbs, will do whatever they have to to get high. For many this means selling their bodies, even though they know that they could get AIDS. Some experts now rate crack smokers as the group with the fastest growing incidence of AIDS. The smokable methamphetamine called ice may soon have a similar distinction, since its effects and addictive power are similar to crack's.
- If you are a health worker or laboratory worker **protect yourself from needle pricks** and other exposure to blood and blood products and other body fluids.
- **Don't engage in sexual intimacies with people infected with HIV** or possibly infected due to present or past IV drug use, smokable cocaine or amphetamine use, or promiscuous sexual behavior, heterosexual or homosexual.
- If you have some doubt about a new sex partner, but not enough to avoid sexual intimacy, **practice safe sex** until you are sure. That is, avoid exchange of bodily fluids and direct genital to genital contact and oral-genital contact by using condoms and dental dams (which go over female genitals during oral sex).
- From a public health perspective, **it is extremely important that these preventive principles be taught to young people** before they become sexually active or experiment with drugs.
- Hope for the future: **Experimental vaccines are being developed and tested.** An effective one may eventually emerge.

Who Should Be Tested for AIDS?

Current testing for HIV infection detects antibodies against the virus. Since it can take weeks or even months for these antibodies to show up, such testing has a built-in error for those who were recently infected. New tests that detect the virus itself may solve this problem.

If you are not in a high-risk group, there is no reason to be tested. It is a waste of resources for thousands or millions of people to be tested when they run essentially no risk. Moreover, there are occasional false positives that can be psychologically devastating. They can also be costly, since further testing must follow.

 If you do belong to a high-risk group, or feel you may have been exposed to the virus, discuss the possibility with your doctor. Your conversation and any test results are confidential by law. You can also be tested anonymously through state health agencies. If you test positive, confirmatory testing will be done. If you are HIV positive, report this to your doctor without delay. Early treatment may forestall full-blown AIDS and prolong life.

If you belong to a high-risk group and experience certain symptoms you should consult a physician and be tested. The symptoms include swollen lymph nodes, night sweats, chronic fatigue, chronic diarrhea, weight loss, persistant mouth sores, and white patches in the mouth.

See a physician immediately if you are HIV positive and develop difficulty breathing, seizures, or severe headache with fever or confusion.

TREATMENT

Only one drug, zidovudine or AZT, has been shown to have any effect on HIV; in some cases it appears to delay the onset and slow the progress of AIDS after infection occurs, but it is quite toxic, so the risks must be weighed against the benefits. Better drugs may be available soon. Other treatment depends on which specific infections or malignancies occur, and may include antibiotics and other medications.

While each manifestation of the disease must be specifically treated as it occurs, two general factors can be applied to strengthen the body and the will to live, which may falter in those who are very sick and feel abandoned. One is proper nutrition. There is no special diet, but AIDS patients should be encouraged to eat nutritious, balanced meals to the extent possible. They often need help in getting, making, or affording healthful and appealing food. The other factor is emotional support. One of the worst things that can happen to an AIDS patient is to be shunned by friends and family. For this reason we emphasize that there is no danger in casual contact with an AIDS patient.

Beware of AIDS Quackery

There are hundreds of unscrupulous operators now running shameless and ruthless scams to rob AIDS victims of their resources. Their products range from nutritional supplements and worthless herbs to hydrogen peroxide and homeopathic remedies. All treatments not recommended by a medical doctor specializing in AIDS should be avoided.

Allergies

An allergic reaction is an inappropriate response of the immune system, which produces antibodies (proteins that bind to other molecules) against harmless substances. The antibodies combine with the offending substance (antigen), and the combination causes histamine and other chemicals to be released into the tissues causing swelling, redness, itching, respiratory distress, or gastrointestinal symptoms. Symptoms range in severity from mild hives to severe wheezing, cardiovascular collapse, and shock. Death, a rare symptom, is most likely in allergies involving the respiratory system.

The hereditary factor is strong. The predisposition to allergies in general (though not specific allergies) tends to run in families. Emotional stress, tension, anxiety, and fatigue increase sensitivity. In some cases extreme temperatures may also predispose people to attacks. Over a lifetime the intensity of allergic symptoms can vary dramatically. Childhood allergies are apparently outgrown, only to return years or decades later.

An allergy can usually be diagnosed by the symptoms, but identifying the culprits is often difficult and time consuming. We know when we have hay fever, hives, or asthma, but we don't always know what triggers it. The methods used include a careful search for associations between symptoms and the environment, skin tests in which small amounts of suspected allergens are introduced into the skin, and other tests.

Preventing the Onset of Allergies

A strategy of early avoidance of allergens may reduce the risk of allergies developing. This involves very careful control of what infants eat and breathe for the first year or so of life. Breast-feeding for several months may make food allergies less likely. The lining of the newborn's digestive system is somewhat permeable to undigested proteins. When these are absorbed, whole antibodies may form and the body then becomes sensitized to the food. New foods should be introduced slowly, in small amounts, and not too early. Children of allergic parents should not be fed eggs, cow's milk, or other commonly allergenic foods, or be exposed to wool, fur, or feathers for the first year. House dust and cockroaches should be reduced as much as possible. Care should be taken not to expose children to drugs through breast milk, especially if allergies run in the family. Breast-feeding mothers should avoid all unnecessary drugs.

124 Common Allergies

Allergic Conjunctivitis. Airborne particles such as pollen, animal dander, dust mites, and wool can land on the surface of the eye and trigger an allergic response. The eyes become itchy, watery, and red. Rubbing the eyes becomes irresistable, but it causes more irritation. Excessive rubbing can damage the surface contour of the eyeball. Consult a physician if you frequently have symptoms resembling allergic conjunctivitis.

Allergic Cough. Like the skin, eyes, nasal membranes, gastrointestinal tract, and other tissues, the lining of the upper respiratory system can become inflamed by contact with allergenic substances. Mucus production increases and an itchy sensation develops that triggers coughing. Sometimes the process is initiated by a cold or the flu that injures the tissue and makes it more sensitive to allergens. Antihistamines and cough medicines with dextromethorphan sometimes help.

Asthma. See separate entry, below.

Hay Fever. This allergic reaction, also known as allergic rhinitis, with sneezing, running nose, and itching eyes, nose, and ears is brought on by contact with pollens of ragweed, grasses, and trees (especially deciduous, rarely evergreen), mold and fungus spores, house dust, and animal dander. Symptoms may also include headache, insomnia, loss of appetite, and fatigue. Coughing and wheezing may also occur.

Prevention and Treatment of Hay Fever

Avoid the allergens as much as possible. Knowing the seasonal variation of the symptoms and the pollination period of the local plants can help pin down the specific allergens, and may help you in avoiding them. Use air filters to keep pollens, fungi, and molds out of the house. If a humidifier is used it should be regularly cleaned since it may harbor molds and spread their spores throughout the house. Control house dust with damp mopping and dusting; avoid sweeping and regular vacuuming, which kick up and spread as much dust as they clean up. Water-filter vacuum cleaners are good.

If practical, get rid of all carpets. They harbor acres of mites and dust that are kicked into the air with every step. Nontoxic sprays may soon be available to kill the insects and render their bodies nonallergenic.

If you must have carpets, choose short-nap ones made of synthetic fibers. Get rid of, or avoid contact with, offending pets, feather pillows, wool rugs, and the like. Foam pillows and mattresses often contain traces of formaldehyde, which is an allergen to many people. Avoid cigarette smoke, aerosol sprays, and volatile household chemicals that irritate the upper respiratory system. Don't overlook gas leaks and fumes from stoves and furnaces. An air conditioner in the bedroom makes a good filter and you might be able to claim the expense as a medical deduction.

Try a saline nasal rinse as a routine hygienic measure, as it is among many Hindus. Mix ¼ teaspoon salt in a cup of warm water. Pour some into one hand, close one nostril with the other hand, tilt your head back, and slowly pour the water into the open nostril while gently sucking through that nostril. Spit the water out of your mouth and blow it out of your nose (gently). Do each nostril two or three times. This removes dust, pollen, and other irritating airborne particles.

If you can't adequately avoid the allergens you might benefit from medication. If so, it's best to see a physician rather than to treat yourself with nonprescription products. For example, nasal and oral decongestants may relieve a stuffy nose for three days or so, but rapid development of tolerance leads to severe rebound congestion; antihistamines can help, but they tend to cause drowsiness; vitamin C may relieve hay fever symptoms, but an adequate dose will probably cause diarrhea. The most effective drugs require prescriptions. Besides, a doctor might be able to help in other ways.

Skin tests and desensitization shots are often tried. Once the allergens are identified, increasing amounts of them are injected under the skin once or twice a week, sometimes for years. These procedures are time consuming, expensive, and of dubious value in many cases. They seem to work better against allergies to plants than allergies to animals.

Food Allergies. Allergic reactions to foods may cause abdominal pain, nausea, vomiting, diarrhea, asthma, headaches, nasal congestion, hives (clusters of itchy red bumps), possibly bed-wetting and ear infections in children, and even anaphylactic shock, a life-threatening reaction with bronchial spasms, suffocation, and unconsciousness. There is some evidence that food allergies may provoke rheumatoid arthritis flare-ups, but this is controversial and probably rare. Severe food allergies, especially when the allergen is unknown, can lead to anxiety about eating, loss of appetite, and consequent anemia, weight loss, and other signs of malnutrition. The most common food allergies are to eggs, wheat, peanuts,

 nuts, peas, soy products, dairy products, shellfish, and whitefish.

A wide variety of other conditions are commonly confused with food allergy. These include: food intolerance due to enzyme deficiency, like lactose intolerance due to lactase deficiency; hypersensitivity reactions like chest pain and headache after consuming MSG and headache from nitrates; food poisoning; seafood toxicity, like scrombroid or ciguatera; bacterial and viral infections from food; contaminants like pesticides in food; and pharmacologic effects of substances naturally present in foods such as histamine in beer, wine, and chocolate (for discussion of many of these, see Section One).

Food allergies are somewhat more common in children and can lead to poor growth, fatigue, insomnia, poor school work, irritability, and difficulty getting along with others. An aversion to a food is not necessarily a whim and should be taken seriously, especially if there is a family history of allergies, including asthma and hay fever. Fortunately, children tend to outgrow food allergies.

The best test for food allergy is the blind challenge. Capsules of the suspected food or a placebo are swallowed and adverse reactions noted. Testing is done over several days, sometimes with the food, sometimes with the placebo. Neither the person being tested nor the person giving the capsules should know if they contain the suspected food or the placebo.

Cytotoxic testing is a heavily promoted method of diagnosing food allergies. Blood is incubated with food extracts and the effects on blood cells noted. Allergies are "diagnosed" and blamed for every disorder the client might have. Supplements that magically fight the allergies are then prescribed and sold to the clients. Allergy experts and nutritionists consider it all quackery—sophisticated exploitation of the gullible and desperate. Consider calling your local medical society or the FDA if someone offers you such testing.

Prevention and Treatment of Food Allergies

The allergens may be identified by keeping a careful diary of foods eaten and symptoms or by trial diets that eliminate suspected foods. Avoid the allergen if possible. This is often difficult because so many prepared foods have small amounts of eggs, milk, wheat, or other commonly allergenic foods. Additives may also be the source of the problem, so read labels. Insecticide residues are sometimes to blame. This can be very difficult to recognize and deal with, but, fortunately, seems to be rare.

Consult a physician if you suspect you have a food allergy, especially if symptoms are severe and the food is important in your diet. If possible, save portions of any food you think you had an allergic reaction to, since it may not be an allergy, but food poisoning, which is much more common.

Drug Allergies. Allergies can occur with any drug, but they are more likely with some than others. A reaction can be immediate, producing hives, fever, or severe anaphylaxis (with wheezing, pallor, low blood pressure, stupor, coma, and even death); or it may become apparent only after weeks or months of using a drug. Allergies to some drugs can cause destruction of red blood cells. Whatever the reaction, it usually subsides promptly after the drug is withdrawn but sometimes lasts for weeks or months.

Drug reactions may occur after eating foods (especially meat or milk, or even mother's milk), contaminated with drugs like penicillin. Sometimes the first medical dose causes a reaction, the person having been previously exposed to the drug in food and thereby sensitized to it.

Prevention and Treatment of Drug Allergies

People with any allergies or even a family history of allergies should always mention the relevant facts to doctors and nurses treating them, and carefully avoid drugs they have had allergic reactions to, as well as related drugs.

See a physician immediately if you experience an apparent allergic reaction to any drug. You may develop a rash, hives, or breathing difficulties. Immediate injection of epinephrine is the treatment of choice in severe cases. Oral antihistamines and corticosteroids help control prolonged reactions. Of course, the offending drug must be withdrawn.

Contact Dermatitis. In this type of allergy inflammation with itching and burning occurs where the offending substance touches the skin. To test a suspected allergen, put a little on the skin and cover it with a bandage. Check it in a day or two for a small rash. Poison oak and ivy reactions are common and typical examples.

Prevention and Treatment of Contact Dermatitis

- **Wash any affected area** thoroughly to remove the allergen, being careful not to spread it to other parts of the body.
- **Avoid the offending substance.** Poison oak and ivy are almost universal allergens. Others are not so obvious and alertness is often required to determine the cause of the problem. Common

offenders include other plant oils and resins, hair dyes, curling chemicals and rinses, soaps, detergents, shampoos, cosmetics, toothpastes, mouthwashes, nail polishes, perfumes, insect sprays, nasal sprays, furs, leather, fabrics, condoms, douches, toilet paper, antiperspirants, deodorants, lipsticks, rectal suppositories, eyeglass frames, hairbrush bristles, shoes, socks, and various metals and plastics such as nickel and others frequently used in the manufacture of earrings, wristwatches, telephones, and ballpoint pens.

Eczema (Atopic Dermatitis). Eczema is an allergic condition that causes dry, itching skin. In chronic cases with frequent scratching the skin weeps and may become infected; it may eventually become thickened and rough.

Eczema runs in families prone to hay fever and asthma, and can be aggravated by emotional stress, sweating, infection, and food allergies. Common sites in infants and children are the cheeks, arms, and legs. Adults have more trouble with their hands, especially if they are often wet; this removes natural oils and dries out the skin.

Prevention and Treatment of Eczema

- **Avoid dressing too warmly,** as it causes sweating and may aggravate itching. Wool clothing should be avoided.
- **Avoid bathing with soap and water,** which tend to dry the skin. Look for cleansers with cetyl alcohol.
- **Avoid oily creams,** which may increase sweat retention and itching.
- **Use aspirin to relieve severe itching,** but do so sparingly to avoid side effects.
- **Prescription steroid creams can relieve severe itching,** but a physician's supervision is necessary to prevent thinning of the skin.
- **Reduction of emotional stress** is sometimes the most important remedy, perhaps partly because stress increases sweating. Caffeine may increase both emotional stress and sweating.

Insect Sting Allergies. Severe allergic reactions to the venom of *Hymenoptera* insects (bees, wasps, yellow jackets, hornets) can cause shortness of breath, heart palpitations, wheezing, coughing, anaphylactic shock, and death. Mild reactions involve swelling and tenderness or numbness of the area around the sting.

Learn to avoid getting stung or bitten, especially by the insects you are allergic to. Learn about the habitats and habits of your "enemies." Avoid disturbing their nests, and don't step on them. You should particularly stay clear of yellow jackets as they will attack without provocation and have very nasty stings. They should not be allowed to nest around homes. Fire ants, a serious and growing problem in southern states, can inflict hundreds of stings in one swarming attack on a bypasser. They should be kept away from homes and popular recreation areas.

Bees and most wasps, on the other hand, are not very aggressive and will usually leave you alone if you leave them alone. Bees, of course, pollinate flowers, and wasps help control undesirable insects; unless someone is severely allergic to their stings, there is usually no reason to eradicate them around the home. When outdoors wear shoes; wear light-colored clothes with muted colors; don't wear perfumes, aftershave lotions, hairsprays, or any other scented cosmetic; and be wary of all possible habitats such as tall grass, abandoned buildings, attics, picnic areas, and rotting trees.

If you get stung remove the stinger (in the case of honeybees), apply ice, a tourniquet (for no longer than 15 minutes), or both, and avoid moving about since muscular activity increases absorption of the venom. If it's necessary to go for help, walk, don't run; but it's better to sit still while being taken to a physician.

Epinephrine should be given subcutaneously (injected just below the skin), or, if the victim is already in shock, intravenously. Anyone with this very serious allergy should get a kit with epinephrine or a similar drug; ask your physician.

Consider immunotherapy treatments (desensitization shots); they are often effective and could save your life. In this therapy injections of tiny amounts of the allergenic substances are given every week or so. The dose is gradually increased until an effective level is reached. The treatments apparently work because the injected substances saturate the antibodies and keep them from overreacting.

If you ever have a very serious reaction to an insect sting, with unusual swelling, pain, sweating, nausea and weakness, BEWARE! The next time could be worse. See an allergist.

If you are allergic, and at high risk of getting stung some day, **consider wearing an identification bracelet** with medical information for emergency purposes.

130 Asthma

Asthma is a disease characterized by susceptibility to asthma attacks. An asthma attack occurs when the soft muscular walls of the bronchial airways go into constrictive spasms and the delicate lining of the walls (the mucosa) becomes inflamed and pours mucus into the airways. The mucus forms plugs that block the tubes. Breathing is difficult and loud. Attacks vary in severity and may last minutes, hours, or days. Extreme attacks can end in death.

Many children who have asthma outgrow it by late adolescence. A few continue to suffer attacks throughout life, particularly if they had eczema in infancy. Adult-onset asthma also tends to improve with age, but sometimes the disease becomes chronic. Unless complications develop, asthmatics are not sick or incapacitated except during an attack.

CAUSES

Asthma attacks are triggered by a wide variety of irritants, infections, allergies, and combinations of these things. Examples include physical exertion, colds, influenza, aspirin, ibuprofen, sulfites, tartrazine (yellow dye no. 5), solvent fumes, industrial pollutants, sawdust, and flour dust, as well as allergic reactions to grass and tree pollen, mold and fungi spores, animal dander and feces dust, and house dust with fragments and feces of microscopic mites and cockroaches. Allergic reactions to foods (particularly peanuts, milk, and fish) sometimes cause asthma attacks, but this is not common.

Susceptibility to asthma runs in families. If both parents have asthma or many allergies their children have about a 50 percent chance of developing asthma.

PREVENTING ASTHMA

Breast-feeding for at least four to six months may help prevent asthma itself, as opposed to preventing asthma attacks. New foods should be introduced in small amounts, slowly and not too early. Children of allergic parents should not be fed eggs, peanuts, nuts, cow's milk, or other commonly allergenic foods, or be exposed to wool, fur, or feathers for the first year. Minimizing exposure to dust, smoke, and fumes may also help.

PREVENTING ASTHMA ATTACKS

- **Don't smoke.** Avoid air pollution.
- **Avoid irritants and allergens.** Reduce house dust, especially in the bedroom. Control home ventilation to reduce pollens. Avoid chemical fumes; fresh paint; hairsprays; pets and their hairs, feathers, and dander; and animal hair and feathers in pillows and furniture. Keep home humidity around 50 percent and not too cool. Always keep warm. Dress well from head to toe in the cold and try not to breath cold air. Get rid of carpets or install the low-nap type and keep them clean. Use the baited roach-control disks to lower your roach population; they are often very effective.
- **Follow the prescribed drug regimen** very carefully. Inadequate doses are ineffective, and overdoses are dangerous. If side effects are severe and success minimal, consider consulting an asthma expert. New drug treatments focusing on reducing chronic inflammation in the lungs are proving very successful in reducing incidence and severity of attacks. Some nonspecialists may not be up on the latest advances in asthma control.
- **Eat moderately,** slowly, and preferably not just before going to bed; digestive disturbances increase the likelihood of an attack. Eat a balanced, nutritious diet to help maintain resistance to infections.
- **Avoid aspirin and other anti-inflammatory drugs** if you are intolerant; they cause attacks in about a fifth of all asthmatics. Other drugs may also, so consult your doctor.
- **Avoid excessive emotional stress** and overexcitement. Anger can provoke an attack, so parents of asthmatic children must delicately balance firmness and leniency. Relaxation training has also been reported helpful.
- **Exercise programs may help increase breathing efficiency** by building up the diaphragm and other breathing muscles. Deep breathing with complete exhalation lets stale air out of the lower lungs and loosens and strengthens breathing muscles. Whistling and blowing bits of paper across a table are often recommended.

  Playing a wind instrument such as a clarinet, recorder, flute, trumpet, or tuba is among the most beneficial of the exercises. This can increase vital capacity, improve lung function, and help promote relaxation. Perhaps most important, especially for child asthmatics, is the psychological benefit of being active, normal, and "included."

Exercise can also be helpful, but strenuous activity for too long can provoke an attack in some, including a few nonasthmatics. While vigorous exercise is okay for most asthmatics, some will have to limit it to short spurts up to two or three minutes. Hiking, baseball, and swimming are generally better than basketball, tennis, or marathon running, though the latter are certainly not ruled out.

- **Immunotherapy (desensitization shots)** is sometimes recommended. It may help, but the expense, discomfort, and frequency of failure make it a questionable procedure for many asthmatics. The shots are generally most successful against allergies to mold spores, dog and cat dander, and house dust mites.

  Skin testing is done so the shots can be customized for the individual. If this treatment is recommended ask for complete information on cost, treatment schedule and duration, probability of success, and the degree of success possible if the treatment works.

TREATMENT

All known allergens should be removed from the person's vicinity. He or she should try to rest and stay calm. Children should be comforted and reassured. Attacks can usually be aborted by promptly inhaling bronchodilator aerosols, which relax the bronchial muscles. It is important that they be used correctly for the most benefit with the fewest side effects. It is not a good idea to treat yourself with nonprescription asthma drugs or herbs.

In severe cases doctors often turn to oral cortisone-type drugs to suppress the allergic reaction. They are usually quite effective, but long-term therapy is fraught with dangers including growth suppression, increased susceptibility to infections, impaired wound healing, skin problems, and psychological disturbances. A major advance is the development of cortisone aerosols that act directly on the airways to decrease chronic inflammation without dangerous increases in blood levels, but they must be used preventively. Proper application of the preventive measures above can help prevent the necessity of more dangerous therapies.

Atherosclerosis

Atherosclerosis, the presence of atheromas (fatty streaks and plaques on the inner walls of the arteries), causes or contributes to more deaths in the United States than all other diseases and accidents combined. The gradual injury to and clogging of the arteries feeding the heart muscle, the brain, and the kidneys leads to heart attack, stroke, and kidney failure.

There is a spectrum of disorders, depending on the extent of artery damage. In the case of coronary artery disease (CAD), in which the vessels feeding the heart muscle are diseased, angina pectoris may be the first sign of trouble. This is pain in the chest upon exertion due to the lack of sufficient blood and oxygen supply to the heart muscle. It may last a few seconds to several minutes, and may or may not progress to a myocardial infarction (MI), a heart attack. In an MI the heart muscle is deprived of blood for so long that a portion of it is permanently damaged. Recovery depends on the extent of damage and the adequacy of treatment; some die and some go on to lead normal lives.

Atherosclerosis often begins early in life, sometimes before puberty, though the disease usually remains silent, producing no signs or symptoms until after age forty or fifty. The earliest change is believed to be a slight injury to the inner lining of an artery, which allows blood to penetrate into the artery wall. There, in a complex series of events involving platelets (small blood cells that initiate clotting), the muscle cells of the artery wall accumulate abnormal amounts of cholesterol. These cells swell to form large plaques (atheromas) that protrude into the artery channels and impede the flow of blood. The atheromas also make the artery wall rigid, so it doesn't contract and dilate normally, and they roughen the surface of the inner wall, increasing the likelihood of clot formation. A clot can plug an artery and cause a heart attack or stroke.

The exact nature of the initial lesion that allows the blood and cholesterol to enter the artery wall is not fully understood, nor is the continuing artery destruction. Whatever the details of the pathology, a great deal of data gathered over decades of research around the world incriminate several risk factors and point to some protective measures. Each risk factor moves the danger of heart attack due to coronary artery disease up a notch. For example, having a high cholesterol level plus high blood pressure plus smoking is three times as dangerous as just one of these. Reducing or eliminating these factors is important in both preventing and treating atherosclerosis and its serious consequences.

Risk Factors

- **Smoking tobacco** (and possibly marijuana). Smokers have about three times the chance of suffering a heart attack as nonsmokers. Smoking causes a lot more heart disease than lung cancer. Heavy marijuana smoking is suspect because it can drive up blood levels of carbon monoxide and other harmful substances.

- **Hypertension.** High blood pressure increases the risk of developing atherosclerosis, probably by promoting injury to the artery walls, forcing blood into the slightest lesion, and inhibiting the healing of lesions.
- **Abnormal levels of blood lipids (cholesterol)** constitute a major risk factor for atherosclerosis and heart attack. Cholesterol is a fatlike substance necessary for the production of cell walls as well as for adrenal and sex hormones. It is synthesized in the liver and so is not needed in the diet. A high level of LDL-cholesterol, which is cholesterol attached to low-density lipoproteins for transport to and deposit into cells, is associated with a higher risk of atherosclerosis and heart disease.

  HDL-cholesterol is a less abundant form attached to high-density lipoproteins. It is believed to collect excess cholesterol, possibly even from cells, and transport it to the liver for excretion. High levels of HDL-cholesterol are apparently favorable to the health of the arteries, but much less is known about this than about the hazards of high levels of LDL-cholesterol. Nevertheless, it appears that when the LDL level is borderline, the HDL level can determine the risk.

  Another measurement of interest is the level of triglycerides, which are fats unattached to protein or cholesterol.

  The following are generally considered desirable levels:

LDL-cholesterol	130 mg/dl or lower
HDL-cholesterol	45 or higher
Triglycerides	150 or lower
Total cholesterol	200 or lower

  Some experts say the ratio of total cholesterol to HDL-cholesterol should be 4.5 or lower, but this is controversial. However, it is clear that total cholesterol can be misleading in someone with a low HDL-cholesterol level, and that LDL-cholesterol is the most important measurement.

  The presence of a risk according to any of these numbers does not necessarily mean treatment, either dietary or otherwise, is necessary. It all depends on the total risk, age, general health, lifestyle, and emotional and psychological factors.
- **Diabetes.** Many diabetics die prematurely of heart attacks. Blood vessel injury seems to be a basic aspect of diabetes, though it

can be minimized by good control of blood sugar.

- **Obesity.** This condition is often associated with hypertension, elevated blood fats, low HDL-cholesterol, and diabetes, all of which predispose one to atherosclerosis and heart disease. Although some obese people are healthy and have clean arteries, as a group obese people are less likely to be free of atherosclerosis than lean people.
- **Poor Physical Fitness.** Lack of exercise is consistently associated with higher levels of LDL-cholesterol and triglycerides and lower levels of HDL-cholesterol. Regular exercise helps maintain normal blood lipid levels. Moreover, fitness increases heart-lung capacity, which is inversely related to heart attack risk.
- **Personality** may contribute to atherosclerosis and heart disease, but this is still unproved. Advocates of this theory describe the personality type they believe to be the most prone to heart disease (type A) as a hard-driving, impatient, irritable person who walks, talks, and eats fast and feels guilty about relaxing. They call this condition "hurry sickness" and say it results in hormonal changes like increased adrenalin and insulin that may promote atherosclerosis. They say that such harmful behavior patterns can be changed, and they provide exercises designed to help people slow down, calm down, and reduce their "floating hostility."

  There are several problems with this theory. Behavior is difficult to measure, and it is usually not clear whether someone is a type A. Moreover, large-scale studies have not clearly linked personality types with risk of heart disease as has been done with cholesterol levels, hypertension, cigarette smoking, and diabetes. While some experts give the theory credence, especially regarding hostility and anger, the risk associated with type A behavior is generally ranked well below the major risk factors.
- **Hormones and Age.** Higher levels of estrogen and possibly certain prostaglandins (hormones derived from fatty acids) seem to reduce the susceptibility of the premenopausal woman's arteries to injury. Young and middle-age men have a higher incidence of atherosclerosis and heart attack than women of the same age. After menopause, however, women tend to catch up with men. Before menopause the most dangerous combination of risk factors for women is smoking and using birth control pills.
- **Genetic predisposition** is a major risk factor for atherosclerosis and cardiovascular disease. Many people are apparently genetically programmed to have high cholesterol levels, high blood pressure, or arteries that are more susceptible to damage and atherosclero-

sis. If a parent or sibling of yours had a heart attack or stroke, or received medical treatment to prevent these, you are at higher risk. Control of the other risk factors is especially important for you.

PREVENTION

Much remains to be learned, but the wealth of information accumulated over the past hundred years or so provides strong circumstantial evidence that the risk of developing atherosclerosis, and of its progressing once it has developed, can be substantially reduced by the following measures.

- **Don't smoke.** If you do smoke, the sooner you quit, the less your risk, but it's never too late to quit.
- **Prevent and control hypertension.** (See **Hypertension,** below.)
- **Control diabetes.** (See **Diabetes,** below.)
- **Keep cholesterol and fat levels low** by following the recommendations for the ideal diet (see Section One), especially in minimizing saturated fat and cholesterol in the diet from fatty meats, butter, cheeses and the like, and eating more of whole grains, beans, fish, fruits, and vegetables. Dietary fibers such as cellulose, pectin, lignin, and other indigestible components of whole grains, legumes, fruits, and vegetables apparently reduce cholesterol absorption. Many common foods, such as oatmeal, carrots, apples, and beans are useful in controlling cholesterol levels. Fish oils and polyunsaturated fats help by other mechanisms. Eating a wide variety of these foods also assures an adequate intake of potassium and magnesium, deficiencies of which may cause heart arrhythmia, angina, and heart attack. It may also help to eat smaller meals more frequently. "Grazing" tends to result in lower cholesterol levels than eating one, two, or three large meals.
- **Keep fit and prevent obesity** with regular exercise and a balanced diet without excessive calories.

Who Should Be Screened for Cholesterol Problems?

Children and adults at high genetic risk are those with siblings or parents who have had a heart attack, stroke, or coronary bypass surgery before age fifty-five. They are less than 2 percent of the population, but they will account for about half of all early heart attack deaths (unless, of course, they or their parents take preventive measures). These people should have blood lipids checked at age two or three, and then once every three to five years. They may have to be very careful about dietary fat and other risk factors, but dietary restriction should not be imposed unless blood studies confirm a problem, and not without extensive consultations with a physician or nutritionist.

Children at average risk should have their blood lipids checked at about age ten. They should be taught the dangers of atherosclerosis and the importance of eating right, not smoking, and keeping fit. Atherosclerosis prevention should be a major focus of health and physical education classes in primary and secondary schools.

Adults should have their blood lipids checked every three to five years, or as suggested by their physicians. The frequency of testing and the likelihood of treatment depend heavily on the number of other risk factors present. For example, if you smoke, have diabetes or hypertension, or if a parent had abnormal lipids and a stroke or even a mild heart attack before age sixty, maintaining normal lipids is all the more important for you. If a physician is not aware of your multiple risk factors, point them out and ask about blood lipid testing.

Postmenopausal women at risk for atherosclerosis should consult their physicians about estrogen replacement therapy, especially if they are also at risk for osteoporosis.

Controversial Issues in Heart Health

Is all the current cholesterol testing and treatment really necessary? Has it been proved to save lives? Some critics say no.

It seems to us that the epidemiological and clinical evidence is simply overwhelming. Close attention to all the risk factors, including abnormal lipids, clearly decreases the risk of atherosclerosis and heart attacks. Even critics admit this, but they say that it has not been proved that large-scale lowering of cholesterol levels has lowered the death rate. Well, it has never been proved that traffic safety laws and education programs lower overall mortality rates either. Yet we all agree we should do whatever we can to avoid getting killed or crippled by a vehicle. For millions of Americans abnormal lipids are equivalent to a truck bearing down on them. It doesn't make sense not to try to get out of the way or stop the truck. While a case can be made that some doctors are a little too quick with the cholesterol-lowering drugs, and that food promotions based on cholesterol claims have gotten completely ridiculous, it's still true that too many people have not been evaluated for their level of risk, and counseled or treated as needed. Ferreting out potential heart attack victims and reducing their risk will be a cornerstone of preventive medicine for a long time to come. DNA testing will soon make this process more precise and cost effective.

Some critics agree with this but question the broader public health measures, especially the sweeping recommendations about diet. However, so many can benefit from less fat and more fiber in the diet for so many reasons that it makes good public health sense to try to nudge the national diet in that direction. Extremes, of course, must be avoided. Infants for example, should not have fats or cholesterol restricted (see **Infant Nutrition,** Section One). And children should be given plenty of starch and protein if fat intake is moderately restricted; calories should never be restricted in children unless obesity is medically diagnosed.

In short, both the individual and public health approaches are necessary: We need to find those at risk and counsel or treat them; and we need to educate the general public about good eating habits.

If there is a serious problem with cholesterol screening efforts, it is that too many people are getting treated, or not treated, based on inadequate blood studies. There are seasonal variations in cholesterol levels (they tend to increase in winter) and a certain amount of error in the lab results. Therefore, for people with high cholesterol, repeated measurements at different times of year are necessary to determine the degree of the problem. And treatment, especially with drugs, should never be based on one blood test. Similarly, you shouldn't be complacent just because one blood test finds normal cholesterol. It could be a lab error or a seasonal low, so you will probably need to get checked again in a few months, especially if you have other risk factors.

Nonprescription Remedies

Several common items have real potential as prevention and treatment measures. One is a nonprescription drug; one is a food, or at least a spice; one is a vitamin; and two are derived from foods or potential foods. You don't have to consult a physician before using these products, but should you?

Aspirin has an anticlotting effect that provides some protection against heart attacks and strokes in those with atherosclerosis. Small amounts are used. As little as a quarter tablet a day may be beneficial for some. However, the drug can produce serious side effects in some and should not be used for this purpose without consulting a physician. In some people aspirin will prevent a heart attack but cause a stroke or stomach bleeding, so talk to a doctor about the risks and benefits for you before you start taking aspirin.

Fiber laxatives are made from a variety of plant materials. One popular ingredient is psyllium hydrophilic mucilloid, a preparation made from psyllium seeds that has been found remarkably effective in lowering cholesterol levels. Carrots, oats, beans, and many other high-fiber foods have a similar effect, and your money might be better spent on them since these laxatives are quite expensive. Moderate use is safe, but don't get carried away or intestinal symptoms (gas, cramping, annoying bowel rumblings) and excessive mineral excretion may occur. Inadequate water intake during fiber supplementation can result in intestinal dehydration and blockage.

Eating fish helps normalize blood lipids, and that is one reason we recommend it. Now fish oil capsules are heavily (and often contrary to FDA regulations) promoted as a preventive and cure for atherosclerosis and heart disease. Should you stock up and start taking them? Absolutely not, unless your doctor recommends or okays them. One problem is that these products have varying amounts of oils, cholesterol, vitamins A and D, and other components. You might spend a lot of money for small amounts of desirable oils, some cholesterol, and excessive vitamins A and D.

Moreover, these products are sold in pill form and marketed as drugs in every sense of the word, yet they don't conform to the standards of quality control that drugs are normally held to; in short, you don't always know what you're getting or what it will do. Your money would be better spent on fish, or on consultation with a nutritionist. If you don't like fish and have abnormal lipids, ask your doctor to recommend a fish oil product; don't choose one based on hype. Another consideration is that fish oils, like aspirin, can increase the risk of stroke in some people. So before you start taking fish oil capsules, talk to a doctor about the risks and benefits for you personally.

Garlic may help lower blood pressure and cholesterol levels, but it takes a lot. Onions and cayenne pepper may have similar but even weaker effects. Overconsumption of these foods can cause burning in the mouth and stomach, irritation of the rectum, diarrhea, and painful defecation ("exhaust pipe syndrome"). The health significance of moderate consumption is not known. Garlic extracts and oils are generally worthless, in spite of the wild claims made for them. If you are under a physician's care for any kind of cardiovascular or lipid disorder, let him or her know if you eat large amounts of garlic, onions, or red pepper.

Niacin, or vitamin B-3, helps reduce blood cholesterol in many cases, and popular books recommend it as self-medication for prevention and treatment of atherosclerosis. The problem is that the doses that work are often toxic, or close to it. The RDA is less than 20 milligrams, but people are self-prescribing thousands of milligrams a day, up to five hundred times the RDA, and they often suffer severe stomach upset, flushing, itching, dizziness, and sometimes liver dysfunction and heart arrhythmias. Large doses are dangerous to those with ulcers. Unfortunately, even though niacin is a nonprescription product, large doses can be more hazardous than some of the prescription cholesterol-reducing drugs. We recommend against taking niacin to prevent or treat abnormal blood lipids without consulting a physician.

TREATMENTS

Treatments for atherosclerosis and its manifestations include balloon angioplasty, in which a tiny balloon is used to widen the area narrowed by atheromas; bypass surgery in which an artery made from another of the patient's blood vessels replaces the damaged one; and the use of various drugs. Treatment also includes diet, treating high blood pressure and diabetes, and not smoking—measures which might have prevented the problem if started some years sooner.

Backaches (Low Back Pain)

Chronic low back pain is extremely common. The majority of Americans have an episode at least once in their lives. The muscles, ligaments, tendons, and intervertebral discs (cartilage cushions between the vertebrae) responsible for supporting the spinal column, if injured, can cause mild to severe pain, sometimes for many months.

CAUSES

The great majority of low back pains are caused by strained and torn muscles, ligaments, and tendons. Disc injury is less common, but generally more serious. The injury may be apparent immediately (especially disc injury), or there may be no pain until hours later. Sometimes the muscles around the injured part go into prolonged contractions or spasms. This may help immobilize the area and prevent further injury, but the spasms themselves may cause severe pain. Disc injury often causes pain to radiate down one leg. This is known as **sciatica,** irritation of the sciatic nerve near the spine due to pressure from the prolapsed disc.

Injury to the tissue is usually caused by excessive stress in lifting, twisting, throwing, or other activity. Poor posture, often a result of weak back muscles, can cause excessive stress on the discs and ligaments and contribute to their injury. Poorly designed chairs, couches, beds, and car seats are often to blame. Obesity and pregnancy put a great deal of added stress on back tissues. Closely spaced pregnancies are especially hard on a woman's back, not only from the added weight of the pregnancy, but from lifting children. Simply standing or sitting for long periods can stress and injure back tissues.

Sometimes symptoms of sciatica can be caused by keeping a wallet in the hip pocket and sitting on it for extended periods. Sitting cross-legged carries the same risk.

PREVENTION

- **Keep your back fit;** exercise it and move it in all possible directions every day to keep the muscles strong and all the connective tissues well-nourished. Keep the abdominal muscles strong too. Walking, swimming, bicycling, and walking in chest-deep water are especially good exercises.
- **Don't indulge in occasional bursts of activity.** If you have been inactive for a couple weeks or more get back into shape gradually and carefully. Warm up slowly before exercising hard.
- **Maintain cardiovascular fitness.** Even without specific back or abdominal exercises, aerobic exercise decreases the risk of back injury.
- **Lift objects properly,** and if you cannot manage with ease don't even try. When lifting things, don't bend at the waist; bend your knees and use your leg muscles, keeping your back straight. Don't twist your upper body when lifting or setting down a heavy object. Don't be afraid to ask for help in lifting.
- **Sit up straight;** don't slump or slouch. Aim for vertebral alignment and a slight lumbar (lower back) curve. Place a small pillow behind you if your chair or car seat does not provide lumbar support. Knees should be slightly higher than hips. Most important, take frequent breaks from sitting. Even proper sitting is harder on the back than standing.

- **Don't wear high heels if they seem to cause pain in your back.**
- **Lose fat if you are obese** (see **Obesity,** below).
- **Avoid sleeping on your stomach,** flat on your back, or on an overly soft or sagging mattress. It's best to sleep on your side on a firm mattress.
- **If you must stand for long periods,** rest one foot on a small lift. Shift feet often.
- **Lie down** for a few minutes several times a day if you can.
- **Don't sit for long periods with a wallet in your back pocket** if you have ever had sciatica. If you sit with your legs crossed alternate them frequently.

SELF-CARE

The most important treatment for most low back injuries is complete bed rest on a firm mattress for one to several days, followed by a gradual return to normal activities. Roll out of bed carefully. Walk around a little, but avoid sitting, lifting, and all the aggravating factors mentioned above. Take care not to stress the injured part: It must heal naturally and this takes time.

On the other hand, too much rest can be counterproductive and prolong the pain. Resting muscle fibers start to shorten and stiffen within days. Moreover, as little as two weeks of bed rest can cause demineralization of your bones; their return to normal can take many months. Therefore, unless the pain is very severe you should start careful movement and mild exercise within a few days. More serious injuries, such as a herniated disc or torn muscle, may require two weeks to two months of rest.

Aspirin or ibuprofen may relieve pain, but beware of stomach irritation. Antacids can minimize side effects.

Light massage may relieve pain some, but vigorous manipulations like twisting and cracking the back can aggravate the injury. An ice pack may help reduce pain, particularly in the first couple of days. Later it's a tossup between ice and a heating pad; you should use whichever you prefer.

Be sure your nutrition is adequate. Vitamin C, which is critical in collagen formation and connective tissue healing, may be especially important. If your intake has been borderline for a long time, supplements of 100 to 200 milligrams per day may be in order for a few weeks or until you improve your diet.

About 90 percent of people with back pain recover without consulting a physician. About 90 percent of those who do seek help improve within two months, most of them within one week. Less than 2 percent end up needing surgery.

Spinal flex and extension

Sit with your hands together and bend your back and neck so your head touches your chest. Come up until you are looking straight up with your hands directly overhead.

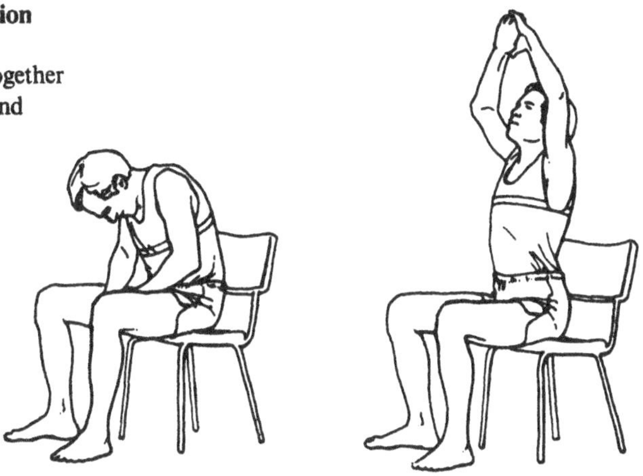

Trunk rotation

With hands on knees, rotate in a circle from the waist.

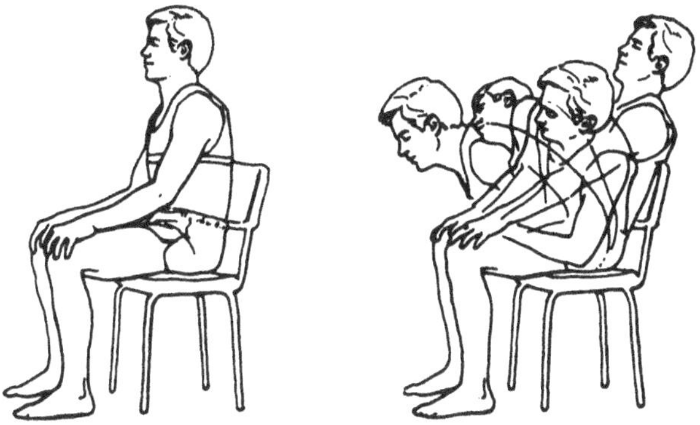

Trunk twist

Twist at the waist and turn your head to one side, then the other.

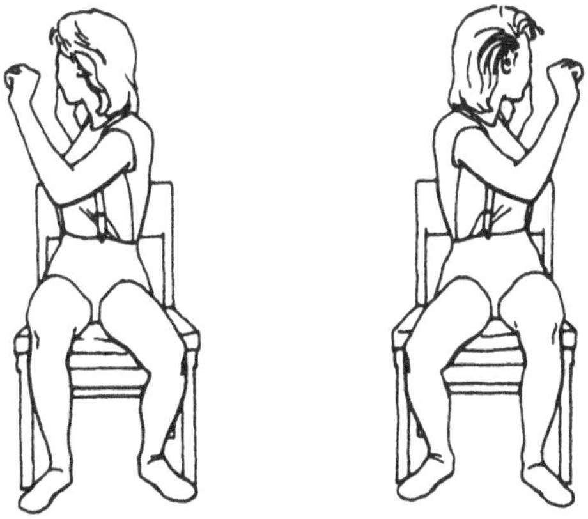

The cobra

Lie flat on your stomach with your hands about even with your shoulders. Slowly push your torso up while keeping your pubic bone on the ground. Pull your head back and look up. Hold for several seconds; rest; repeat.

This exercise, which stretches the abdominal and hip flexor muscles, can be harmful in certain back conditions; if you are being treated for a back problem, ask your physician before trying this.

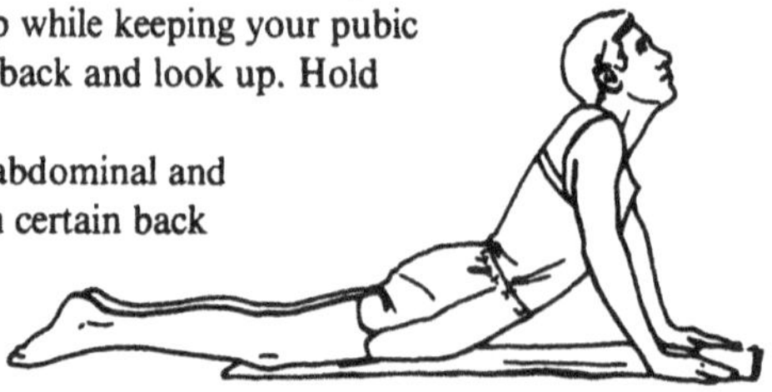

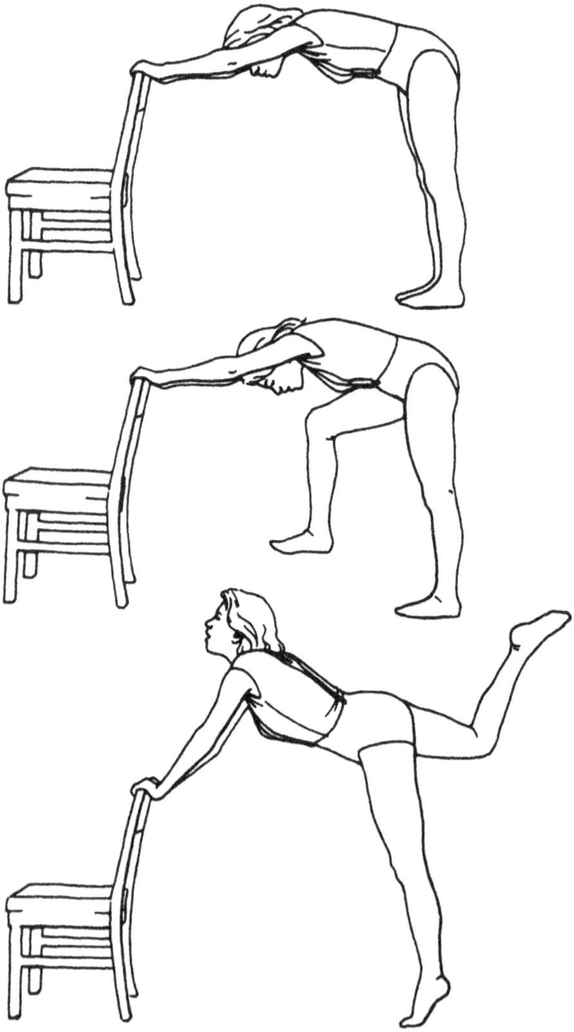

Whole body stretch and flex

1. Feet flat, head even with the arms
2. Bring head down, leg forward
3. Swing head and leg up while coming to your toes
4. Swing head and legs down to #2 position
5. Repeat

See a physician immediately if you develop weakness or numbness in a leg that is clearly more than the common sensation of one's leg "falling asleep" from sitting too long.

See a physician promptly if back pain is accompanied by fever or by urinary problems.

Consult a physician soon if back pain has not improved after three days of bed rest.

MEDICAL CARE

The physician will evaluate your symptoms to determine the location and extent of injury. In most cases advice similar to that above will be given. In severe cases pain relievers and muscle relaxants may be prescribed. Pain can sometimes be relieved by a TENS device—transcutaneous electrical nerve stimulation, a form of counterirritation applied to the skin. Acupuncture and massage may help on the same principle.

The best bet for most stubborn chronic cases is education and behavior modification. Ask your physician to refer you to a pain clinic, a "back school," or a patient education course. You can learn specific exercises that fit your needs and techniques for daily living that minimize stress on your back.

As a last resort surgery must be considered. Discuss the options, their risks, and benefits with your doctor.

Sometimes back pain is more serious than a pulled muscle, strained ligament, or ruptured disc. It could be arthritis, an infection, osteoporosis, a tumor, or a disease of the muscles, nerves, or kidneys. Therefore, it is prudent to discuss persistant or unusual pains with a medical doctor.

Birth Defects and Sickness in the Newborn

Routine Prenatal Care

Once pregnancy is confirmed, a woman should select a physician or nurse-midwife with whom she feels she can work for about a year. Accessibility, responsiveness, readiness to answer all questions, and personal and philosophical compatibility are important considerations. A nurse-midwife should be certified by the American College of Midwifery and have a physician on call for backup. The advantage of a nurse-midwife is that she is frequently very knowledgeable about, and available for dealing with, the many normal but often distressing symptoms of pregnancy. She can often provide more thorough and personalized coaching in exercises and other preparations for birth. She can also usually labor sit, that is, be at the woman's side through most or all of the labor and later coach her in breast-feeding.

Routine care during pregnancy, which requires an obstetrician or gynecologist, will include a complete medical history and physical examination, a pelvic exam, a Pap test, blood pressure checks, testing for Rh factor, blood count, weight checks, urinalysis, urine culture, blood typing, determination of nutritional status, and screening for diabetes, rubella, and several sexually transmitted diseases. Genetic disorders common to certain ethnic groups are checked for. Certain women should be tested for alpha-fetoprotein to detect neural tube (from which the fetal brain and spinal cord form) defects. Amniocentesis for diagnosis of chromosomal disorders (especially Down's syndrome) is recommended for women over thirty-five and others at high risk. In some cases testing for tuberculosis and other infectious diseases is recommended. Although it is not routinely recommended, after about twelve weeks the fetal heartbeat can be monitored and the fetus visualized with ultrasound.

Nutritional considerations are very important during pregnancy. A balanced diet with adequate amounts of all the essential nutrients and adequate calories is crucial to the health of both the mother and the developing fetus. Pregnancy is no time to go on a diet to lose weight; the mother-to-be really must eat for two people. How much weight should she gain? Through most of the twentieth century, up until about the mid-sixties, weight gain was strictly controlled with diet, salt restriction, and sometimes diuretics and even appetite suppressants in the belief that this would help prevent preeclampsia and toxemia of pregnancy (see **Toxemia,** below). This practice generally results in smaller, less healthy babies and has been largely abandoned. The consensus now is that the optimal weight gain is about twenty-five to thirty pounds. A little more may be all right for some women, but too much may predispose a woman to hypertension, diabetes, and fatigue.

There is no special diet recommended for pregnancy, but it is more important than ever to eat as well as possible, and substantially more than usual (see Section One for guidelines to a balanced diet). The nutrients most likely needing attention are calories, protein, iron, folic acid, and calcium. The requirements for these increase by 50 to 100 percent. The intake of **high protein** and **high calcium** foods should be increased substantially. Supplements of **iron** and **folic acid** are usually advisable. Other vitamin and mineral supplements may be taken, but it is best not to exceed the RDAs, especially for vitamins A and D. Special care should be taken to avoid potential sources of natural toxins such as moldy foods and sprouting potatoes.

PREVENTING BIRTH DEFECTS AND MENTAL RETARDATION

It is a great tragedy that 3 to 4 percent of all children born to normal parents develop serious birth defects, genetic disease, or mental retardation. This is about one hundred thousand per year in the United States, which already has over six million retarded persons. Millions more will later develop inherited diseases that cause early death or disability. Contrary to common belief that birth defects are more common now, the vast majority of birth defects are about as common as they were a generation ago, though babies with certain serious problems are more likely to live now. The incidence of neural tube defects and Down's syndrome are much lower than they were two decades ago, but the reasons for this are unclear.

It is one of the great hopes of preventive medicine that most of these tragedies can eventually be prevented by the application of medical genetics and good prenatal care. Progress has been slow, however, because the cause of most birth defects is unknown. About 25 percent are caused by defects in chromosomes and genes, and another 5 to 7 percent are caused by drugs, chemicals, infections, and other known environmental factors. It is only these cases, which comprise approximately one-third of all birth defects, that we can theoretically prevent, at least until we know more about the other causes.

This is an important point to understand because mothers often blame themselves and suffer needless and unjustified guilt in the false belief that if they had done something different the child might have been healthy. Similar considerations hold for miscarriage which is, contrary to popular belief, almost *never* caused by physical or emotional stress, travel, or exercise. Most miscarriages are the result of a genetic or anatomical abnormality of the fetus that cannot be prevented with our present knowledge.

Chromosome defects, such as having too many or too few, are responsible for Down's syndrome (mongolism), hermaphroditism, and other disorders. Effective contraception for women over age thirty-five probably accounts for some of the decrease in incidence of these disorders, which are more common in infants born to older women.

Molecular diseases, also known as inborn errors of metabolism or genetic diseases, include phenylketonuria (PKU), sickle-cell disease, Tay-

 Sachs disease, galactosemia, hemophilia, and hundreds more; they account for almost one-third of chronically institutionalized children in the United States. These disorders are often due to a single defect in a single gene that blocks the metabolism of amino acids, fats, carbohydrates, or other biochemicals. The unmetabolized substance then accumulates to toxic levels and damages the brain, eyes, or other tissue. In other cases the metabolic block prevents the formation of a necessary protein, or the removal of a waste product. Mental retardation, blindness, anemia, and other severe problems can result. Sometimes early recognition of the defect and proper treatment from birth or even before can prevent the worst. In most cases genetic counseling of those affected and close relatives is recommended.

Other genetically determined defects include clubfoot, hip dislocations, cleft palate, and pyloric stenosis (an abnormality of the opening between the stomach and intestine). More complex genetic disorders include cystic fibrosis, dwarfism, gout, Wilson's disease, progressive muscular dystrophy, and some types of hypercholesterolemia (high cholesterol levels that can lead to early heart attacks). Most of these conditions can be treated to improve the quality and length of life.

Drug use during pregnancy can cause serious birth defects and mental retardation. A fetus can be harmed at *any time* during pregnancy, and care is always in order. However, it appears that the *most critical period,* during which the fetus is most sensitive and vulnerable to harm, is from day eighteen to day twenty-eight, approximately the third and fourth weeks of pregnancy. Therefore, this is a reasonable rule of thumb: A woman should assume she is pregnant from the day she has had intercourse without protection or from the first day her period is due until her period starts. During this time she should avoid anything that has been implicated as a cause of birth defects.

Drugs known to cause fetal harm include alcohol, diethylstilbestrol (DES), heroin, nicotine and other constituents of cigarette smoke, some anticancer and anticonvulsant drugs, methadone, lithium, testosterone and related steroids, progestins, and large doses of vitamins A and D.

Drugs suspected of causing fetal harm include some antibiotics, aspirin, cortisone-type drugs, various diuretics, oral diabetes drugs, various tranquilizers, LSD, marijuana, and excessive doses of iodine and trace minerals. Extremely high doses of the B vitamins and other nutrients might also be harmful. Because so many drugs and nutritional supplements (in excessive doses) are known or suspected culprits, the safest policy is to avoid any not prescribed or recommended by your physician.

The question of alcohol use during pregnancy deserves further comment. Fetal alcohol syndrome, with such symptoms as a flat face, a short, upturned nose, small eyes and head, facial asymmetry, and lower intelligence, was only recognized in the 1970s after more than twenty-five centuries of alcohol use. This is not because we have all been too drunk to notice, but because the effect is too rare to detect without careful statistical analysis of expertly obtained data.

The question of how much alcohol during pregnancy may cause the syndrome is still hotly debated. Since no safe level of intake has been firmly established, many physicians say the less the better and none is best. Others say this is going too far, that it is unnecessarily restrictive since there is no evidence of harm from light, occasional drinking; meaning the equivalent of a beer or two a few times a month. However, light drinking plus cigarette smoking appears much riskier than either alone.

Hot tubs, saunas, and steam baths should be avoided or used with care, especially during the first trimester of pregnancy. If the body's core temperature exceeds 102° F, the fetus may suffer brain, nerve, or other damage.

Occupational hazards to the fetus include exposure to benzene, cadmium, lead, chloroprene, various insecticides, and possibly surgical anesthetics. All due care should be taken, but there is no cause for alarm at the increasing numbers of women in the work force; there has not been the associated epidemic of birth defects, that some feared might occur.

X-rays during early pregnancy, especially large doses to the bowel, back, or kidney, may cause fetal defects. They should be avoided when there is any possibility of being pregnant, except for the most urgent medical reasons.

Some infections during pregnancy can cause very serious birth defects. Often the mother is only mildly ill with slight malaise and low-grade fever, or none at all. The main culprits are rubella, cytomegalovirus (a herpes-type virus), herpes virus, and toxoplasmosis from cats, birds, or undercooked beef or pork. Any woman who is pregnant or may be pregnant should avoid handling cats and birds and their litter, and avoid eating undercooked meat. They should not attend infants or children with rubella or undiagnosed illnesses. Girls should be vaccinated against rubella before the onset of menstruation, not while pregnant or possibly pregnant. If she has a history of vaginal herpes, the mother must be checked frequently for a recurrence near delivery time.

Toxemia of pregnancy, also known as eclampsia, is a serious complication of pregnancy. In the early stage, known as preeclampsia, there is high blood pressure, excessive edema (swelling) of the hands, feet, and face, and protein in the urine. These are dangerous signs. If they progress to eclampsia, blood pressure soars and there may be visual changes including partial blindness, severe headaches, dizziness, vomiting, kidney and liver damage, convulsions, shock, coma, and death of the mother and fetus. If the infant survives it may be small, even if fullterm, and may suffer varying degrees of brain damage and possible mental retardation, epilepsy, cerebral palsy, or other neurological disorders. The cause of toxemia is unknown, but good care seems to minimize the danger.

Rh disease. The Rh factor is a protein found in the blood cells of about 85 percent of the population. If the mother is Rh-negative and the father is Rh-positive, the fetus may be Rh-positive and its blood may sensitize the mother's immune system, that is, prime it to react against the fetal Rh-positive blood. In subsequent pregnancies this could cause a serious, even fatal, reaction in an Rh-positive fetus. Blood transfusions in the uterus and at birth may save the infant's life and prevent retardation.

Rh disease can be prevented in Rh-negative women by an injection of immune globulin after any incident in which Rh-positive cells may have entered her blood, including giving birth to an Rh-positive child, an abortion, miscarriage, ectopic pregnancy, or amniocentesis for chromosome testing. The immune globulin prevents the woman from developing antibodies to Rh-positive cells in her blood by destroying the cells quickly.

Incest and inbreeding greatly increase the risk of birth defects. Most people carry about three to six defective genes. Such genes are recessive and may be carried for generations without showing up as a disease or malformation. But if two people with the same defective gene mate, the children have a much higher chance of developing the defect. Naturally, the chances of having the same defective recessive gene are much greater with blood relatives. Groups that are isolated geographically or culturally, like the Amish and certain communities in the Appalachians, have a high incidence of inbreeding and high rates of mental retardation, congential deafness, dwarfism, and other genetic disorders.

Because many of the recessive genes are much more common to some ethnic groups than others, marrying outside the group may decrease the probability of these disorders occurring. The evidence in favor of outbreeding, hybridizing, and inter-ethnic marriages is infinitely stronger than arguments for "racial purity."

A high-risk pregnancy is one that occurs in a woman in such poor health that the pregnancy carries a much higher than average risk of harm to the mother and the child. Women in the high-risk groups should consider the hazards carefully before deciding to have a child, and should carefully follow their doctors' advice should they become pregnant. High-risk conditions include alcoholism or any other kind of drug addiction, cancer, diabetes, hypertension, kidney disease, heart disease, and congenital anemias like sickle-cell disease.

Exercise during pregnancy is important to maintain general fitness, to improve circulation, to relieve swelling, to prevent back pain, and to prepare for the physical stress of childbirth. The same activities enjoyed before pregnancy can usually be continued, but with extra care not to fall, especially in the later months. Walking, swimming, and abdominal exercises (such as sit-ups with bent knees) are particularly good. Moderation is recommended. Very heavy exercise may deprive the fetus of some blood flow and nutrients, and some evidence suggests that runners who train hard during pregnancy may have smaller babies. Any exercise should stop if it causes breathlessness, palpitations, dizziness, nausea, chest pain or tightness, decreased fetal activity, vaginal bleeding or leaking, uterine contraction, or any unusual pains.

Sexual intercourse during pregnancy is generally safe, but not if there is a risk of the woman contracting a venereal disease. Also, she should urinate after intercourse to lessen the risk of a urinary tract infection.

Home delivery is an attractive option to many women because of the warm congenial atmosphere compared to the often cold, uninviting air of the labor and delivery rooms. Unfortunately, home delivery is risky even in healthy low-risk pregnancies because serious complications, like hemorrhage or fetal distress, can occur without warning. Hospitals are equipped to save lives in such emergencies. While the odds are against complications if the woman is healthy, if the baby or mother is harmed it will seem a very high price to pay for the luxury of a home birth. A better alternative is a family-oriented childbirth center with a homelike atmosphere, which many hospitals are setting up. Husbands and other partners are encouraged to participate. If home delivery is nevertheless preferred, backup arrangements should be made with a nearby hospital and transportation should be planned.

152 Sickness in the Newborn

Sudden Infant Death Syndrome (SIDS). In SIDS an infant of usually less than six months of age, for no apparent reason, suddenly stops breathing, the heart stops, and death ensues. In the United States there are about two cases per one thousand live births. The vast majority of infants are not in danger, but the problem causes a great deal of anxiety because of its seeming arbitrary nature.

SIDS, by definition, cannot be treated, for death is final. However, progress is being made in preventing it. This is possible because the syndrome is not as arbitrary as it seems; some infants are much more at risk than others. These include siblings (especially twins) of SIDS victims, premature or unusually small infants, and those with a history of "almost SIDS," that is, one or more episodes of cessation of breathing (apnea). Such infants can be monitored at home with electronic equipment on loan from a hospital. Parents should be alert for breathing problems, prolonged staring spells, feeding difficulties, sleep disturbances, rigid posturing, and pallor or a gray appearance. If any of these occur, a physician should be consulted.

The risk of SIDS can be reduced by the mother avoiding smoking during pregnancy and in the presence of the infant, and by protecting the infant from cold and flu germs. SIDS is most likely to occur after a recent virus infection, during winter months, and at two or three months of age. In fact, many cases of so-called SIDS turn out to be infections, heart abnormalities, allergic reactions, or suffocation. Regarding the latter, ongoing research should clarify the question of whether it's best to put an infant to bed on the back or stomach. It is clear that an infant should *not* be left alone on a waterbed.

HIB, scourge of the very young. A major cause of mental retardation as well as visual and hearing impairment strikes not during gestation, but a few months or years after birth. This is Hemophilus influenza type b (HIB), a very severe bacterial infection that can cause meningitis and other severe complications, and even death. Brain damage and mental retardation can result. This infection was misnamed when it was mistakenly associated with the influenza epidemic of 1892. HIB was believed to cause influenza until the 1918 flu epidemic when scientists learned it was a very different "bug" from the flu virus. However, like common childhood viral diseases, it is highly contagious because the bacteria are spread through the air; day-care centers can be virtual breeding grounds for HIB. A vaccine is available and strongly recommended to be given to all children at eighteen months.

Cancers

Cancer is an abnormal, excessive growth of cells. Each type of cancer has its own characteristics depending on the tissues and specific cells it originates from. Some grow slowly and stay put; others grow rapidly, spread to distant organs, and interfere with vital organ functions. About one in four Americans now living will eventually develop at least one form of cancer. Tremendous efforts in recent decades have led to significant improvements in the detection and treatment of the disease, but it is still among the major causes of death and disability and, with the possible exception of AIDS, the most feared disease in the United States.

A consensus is developing that much more emphasis must be placed on cancer prevention. We already know enough to prevent or significantly delay about two-thirds of all cancers. Now we need to apply our knowledge. The following is a summary of the most important factors involved in cancer development and cancer prevention. Early detection is also very important. It is summarized at the end of this section and discussed in detail in Section Three.

Cancer Promoting Factors in the Diet

Dietary Fats and Cancer. One of the most significant developments in preventive medicine since the discovery of the links between smoking and lung cancer, and diet and heart disease, is the discovery of strong correlations between dietary fat and cancer of the breast, prostate, and colon, all major killers in the United States. Other cancers may also be linked to diet. The evidence is strong enough for the American Cancer Society and the National Cancer Institute to issue dietary guidelines recommending less fat and more fruits, vegetables and other high-fiber foods. The recommendations are consistent with those of the National Research Council, the Surgeon General, and other responsible agencies and authorities. They are also consistent with the diet long recommended for reducing atherosclerosis and heart disease.

The conclusions are based on epidemiological and biochemical studies. For example, in dozens of countries studied, the per capita rates of breast, colon, and prostate cancers are directly proportional to dietary animal fat intake. American blacks, who eat much more animal fat than Africans, have two to three times the rate of these cancers. Japanese who move to Hawaii, where they eat more meat, develop more of these cancers. If they move to California, where they eat still more meat, these cancers increase further. Seventh Day Adventists in the United States eat much less meat than average Americans and have much lower than average rates of these and other cancers. Those who are strict vegetarians have the lowest rates.

On the biochemical side, dietary animal fat appears to increase the levels of female hormones that promote breast cancer. Vegetarians, who eat less animal fat and are less likely to get cancer, produce much less of the bile acids (secreted by the gall bladder) than nonvegetarians. Some bile acids are proved carcinogens (cancer causers) and would be banned if they were food additives. The production of known mutagens (very likely carcinogens) in human stools can be greatly decreased by reducing dietary fat. Another strike against dietary fat is that obesity, which is promoted by fat in the diet, increases the risk of uterine and possibly other cancers.

Broiled, charred, and smoked meats have large amounts of cancer-causing substances.

What About Vegetable Oils? Some animal studies have shown a cancer-promoting effect from very large amounts of polyunsaturated vegetable oils in the diet. Results of human studies have been inconsistent, but moderate amounts of corn oil, safflower oil, and the other highly unsaturated oils are probably perfectly safe. However, olive oil is probably safer for very heavy oil users. Rancid oils of any type may promote cancer as might vegetable oils used over and over for deep frying.

Nitrates and nitrites, used for centuries to preserve various processed meats, are suspected of combining with amines (amino acid fragments) to form carcinogenic nitrosamines. Eating vitamin C foods with those that contain nitrates probably greatly reduces the cancer risk.

Natural Plant Carcinogens. Many people are concerned about pesticide residues in food and believe they are causing many cancers. So far these fears appear to be unfounded. While heavy exposure to some pesticides may promote some cancers in farmers and chemical workers, there is no evidence that the traces found in foods can cause disease. However, many edible plants contain natural pesticides, many of which are mutagenic and carcinogenic. The levels of the toxins are especially high in plants bred to resist insects and fungi; some new varieties have been banned for this reason. Overall, our consumption of carcinogens from nature is probably much greater than that from synthetic pesticides. (This conclusion should not discourage proponents of nonchemical, organic farming; there are other important reasons to avoid or minimize farm chemicals, including hazards to workers, water pollution, harm to wildlife, and soil erosion due to low content of organic matter in soil.)

The task of identifying the toxins and estimating their potential for harm has only just begun. Many food plants contain both carcinogens and anticarcinogens, like vitamins A and C, and their net effect is beneficial. Others will be shown to have such high levels of toxins that prudent people will use them in moderation, if at all. Until more details are available, the best advice is to eat moderate amounts of a wide variety of foods, favoring those with known or suspected anticancer potential. This will minimize the intake of any given toxin.

The following examples illustrate the problem. Safrole and related compounds known to cause cancer in rats are present in sassafras (used for herb tea and root beer) and black pepper; hydrazine and related carcinogens are present in large amounts in edible mushrooms, including the popular false morel and common commercial mushrooms. Psoralen derivatives are carcinogens present in celery, parsley, and related plants. Gossypol, a probable carcinogen, is present in large amounts in cottonseed oil, which is added to some margarines, cooking oils, and sesame butters; and nitrates, which form carcinogenic nitroso compounds, are present in beets, celery, lettuce, spinach, and other vegetables.

The bracken fern is so toxic that it has been compared to the fictional plants from the horror movie, *Day of the Triffids.* In the film triffids proliferate, chase people, and eat them. Bracken fern is one of the world's six most common plants and it thrives on all continents except Antarctica. It emits several known carcinogens as well as potassium cyanide. These toxins poison the soil, inhibit other plant growth, and promote bracken fern proliferation. Cattle, sheep, and deer that graze on the plant develop cancers of the mouth and stomach. People who drink milk from cows that eat bracken have a higher incidence of stomach and esophageal cancers. People who drink water from bracken-covered slopes or breathe the spores released in the summer and fall are exposed to the toxins. Some experts recommend that forestry workers and hikers who frequent bracken-infested areas wear face masks.

Nutrition Against Cancer

Several food elements are believed to boost resistance to cancer when provided in adequate amounts. Nonetheless, there is no evidence that very large doses provide extra protection, and in some cases such doses can be dangerous.

- **Carotene,** a precursor of vitamin A, and other carotenoids have been shown to be anticarcinogenic in rodents and appear to provide some protection from lung cancer in humans. These substances are present in all plants with chlorophyll.

- **Vitamin C** may help prevent the formation of carcinogenic nitrosamines if taken with foods containing nitrites. The amount required is believed to be small. Eating some vitamin C food with every meal is a good idea. The general increased consumption of vitamin C foods in the past few decades may be largely responsible for the plummeting stomach cancer rate in the United States.
- **Vitamin E** is a scavenger of free radicals, highly reactive atoms that can damage DNA, and may also provide some protection from cancer initiation.
- **Selenium** inhibits the induction of many kinds of tumors in animals and is believed to be an important anticancer factor in the diet. Whole grains are usually a good source.
- **Deficiencies of vitamin B complex and iron** have been linked to a precancerous condition of the mouth, pharynx, and esophagus known as Plummer-Vinson syndrome.
- **Miscellaneous vegetables,** including broccoli, Brussels sprouts, cauliflower, cabbage, and turnips have been reported to stimulate liver, intestinal, and lung enzymes that detoxify carcinogens in animals and increase their resistance to cancer. Cabbage, asparagus, radish, and other vegetable juices have been reported to inhibit the ability of tobacco smoke to cause mutations (genetic changes that likely cause cancer).
- **Fiber** in the diet may help protect against cancer. People with lots of fiber in their diets tend to have lower rates of colon cancer. It is theorized that fiber exerts its protective effect by creating bulk as it absorbs water in the intestine and thereby dilutes carcinogens and speeds transit through the bowel. It may also favorably influence intestinal flora (bacteria in the intestines) and decrease the conversion of bile acids to carcinogens.
- **Vitamin D and calcium** may provide some protection against colon cancer. This has not been firmly established, but some experts recommend two to three glasses of vitamin D-fortified skim milk as a potential cancer preventive.
- **BHA and BHT,** the antioxidants used as food preservatives, have been shown to inhibit some chemically induced cancers in animals and may have contributed to keeping the stomach cancer incidence low in the United States. They are still under suspicion as possible liver toxins, however, and should *not* be consumed as "supplements" or herpes medicines as recommended by some writers.

Drugs That Promote Cancer

A number of drugs and hormones have a tendency to cause or promote various cancers. Tobacco is the most important of these.

- **Tobacco.** Smoking, snuffing, and chewing tobacco have long been linked with mouth, nasal, lip, esophageal, laryngeal, lung, bladder, and pancreatic cancers. Other cancers may also be involved. The use of tobacco increases the risk of these cancers by up to ten times. Cigar and pipe smoking are about one-third to one-half as risky as cigarette smoking. Snuffing and chewing tobacco are less risky than smoking, but can cause oral cancer. The danger of smoking is significantly increased by exposure to many environmental and occupational pollutants such as asbestos, coal, rubber, textiles, dust, chemicals, and uranium.
- **Marijuana** smoking may carry a significant risk of developing lung, mouth, and throat cancers, and possibly others (see **Marijuana,** Section Four).
- **Alcohol.** The risk of esophageal cancer among alcoholics is about seventeen times the average. For heavy drinkers, those who average about six beers, five small glasses of wine, or two ounces of liquor every day, the risk of cancer of the mouth or esophagus is two to five times the risk for nondrinkers. The risk of pancreatic cancer is also higher for drinkers. In addition, alcohol promotes the cancer-causing effects of tobacco.
- **DES (diethystilbestrol),** the synthetic estrogen, was used in the 1940s and 1950s for menopausal symptoms, pregnancy testing, pregnancy nausea, and threatened miscarriage. By 1971 it was clear that exposure in the uterus fifteen to twenty years earlier was the cause of a series of cases of the very rare adenocarcinoma of the vagina in young women. Hundreds of thousands of women born in the United States between 1947 and 1971 have been exposed and are considered at risk; they should have semi-annual checkups. DES mothers may also be at risk; they should have an annual pelvic examination and Pap test and should minimize further estrogen exposure.
- **Postmenopausal estrogens** may increase the risk of endometrial cancer (cancer of the lining of the uterus) in some women. However, new dose regimens and estrogen given in combination with progestins seem to have a protective effect, especially against breast cancer. Discuss the risks and benefits with your physician.
- **Anabolic steroids,** the testosterone analogues that are widely used

by weight lifters, body builders, and other athletes, may promote liver and other cancers.

- **Other drugs,** including some tranquilizers, antibiotics, and antihistamines, have been linked with various tumors in laboratory animals. However, these studies are suggestive only and do not prove these drugs cause cancer in humans; nonetheless they do provide another reason to keep drug intake to a minimum.

Occupational Cancer Hazards

It is estimated that somewhere between 5 and 20 percent of all cancers in the United States are due to exposure to cancer-causing substances on the job. The list includes radioactive substances, arsenic, coal tar pitch, dry cleaning chemicals, gasoline, benzenes, benzidine, asbestos, PVC (polyvinyl chloride), nirobiphenyl, wood dust, and coke-oven emissions. If you work in an industrial, chemical, or nuclear plant, or uranium or other mine, it is very important to follow all the safety rules and to report violations to your union or to the Occupational Safety and Health Administration (OSHA). Keep in mind that simultaneous exposure to cigarette smoke and asbestos greatly increases the already high risk of exposure to either. The same may be true of smoking and other industrial carcinogens.

X-Rays and Cancer

It has been known for decades that radiologists have a high risk of developing leukemia if they don't take precautions to reduce their exposure to X-rays. We also know that infants exposed to X-rays while in the uterus are more likely to develop cancer. There is no doubt that X-ray exposure promotes the development of cancer and should be minimized to the extent possible without risking health. The FDA has been trying to reduce that exposure, and it recommends the discontinuation of the following:

- all routine chest X-rays made to uncover diseases (like tuberculosis, lung cancer, and heart problems) in apparently well people,
- all routine prenatal screening examination by X-ray,
- routine chest X-rays given solely because of admission to a hospital,
- mandatory chest X-rays for employment,
- repeated X-ray examination of TB reactors (those with positive tuberculosis skin tests), asymptomatic TB patients, and people in nursing homes and chronic disease hospitals.

Dentists are also guilty of unnecessary exposure. Full mouth X-rays are rarely necessary more often than once every five to ten years, but many dentists take them far more often.

Chiropractors use X-rays without cause and expose people unnecessarily. Some even offer them free as an inducement to make an appointment.

It is a good idea to always ask the physician or dentist who proposes an X-ray to explain its benefit and whether a previous film might suffice. Keep a record of your exposure, including the name of the doctor, the type of exam, and the purpose. Request a copy of the X-rays if you are moving or going to another doctor. If you must be exposed to an X-ray:

- cooperate with the operator during exposure to avoid the need for retakes;
- beware of old X-ray machines, the type with the short, pointed plastic cone, as they may emit excessive X-ray energy. If in doubt ask whether the equipment has been inspected by a licensing agency or professional organization. The results of these inspections are open to the public. For more information, ask your State Radiological Health Agency;
- be sure to tell your doctor if you are pregnant or might be.

These considerations should not frighten you away from prudent X-ray use. For example, mammography delivers very low doses and the benefits are much greater than the risks for women over thirty-five.

Nuclear Radiation and Cancer

Nuclear radiation has long been known to cause cancer by damaging cellular reproductive and control mechanisms. Japanese survivors of the atomic bombing of Hiroshima and Nagasaki have been dying of leukemia and other cancers at a very high rate for thirty years. Should nuclear war occur, many survivors would die of cancer in the following years. The widespread construction of nuclear power plants, particularly plutonium breeder reactors, could greatly increase the cancer risk if containment is not perfect. Plutonium remains deadly for a half million years.

Air and Water Pollution and Cancer

The dumping of industrial wastes into the nation's air and water supplies has increased the cancer risk in some areas. Cigarette smokers in cities downwind from sulfur-emitting power plants have a greater risk of developing lung cancer than smokers in less polluted areas. Some researchers believe that the sulfuric acid increases the cancinogenicity of cigarette smoke.

Pesticides and herbicides in water supplies are a source of constant concern. Industrial wastes in the drinking water have been linked to increased cancer mortality in Louisiana and other states. One of the problems is that the chlorine added to water to disinfect it often combines with organic industrial chemicals and decaying plant material to form the carcinogenic chloroform.

The Environmental Protection Agency (EPA) is gradually (some say too gradually) forcing the cleanup of the nation's waters. Individuals can remain alert to political efforts to slow the cleanup, and drink unchlorinated spring water if tap water is chlorinated and contaminated with industrial wastes or decaying plant matter. Small amounts of chlorine without industrial wastes are probably not hazardous. Individuals can also report suspected illegal dumping of chemicals into waterways to the local police or their State Attorney General's Office.

The problem of cancer and other diseases caused by manmade toxins grows steadily with industrialization. Developed nations and those struggling to catch up *cannot* ignore this. Politicians and industrialists concerned about the economic cost of pollution control must include in their calculations the health care costs and lower productivity that result from not controlling pollution.

Asbestos is a hazard not only to those who work with it every day, but to anyone who breathes it. Workers tearing down old buildings should be very cautious with any insulating materials and avoid breathing the dust from them. Trail biking may be hazardous in some parts of the country. The dust churned up on country roads is sometimes almost pure asbestos, a natural mineral fiber.

Radon is a radioactive gas produced in the earth by uranium. Houses built over natural uranium deposits can accumulate the gas in dangerous concentrations, especially if they are tightly insulated. Radon is believed to be responsible for several thousand deaths due to lung cancer each year. It also makes cigarette smoking much more likely to cause lung cancer. If your house is in a known hot spot you should test the radon level with a test kit available at a hardware store. There are two types of tests, a charcoal-absorbent cannister and an alpha-track detector. For accuracy you may want to use them both. It shouldn't cost more than about fifty dollars. Follow the instructions on the labels. If the readings are high get a copy of the EPA's *Radon Reduction Methods* before hiring a contractor. You might be able to make the changes yourself.

Ventilating the basement and caulking some cracks may be all that is necessary. There is a lot of fraud in this area, so move cautiously and don't let anyone scare you or stampede you. If you hire a contractor he or she should be EPA-certified to do radon reduction work. Even in severe cases the cost should be less than two thousand dollars.

The Sun and Skin Cancer

So-called aging of the skin is largely a result of irreversible sun damage, not time. The changes in sun-damaged skin commonly precede malignant changes. Premalignant lesions are usually hard, dry scales on a red base, or a persistant sore or ulcer. They may eventually develop into squamous (or scalelike) cell or basal cell cancer. Untreated, these can extend to the underlying bone and eventually cause death. However, when detected early these cancers are usually successfully treated with surgery, freezing, burning, or chemosurgery.

Basal cell cancer is the most common skin cancer. It usually occurs on the face, neck, and top of the hands. It starts as a small pearly pimple, sometimes with tiny blood vessels on the surface. Later it develops a crust that bleeds easily if irritated.

Squamous cell cancer occurs most often on the head but may occur on the hands or elsewhere. It may look like a basal cell cancer or it may appear as sharply outlined red scaly patches. While sun exposure is the cause of most of these cancers, they can also be caused by exposure to coal tar, pitch, arsenic, paraffin oil, and X-rays.

Malignant melanoma is an increasingly common, often deadly cancer of the melanin-producing cells (melanocytes) of the skin. It may result from the transformation of a mole or by itself. Women get it somewhat more often than men, the older more often than the young, and lighter-skinned people, especially blue-eyed poor tanners who freckle and burn easily, much more often than darker people. Malignant melanoma is usually dark brown or black with irregular borders and surface. It grows and may ulcerate and bleed easily if injured. The original color may turn into shades of blue, red, and even white.

The most common sites of melanoma are the face, head and neck, the back, and the legs. Movement to vital organs occurs early and rapidly; delay in diagnosis and removal can be fatal. Susceptibility seems to be hereditary. Members of affected families often develop dysplastic nevi, moles with a tendency to become malignant. Such moles should be monitored carefully for changes in size, color, and shape, as well as bleeding, scaling, and itching or burning of the surrounding skin.

Sunlight is by far the most common trigger for all skin cancers. Their incidence in populations is proportional to closeness to the equator, to skin exposure, and to skin lightness. Pigment protects the cells from the mutagenic ultraviolet rays of sunlight. Incidence is high among descendents of northern Europeans living in the southern U.S. and northern Australia, especially sunbathers, farmers, fishermen, and laborers who like to work with a minimum of clothing. Sporadic heavy overexposure is more hazardous than smaller exposures every day. Contrary to some reports, fluorescent lights emit too little ultraviolet light to be a hazard.

The fair-skinned sunbather or unprotected worker often suffers **solar elastosis,** a degeneration of the skin that starts as a yellowish mottling, changes to pigmented blotches, and gives rise to malignant changes. Even teenagers can develop solar elastosis. Affected areas should be watched for life for signs of malignancy, especially if exposure to the sun continues. The damage done by ultraviolet radiation to the skin cells is cumulative and cannot be reversed or healed, only prevented from progressing.

PREVENTION OF SKIN CANCER

Avoid excessive exposure to the sun, especially if you are fair skinned. Ignore the tanning fad. "Healthy tan" is an oxymoron; all tanning is cumulative and irreversible toxic injury. Even if it doesn't give you skin cancer it will age your skin and cause wrinkling and sagging. Use protective clothing and a sunscreen, preferably one that blocks both UVA and UVB. Most sunscreens block only UVB, but broad-spectrum products that block both types of ultraviolet rays are appearing on the market. For exposure during the peak hours of 10 A.M. to 3 P.M. the sun protective factor (SPF) of your sunscreen should be at least 15, which means it takes fifteen times as long to get sunburned as it would without sunscreen. Sunscreen should be applied at least one-half hour before going out. Don't neglect to protect yourself when skiing. Snow reflects about 80 percent of UV radiation. Don't be fooled by cloudy days; UV radiation penetrates clouds very well.

Stay away from tanning booths, beds, and lamps. These gadgets emit very high levels of UVA radiation and send about five thousand people a year to emergency rooms with radiation injuries. They also increase the risk of skin cancer, wrinkling, cataracts, blood vessel injuries, eye burns, and phototoxic and photoallergic reactions. Commercial promotions for tanning salons and machines are rife with dangerous misrepresentations about their safety.

Watch for solar elastosis, as described above. See a dermatologist soon if you suspect it. Remember, only an expert can tell for sure if a growth, lesion, or pigmented area is cancerous or precancerous. The latter lesions can often be treated and cancer prevented by application of 5-fluorocil. This powerful drug is available by prescription only. A physician *must* supervise its use. Tretinoin, or Retin-A, another prescription topical drug, may also reverse some precancerous lesions.

Because of the thinning of the ozone layer, population growth in the sunbelt states, skimpier clothing, and growing participation in outdoor recreational and fitness activities, the incidence of skin cancer is increasing dramatically. Because the increase is worldwide (incidence has doubled through the 1980s), ozone depletion is probably the most important factor. Experts estimate that each percentage point of ozone depletion results in some two hundred thousand additional cases of skin cancer worldwide, including fifteen thousand cases of melanoma. Stopping the destruction of the ozone by industrial chemicals known as chlorofluorocarbons (CFCs) should be a major priority of world and national health officials and preventive medicine advocates everywhere. Their efforts should be supported by the public even if it means paying a little more for alternatives to aerosols and refrigerants now widely used.

Sex and Cancer

Hepatitis B and AIDS, both of which most commonly affect homosexual men, can lead to cancers. (They are discussed in detail in their own entries in this section.)

Cancer of the cervix has a strong association with sexual activity: Virgins and celibates have little chance of getting it. Those who start having intercourse before the age of twenty have about twelve times the risk of those who refrain until after twenty. The risk seems to be increased by multiple partners: Prostitutes have the highest incidence of all.

Genital herpes and genital warts may promote cervical cancer. Using a condom or diaphragm probably decreases the risk, but it is no guarantee. Women who have genital herpes or warts should get frequent Pap smears to detect any precancerous conditions that can then be treated with simple cryosurgery (freezing) and other methods. Genital warts that are not removed should be monitored.

Early Cancer Detection

The sooner a cancer is recognized, the more likely treatment is to succeed. It is important to know what cancers you are at risk for, whether you should be screened or examined, and what self-examinations are possible. You should be familiar with the early warning signs and how to look for them. (All this is discussed in detail in Section Three.)

Chickenpox and Shingles

Chickenpox is a highly contagious virus infection that few children escape. It is generally a mild illness with low-grade fever and a rash with clusters of raised red spots. These become blisters that collapse and scab over. New crops of blisters erupt for three or four days. The major complaint is itching. The rare adult case is usually more severe and can even result in pneumonia. The incubation period is about two to three weeks. The virus can be transmitted in the fluid from the easily broken blisters or in droplets from the mouth or throat. It is contagious for about a week after the blisters first appear. The scabs are not contagious.

In otherwise healthy children, complications such as encephalitis and severe bacterial infection of the lesions are very rare. On the other hand, if a child is undergoing treatment for cancer the virus can run rampant and cause fatal infection of the brain and other organs.

Pregnant women who contract chickenpox can pass it on to the fetus or newborn, in whom it can be serious. Therefore, a pregnant woman who has never had chickenpox and develops a rash should consult her physician right away. Treatment can lessen the danger.

One episode of chickenpox confers lifelong immunity against the disease, but in most cases the virus manages to survive in a latent form in the nerve roots and can cause shingles years or decades later. The varicella-zoster (chickenpox-shingles) virus belongs to the herpes family, other members of which also remain latent in nerve roots and cause outbreaks later as they move down the nerves to the skin.

Shingles is a rash with intense, burning pain. It is caused by reactivated chickenpox viruses, usually decades after chickenpox occurred. The trunk and face are the most common sites affected. In most cases only one side of the body is involved. The rash usually clears up in a week or two, but nerve damage may cause pain to last months.

PREVENTION

A vaccine is now available and will be widely used in children with compromised immune systems due to AIDS and cancer treatment. So far it is not recommended for all children because it is feared that the protection it provides may not last a lifetime; instead of the mild childhood disease, many might contract it as adults and get much sicker. However, these doubts are fading and we are edging closer to immunizing all children. Some feel the disease can be eradicated like smallpox was. In any case, susceptible women of childbearing age are certainly candidates for the vaccine.

Until the vaccine is widely available, susceptible women who are pregnant or might be pregnant should avoid exposure to chickenpox and shingles. If they are exposed they should immediately consult their physicians about chickenpox immune globulin, which provides some protection if given quickly enough. The price is high, about four hundred dollars, but well worth it if infection of the newborn is prevented.

TREATMENT

If the fever is high, 103°F or more, bed rest and lots of fluids are essential. Acetaminophen helps reduce fever and itching, but may prolong symptoms by a day or so. Scratching should be discouraged and nails trimmed to prevent bacterial infection. The hands should be washed several times a day and the affected skin kept clean. Bathing with baking soda or colloidal oatmeal in the water may relieve itching.

Although serious symptoms are rare, they can occur. It is very important to **see a physician immediately if** there are convulsions, a stiff neck, severe lethargy or headache, or rapid breathing.

Call a physician if pain is severe or the lesions seem to be infected by bacteria, with large areas of redness or draining pus. Treatment over the phone is preferable to an office visit in order to prevent the spread of the disease.

See a physician if shingles is suspected. Effective drugs are available for pain, inflammation, and even suppression of the virus.

166 Colds

The symptoms of colds are variable but usually include two or more of the following: weakness and malaise, loss of appetite, raspy or sore throat, sneezing, copious nasal discharge, nasal stuffiness, coughing, and sometimes mild fever. Colds rarely last more than a week or so and are rarely serious except in the chronically ill or debilitated.

Is It a Cold or Flu?

The common cold is often confused with influenza (flu), which is generally much more serious (see **Influenza,** below). The confusion causes unnecessary clinic visits for colds as well as delay in seeking help for the flu in high-risk groups. Colds usually come on gradually, do not cause high fever, and produce symptoms mostly in the upper respiratory system. Influenza usually comes on suddenly with fever, muscle pain, headache, sore and red eyes, and a dry cough. Colds occur any time of year, while flu comes in epidemics in the winter, and usually are announced with local publicity.

CAUSE

Colds are caused by **viruses** (more than two hunded types of rhinoviruses, adenoviruses, and others) that escape the action of the cilia in the upper respiratory tract, penetrate the protective layer of mucus, attach themselves to living cells, and inject their genetic material into the cells. The cells' resources are then turned to making more viruses that destroy the cells and burst out to attack surrounding cells.

In self-defense the cells release interferon and other antiviral chemicals, as well as histamines that dilate capillaries and promote congestion and mucus secretion. Nerve endings in the nose and trachea are stimulated by the extra fluid and congestion and initiate a sneeze or cough reflex. The miseries of a cold are primarily caused by the defensive reaction to the infection.

Colds are spread when the viruses are passed on to the mucous membranes of other people. Research suggests that colds are caught with the hands more readily than through the air. A person with a cold sheds millions of the viruses and can easily leave a trail of them on whatever or whomever he or she touches. They can then be picked up by shaking hands, or touching a doorknob, hand railing, money, or other object; then introduced onto the mucous membranes by rubbing the eyes or nose. Cold viruses can probably also be spread by kissing, sharing eating utensils, and inhaling droplets in the air from sneezing and coughing, but these modes of transmission may be less important than hand-to-hand innoculation.

People usually have fewer colds as they get older. Young children, who have no immunity to most of the viruses, average three or four colds a year. Those in their sixties average fewer than one a year, perhaps because they have already been infected by most of the common cold viruses and are at least partially immune to them, or because they have the least contact with young children, who are the most likely to harbor and spread the viruses.

Does Cold Cause Colds? Colds can occur any time of year, in warm weather or cold. One cannot catch a cold by getting caught in a downpour or being exposed to a draft, at least not without being exposed to the virus. Why, then, the common beliefs to the contrary, that are strong enough to give the illness its very name? Perhaps the stress of prolonged exposure to the cold lowers resistance to the virus and makes illness more likely if exposure does occur. Perhaps the viruses survive longer on colder objects. And maybe it's a fallacy.

PREVENTION

Without vaccines against dozens of the most common rhinoviruses there can be no dramatically effective primary prevention of the colds they cause. We are left with general measures that should reduce the risk to individuals and help slow epidemics.

- **Stay away from people with colds,** especially runny-nose toddlers who are likely to be covered from head to foot with cold viruses and spreading them to everything and everyone they touch.
- **People with colds should be aware** that they are shedding millions of viruses that can infect other people. They should wash their hands often and avoid touching others or sneezing or coughing around them. Tissues impregnated with citric acid and other chemicals that inactivate viruses might gain popularity and help reduce contagion.
- **Wash your hands** before touching your eyes, nose, or mouth, particularly if you have been around someone with a cold or in a public building touching railings, door handles, and other objects.
- **Stay in good general health.** Eat right, exercise, and get adequate rest and sleep.

- **Don't smoke and don't expose others, especially children, to smoke,** as it damages the cilia of the respiratory system and otherwise harms the body's defenses.

Does Vitamin C Prevent Colds? Adequate intake of all the essential nutrients is important for optimum resistance to infections, but the evidence indicates that taking massive doses of vitamin C does *not* prevent colds. However, taking large doses several times a day does seem to provide some symptomatic relief. The problem is that the effective dose is usually well into the potentially toxic range. You may be trading a slight reduction in your sniffling and sneezing for stomach distress, diarrhea, and other side effects (see Section One).

TREATMENT

Certain types of interferon (a natural antiviral agent) may eventually be used to cure colds, but for the foreseeable future there will be no cure. Nevertheless, proper treatment is important because it can prevent complications and speed recovery.

- **Heed the symptoms early.** Do not try to brave your way through them or ignore them. Greatly reduce your activity level. Rest, relax, and get extra sleep. In severe cases, stay in bed for a day or two.
- **Drink extra fluids,** especially soups and fruit and vegetable juices. Soups and teas with chicken, cayenne, garlic, ginger, mullein, or peppermint help loosen mucus and clear the nasal passages.
- **Frequent sniffing** to prevent mucus from running out of the nose can promote eustachian tube infection or irritation that can lead to middle ear infection. Yet blowing hard carries similar risks. Therefore, the best bet is to blow your nose frequently, but very gently.
- Regardless of what the commercials may claim for cold pills, **it rarely makes sense to take a pill,** even aspirin, for a cold. The drugs most likely to provide relief of specific symptoms are cough medicines containing dextromethorphan and single-ingredient nasal sprays, drops, and inhalers. The latter should be used sparingly and for no longer than three days. They should *never* be shared, since they may contain viruses sucked into the bottle. (See Section Four for more on nonprescription drugs for cold symptoms.)

- **People with diabetes or diseases of the heart, lung, liver, or kidney** should inform their physicians when they develop symptoms. So should those who have had their spleens removed.
- An otherwise healthy person who develops **a high fever** (101°F or 38.3°C), **has sharp chest pains, coughs up thick phlegm,** or has a severe sore throat or difficulty breathing should see a physician.
- **Children with throat pain** should be seen by a physician, as should adults if there is also pus on the throat or tonsils, fever, swollen glands in the neck, a rash, a history of rheumatic fever, or exposure to someone known to have strep throat. Symptoms other than a runny nose that last longer than a week may be signs of a complication; a physician should be consulted.

Dementia and Alzheimer's Disease

The **causes of dementia** (loss of mental capacity and intellectual functions) include strokes, brain tumors, head trauma, alcoholism and other drug abuse, chronic exposure to chemical solvents, certain vitamin deficiencies, and protein-calorie deficiency. Some forms of extreme depression can mimic dementia. However, **Alzheimer's disease is the most common cause of dementia** in persons over fifty and one of the top four or five contributing causes of death in the United States. It costs individuals, the health care system, and the nation at least thirty billion dollars each year. There are almost 350,000 new diagnoses each year, and these figures are likely to accelerate in coming decades as the population of older people increases.

In Alzheimer's any and all of the typical signs and symptoms of dementia may occur, starting gradually with slight impairment of recent memory, learning ability, and problem solving. Early signs may go unnoticed as habits sustain social behavior, but eventually the mental deficiency becomes obvious to all. The person becomes slow, sloppy, and confused, and has difficulty with complex tasks and unfamiliar situations.

The difficulties often cause angry and frustrated emotional outbursts. Frequently there is depression, apathy, anxiety, a loss of liveliness, and sometimes even delusions and hallucinations. In the late stages of severe cases all mental powers are lost, and the patient does not even know where or who he—or more likely—she is. (Women with the disorder outnumber men two to one.) He or she may suffer seizures and become totally bedridden and dependent on nursing care. Death—due to infections, malnutrion, and other complications of being bedridden—can come within ten years of the onset in severe cases. In some cases, however, the dementia is relatively mild and survival much longer. The most severe cases, those that progress rapidly and have a poor prognosis, are often associated with rigidity, tremors, and other Parkinsonian symptoms.

The diagnosis of Alzheimer's disease is generally by excluding other causes of the symptoms, such as vitamin B-12 deficiency, alcoholism, severe depression, syphilis, and AIDS. This is very important because some of these other causes are curable, whereas there is no effective treatment for Alzheimer's disease. However, diagnostic methods are improving and will be specific sooner or later. CAT scanning is already proving helpful. Magnetic resonance imaging (MRI) is apparently capable of detecting degeneration in certain areas of the brain; it may become widely used in detecting and monitoring Alzheimer's. On the biochemical front, monoclonal antibodies are being developed to detect characteristic plaques and tangles where normal brain cells once were.

What causes the brain degeneration is the subject of intense research and debate. The leading theories include genetic predisposition; infection with a slow virus or perhaps a similar but even smaller organism called a prion; an autoimmune process in which the body produces antibodies to its own brain cells; a toxin, perhaps aluminum or a heavy metal; or a combination of these factors.

It should be noted that if aluminum is involved, it is not simply a matter of exposure or ingestion since Alzheimer patients do not have higher intakes or blood levels of the ubiquitous metal than normal people. But they may have a deficiency, perhaps hereditary, in the transport system of the brain cells that normally keeps aluminum out. The accumulation of the metal in the neurons could lead to damage and malfunctions.

PREVENTION OF DEMENTIA

Prevention of non-Alzheimer's causes of dementia include avoiding and preventing drug abuse, alcoholism, sexually transmitted diseases, head injuries (boxers and motorcycle riders should wear helmets), strokes, and malnutrition. Most of these are discussed in other parts of the book.

To prevent Alzheimer's disease we need to locate the gene and learn how to turn it off or prevent environmental triggers from turning it on. These things can and surely will be done; the question is, when? That is a question of national commitment. Two million Americans already have the disease. With people living longer and the population of elderly growing, can we and will we prevent a greater catastrophe?

The disease is surely genetic, and it is unlikely that a single infective agent is the cause or trigger that activates the gene; there are probably several environmental triggers. Therefore, a vaccine of the traditional type is not likely. However, a new kind of vaccine is being developed against the antibodies that do the damage in autoimmune disorders. Theoretically, early diagnosis and vaccination before much damage has been done to the brain cells could prevent dementia.

Are You at Risk? You are much more at risk if a close blood relative has or had the disease. There is not much you can do about that now, but this may change. Eventually people at risk may be counseled on practical preventive measures, and early diagnosis and treatment may minimize damage.

Should You Avoid Aluminum? Popular articles and books are prematurely blaming Alzheimer's disease on aluminum exposure and creating widespread fear of the metal. However, it is the most abundant metal and the third most abundant of all the elements on earth. It is impossible to totally avoid and trying to do so might be as incapacitating as Alzheimer's. Nevertheless, the metal has no function in the body and large amounts are known to be toxic if they get into the brain. If Alzheimer's disease has occurred in a blood relative it wouldn't hurt to avoid the few sources that can account for 80 percent or more of your intake, at least until we have more information. The most important sources are antacids that contain aluminum (they are constipating anyway), powdered junk foods (read labels), and processed cheese (there are so many better cheeses). Pots, pans, and beverage cans are a relatively minor source of aluminum in the diet.

TREATMENT

All complicating symptoms and health problems, such as nutritional deficiencies, infections, dehydration, and congestive heart failure, need to be effectively treated since they can make the mental condition much worse and accelerate deterioration. Tranquilizers, antidepressants, pain killers, antihistamines, and other drugs are sometimes essential, but their use and dosages must be strictly minimized to the extent possible because Alzheimer patients are often much more susceptible to drug toxicity, which can severely increase the symptoms. All optional drugs should be avoided, and any drug use should be supervised.

Because the patients are often confused and afraid, family members and health professionals involved in their care must be supportive and accepting, and must take the time again and again to explain and reassure. Familiar, pleasant surroundings should be maintained as far as possible. Rearranging the room, changing the wallpaper, or going on a trip are likely to be confusing and upsetting. Obligations and pressures to perform and produce must be minimized in order to prevent confusion, frustration, and emotional outbursts. Every effort must be made to avoid injuries. The home should be made safe with good lighting and the removal of loose rugs, low tables, and anything else that can be tripped or slipped on. Stairs should be blocked.

Dental and Gum Disease

Dental and gum disease, the most common health problem in the United States, is costly, painful, inconvenient, and even deadly. The spread of bacterial infection from cavities to the blood can promote certain kinds of heart disease. Bacteria from gingivitis and generally poor oral hygiene can be aspirated into the lungs and cause a kind of pneumonia. Some people feel that dental health is peripheral to general health and that losing one's teeth is no big problem since dentures can be worn. But natural teeth exert enormous pressures while dentures produce, at best, one-fifth of this biting and chewing force. Considering the nutritional value of whole natural foods that require plenty of chewing, perhaps this is why it is often said that dentures can cost ten years of one's lifespan.

CAUSES

Caries in teeth (decay and decalcification) is caused by an attack and invasion by organized, highly concentrated colonies of bacteria, mostly *Streptococcus mutans* and *Lactobacillus acidophilus*. Disorganized and free-floating, these germs are harmless; the latter may even be beneficial in the intestine. But when they manage to adhere to the surface of the teeth the trouble begins. They excrete a sticky transparent film of dextran, multiply by the millions, and deposit more dextran.

This whitish-yellowish film of germs and dextran is called plaque and feels furry to the tongue. When the plaque is thick enough it shields the bacteria from oxygen and they begin to produce acids that eat away the tooth enamel. Soon a cavity is formed.

When plaque hardens at the gumline, germs colonize beneath it and evolve fermentation products that irritate and inflame the gums. This inflammation is known as **gingivitis.** It can be aggravated by various irritants including broken, malformed teeth, improperly placed or overhanging fillings, poorly constructed crowns and bridges, and inadequate vitamin C in the diet.

When hardened calculus or tartar develops from plaque, its rough surface causes tiny breaks in the gum tissue and gum infection sets in. Pockets of infection form and reach deeper toward the base of the teeth. The tiny connective tissue filaments anchoring the teeth to the gums are attacked and destroyed. This is **periodontal disease** or gum disease, sometimes called pyorrhea. Eventually even the jawbone may become infected.

Genetic susceptibility to dental and gum disease varies substantially. Some people get very few cavities in spite of relatively poor eating habits and oral hygiene, while others who take more care get more cavities. But whatever your given level of resistence, controllable factors determine the degree of damage done. In almost all cases, the disease is totally preventable, though some will have to work more at it than others.

Nutritional factors during tooth development in fetal growth, infancy, and childhood can have significant effects. Poor nutrition leads to weakness in the microstructure of the calcified tissues and vulnerability later in life, in spite of improved nutrition. Clearly, dental and gum disease prevention should begin early in life, preferably in the uterus.

The most important nutrients during and after tooth development, the lack of which commonly cause gum and dental problems sooner or later, are vitamins A, C, and D, and calcium, phosphorous, and fluoride. Vitamin A deficiency in the fetus or during infancy causes abnormal tooth structure, poor calcification, and reduced enamel formation.

Fluoride deficiency causes defective calcification and vulnerable teeth. The mineral is important in tooth formation, and may also be essential in bone growth and development. The widespread fortification of drinking water with small amounts of fluoride is the single most important factor in the dramatic reduction of dental disease in the United States over the past few decades.

Vitamin C deficiency causes weakening of the collagen connective tissue. The gums are spongy, bleed easily, and may ulcerate. Dentin formation is decreased. (Dentin is the bonelike bulk of the tooth, just under the harder enamel, the visible layer.) **Deficiency of vitamin D, calcium, or phosphorous** causes delayed eruption of teeth, poor positioning, decreased dentin and enamel, and increased susceptibility to decay.

 Mild deficiency of B vitamins, most commonly folate and niacin, can weaken the soft tissues and tooth-supporting structures and increase their vulnerability to infection.

Carbohydrates are needed by the bacteria in order to produce the sticky dextrans and the corrosive acids. Whenever a starchy or sugary food is eaten, bacteria metabolize the residue left in the mouth and produce acid. Depending on the food, after about an hour or two (the *clearance time*) the acid level returns to normal. The sugar and starch of candies and breads have the longest clearance times and lead to the most damage.

Saliva is very important in preventing decay; it constantly washes away debris, neutralizes acid with its bicarbonate, ammonia, and arginine, and decreases bacterial acid production with its sialin, a tetrapeptide (chain of four amino acids). It also provides a constant bath of fluoride, calcium, and phosphorous for direct absorption into the enamel.

Animals with their salivary glands removed and humans with low saliva production usually experience a tremendous increase of tooth decay. This may partly explain the known action of some drugs like amphetamines and some tranquilizers in increasing tooth decay. There is some suspicion that marijuana may have a similar effect, since it is known to cause dry mouth. Cigarette smokers have a higher rate of jawbone decalcification and more loose teeth. This is consistent with an increased risk of osteoporosis among smokers. Habitual mouth breathing can also lead to dry mouth and increased dental disease.

Poor dental care itself can promote dental disease. Poorly placed or overhinging fillings and crowns can create crevices and areas vulnerable to plaque build up, gum irritation, and infection.

Thumb sucking generally does *not* cause dental problems unless it continues past age four.

PREVENTION

Long-term studies involving thousands of people prove that we now have the ability to essentially wipe out this serious infectious disease. Here we summarize the necessary steps.

- **Assure the best nutrition** from gestation through old age. Adequate amounts of all the essential nutrients are necessary, but calcium, phosphorous, fluoride, and vitamins A, C, and D are the most important, though intake above the RDA is not helpful.

- **Eat whole natural foods.** Whole grains, beans, and fresh fruits and vegetables, besides providing important nutrients, require plenty of chewing. This exercises, stimulates, and strengthens the teeth, gums, jawbones, and chewing muscles. The coarse fiber in raw produce helps clean the teeth. Lime-soaked tortillas actually help repair tiny cavities, as the calcium from the lime plugs the holes and is incorporated into the structure of the teeth.
- **Presweetened cereals are among the worst foods** for dental health. Some have well over 50 percent sucrose, as well as refined flour, and crunchiness that forces the sticky mass between the teeth. Unfortunately, the largest group of consumers of these products, young children and teenagers, are the least likely to floss the stuff out. Chewy candies and raisins and other dried fruit can cause similar problems.
- **Don't chew gum for more than a few minutes a day.** Teeth and supporting tissues can take about a half hour of chewing each day. Habitual gum chewers may chew for several hours. The resulting trauma on the teeth, jawbone, and gum tissue can be enormous. Children without a full set of adult teeth are especially at risk of serious harm to the teeth and the bite.
- **Use fluoride-containing drinking water,** rinses, and toothpastes. The fluoride greatly strengthens the teeth and even promotes remineralization of early enamel lesions. It also has an antibiotic action against the bacteria that cause decay and infect the gums.
- **Brush and floss carefully** at least once a day, preferably before bed. No matter how well you eat, this is essential. Good, natural foods often have plenty of carbohydrates and long enough clearance times to contribute to plaque build up. Hygiene is also most important during tooth growth. A tooth kept free of plaque and decay in its early months will be less vulnerable years later.
- **The principle of plaque control is simple.** Every surface of every tooth, including areas below the gum line in the sulcus (crevice), surfaces touching other teeth, and fissures on the tops of molars must be scraped clean regularly. Thoroughness is more important than frequency. It would be preferable to brush and floss very thoroughly once each day than to superficially brush three times a day.

  Some tooth surfaces must be cleaned with a brush; others require floss. The toothbrush should be soft. A hard or even medium brush can cause gum recession and tooth sensitivity. Soft polished nylon bristles are best. They soften up under warm water and don't have the sharp, jagged edges of boar bristles that can put holes in your gums and promote infection. Look for the American Dental Association (ADA) seal. Get a new toothbrush every two months or more often.

Toothpaste is not necessary for cleaning, though it is useful for fluoride application. Certainly the highly abrasive type advertised as good for getting teeth very white should be avoided. Teeth are not naturally white but various shades of yellow. Heavy use of abrasive toothpaste can cause enamel thinning and tooth sensitivity.

When brushing, systematically clean as many tooth surfaces as you can. To clean below the gum line, hold the brush at about a 45-degree angle (midway between horizontal and vertical) where the gum meets the teeth. Gently vibrate the brush to dislodge plaque between the teeth and gums.

Then use dental floss or ribbon to clean areas you missed with the brush. Gently ease the ribbon between the teeth and insert it between the gum and each tooth, as far down as it will go. Scrape up and down a couple times. Be gentle with your gums.

Every few months use a disclosing wafer after cleaning (they are available in drug stores) to check how good a job you are doing. The wafer releases a red dye that clings to any remaining plaque and shows areas you may have missed.

While all this may seem like a lot of trouble, if done properly the rewards are enormous: a fresh, clean mouth, and freedom from cavities, gum disease, and all the inconvenience, pain, and expense involved.

- **Plaque Removing Rinses?** A flurry of so-called antiplaque mouth rinses appeared on the market in the late 1980s. Only one, Listerine, has been judged effective by an FDA panel of experts, but the evidence even for it is weak. Your money would be better spent on good toothbrushes and, if your water lacks fluoride, fluoride rinses.
- **Sealants** made from a clear plastic-bonding resin can seal crevices on the biting surfaces of teeth, keep bacteria out, and prevent decay. This is one of the most effective, yet underutilized preventives available. The tooth enamel is etched with acid, the sealant is applied, and light is used to harden it. It is usually applied to molars, whose rough biting surfaces are not always well-protected by fluoride. The treatment is simple, painless, and inexpensive, and can protect for about five years.

- **Water-irrigation devices** are recommended by some dentists in spite of the lack of evidence of benefit. If improperly used, these devices can aggravate and even cause gum disease by weakening the tissue and forcing bacteria and their byproducts into the gum. Those who use such a product should be instructed in its safe use; be especially careful about the higher settings. The spray should never be directed at an area of inflammation, irritation, or pain.
- **Protecting primary (baby) teeth** is important since the last of them don't come out until about age thirteen. Children whose baby teeth rot away early are more likely to have speech problems, psychological problems, and a need for expensive orthodontic treatment. One of the most important preventive measures is to *not* put the baby to bed with a bottle of milk or juice after the teeth start erupting. All too often the fluid pools around the teeth and sits there for hours while the child sleeps. The sugars (including milk sugar) feed the bacteria that destroy the teeth.
- **Chlorinated pool water** is often far too acid and can cause enamel erosion, with gritty, painful, chalky, or transparent teeth, in people who swim laps frequently or otherwise spend a lot of time in the pool. The pH should be read three times a day and kept between 7.2 to 7.8. If you swim often in a pool, do not hesitate to ask the pool manager about pH readings, which are very easy to do. If in doubt, get some pH paper from a drug store, pool supply store, gardening shop, or chemical supply store and do the measurements yourself. The paper is inexpensive and simple to use; just follow the directions on the box.
- **Vaccines** against tooth decay are being tested. The idea is to stimulate the body's production of antibodies against the *Streptococcus mutans* bacteria that are responsible for most tooth decay.
- **See a dentist and hygienist regularly.** Ask for specific instructions on cleaning areas you may not be doing well. Ask about sealants and fluoride treatments, especially for children.

  How often you should visit your dentist is an individual matter. Most children up to about twelve should have their teeth examined and cleaned about every six months. Adults with few problems should see a dentist every year or two. But most adults can profit from twice yearly cleanings because even the most conscientious of us usually have a few isolated areas that are hard to clean where soft plaque can change to hard calculus in a matter of weeks.

EARLY WARNING SIGNS

Any of the following should be discussed with a dentist; they should also remind you to clean your teeth well every day.

- **sensitivity** to heat, cold, or sweets
- **pain when chewing**
- **brown spots or little holes** on a tooth
- **swelling or pus** around the gumline, or gums that bleed or are red or tender
- **a change in your bite,** the way your teeth fit together
- **bad breath** unresponsive to thorough brushing and flossing and not due to sinus infection
- **loose adult teeth**
- **persistant pain** in the mouth or sinus area. Toothaches are rather late signs and require attention within a day or two. The best way to relieve a toothache is to clean out the cavity as thoroughly as possible using a brush and vigorously rinsing. Keep food debris away from the affected tooth. Then, of course, see a dentist.

TREATMENT

Any substantially decayed area of a tooth must be scraped and drilled out, and the hole must be filled. The most common fillings are amalgams of silver, mercury, tin, and other metals; half the United States population has at least one. There is increasing concern about the health problems mercury may cause—not only in those who are allergic to the heavy metal (perhaps 5 percent of the population), but in anyone who has too much mercury in the body from all sources combined. It has been claimed that mercury in fillings can cause all kinds of psychiatric and neurological problems. However, there is no good evidence for these claims and amalgams need not be removed in most cases. Nevertheless, mercury is a toxin that can reach significant levels in dentists and their assistants, so the trend to other materials like plastics and ceramics is a good one.

Proper treatment of dental and gum disease also involves thorough cleaning and instruction in self-care by a dental hygienist. The advice should be carefully followed in order to prevent further problems and costly and painful treatments.

Diabetes

Diabetes mellitus is a disease in which there is insensitivity to or inadequate amounts of the hormone insulin. This leads to disturbances of carbohydrate, fat, and protein metabolism. High blood sugar leads to damage to blood vessels, kidneys, eyes, and nerves, and a tendency to atherosclerosis, especially of the heart, leg, and brain arteries. It also impairs immunity and leads to increased susceptibility to infection.

There are really two types of diabetes mellitus, the insulin-dependent, ketosis-prone *type I* and the noninsulin-dependent, more stable *type II,* often called *NIDDM.* Of course, we are all dependent on insulin; the terms refer to the usual treatment for the two types.

Type I (which can occur at any age but most often begins in childhood) accounts for about 10 percent of the cases and usually has a sudden onset with increased thirst and hunger, weight loss, weakness, fatigue, increased urination, blurred vision, irritability, and other symptoms. There is sugar in the urine (glucosuria) because of excessive sugar in the blood (hyperglycemia). The basic problem is a severe lack of insulin, required for the entry of glucose into muscle and other cells. No matter how much is eaten the glucose does not enter the cells but accumulates in the blood and spills into the urine. Fat is mobilized to feed the starving cells, but their use leaves a flood of breakdown products, the ketones (acetone and others), in the blood. This is *ketosis* and it is responsible for many of the symptoms and complications of the disease.

Type II diabetes usually occurs in genetically prone overweight people over thirty-five. The onset is milder than with insulin-dependent diabetes and may include one or more of the following symptoms: excessive thirst and urination, decreased libido, blurred vision, headache, itching, loose teeth, infection, abscessed gums, weakness, and fatigue. Sometimes there are no symptoms. Tests show hyperglycemia and other signs. The basic problem is insufficient insulin and relative insensitivity to it.

Several million Americans have type II diabetes and don't know it. If you are over forty and overweight, see a physician for a general physical examination, including a blood pressure check and diabetes screening. This is especially important if a close relative has or had the disorder. If you have any unexplained symptoms such as unusual thirst, hunger, or fatigue or frequent infections, let your doctor know. Other indications for diabetes testing are listed below (see **Early Detection**).

CAUSE

The primary cause of insufficient insulin production is not known but is the subject of intense research. Genetic susceptibility is apparently important in both types of diabetes, but environmental triggers probably also play a role. A theory rapidly gaining support is that the insulin-producing beta-cells of the pancreas are damaged by an autoimmune reaction, perhaps triggered by a virus. The abnormal production of antibodies to the beta-cells gradually destroys them until, years after the process began, the disease becomes apparent. This results in type I diabetes. Another theory is that beta-cells are damaged by certain chemicals.

PREVENTION

True primary prevention would involve indentification of those genetically prone to diabetes, followed by intervention in the process of diabetes development by control or elimination of the environmental triggers, perhaps with vaccines against common childhood viruses, or by avoiding certain foods or pollutants. We are inching toward such primary prevention, but we've got several yards to go. In the meantime, there are secondary preventive measures that may delay and reduce the harm the disease does.

- **Avoiding obesity and staying fit** from an early age can be considered a general preventive measure for type II diabetes, whether one is known to be at risk or not. Discouraging obesity as a public health measure can reduce the harm done by diabetes.
- **Breast-feeding** may prove to have a protective effect. If a virus is involved, the antibodies from mother's milk might disarm them and prevent damage to the pancreatic beta-cells.

EARLY DETECTION

Those at risk for diabetes should be identified as early as possible and tested regularly regardless of how well they may feel.

A person should be tested if he or she: has a family history of diabetes; has a history of gestational diabetes; is pregnant; delivered an infant weighing more than 9 pounds; has recurrent infections; is obese; has high blood pressure; has abnormal levels of blood lipids; is over forty; is an American Indian, Hispanic, or black; or has previously had an abnormal glucose tolerance test.

Some of these indications are more important than others. A family history, for example, is more important than being forty. And a combination of indications makes testing more urgent than just one, of course. If you are black, have a family history of diabetes, have high cholesterol, and are obese and over forty, it's much more urgent than if you are just black.

Once diabetes is found, since there is no way of knowing how long it has been present, there should be thorough examinations for complications that might have already developed in blood vessels, nerves, eyes, kidneys, and other organs.

TREATMENT

Choosing your physician is important because the diabetic and the physician must work together for many years and must feel completely comfortable and confident with each other. The basic care involves the proper balancing and timing of food intake, exercise, and medication dose, if any. Too much food and too little exercise or insulin can cause hyperglycemia. Too little food and too much exercise or medicine can cause hypoglycemia and its many complications. Equally important is proper self-monitoring of blood glucose by patients who are able.

Besides understanding these relationships, there is a need for extra care in personal hygiene, prevention and treatment of infections, and avoidance of cigarette smoking and excessive alcohol consumption. Attention to proper nutrition and exercise is believed to be critical to minimizing complications.

In type I diabetes replacement of insulin is usually necessary for life, and the doses must be carefully timed and balanced with eating and physical activity. Guidance from a registered dietician is very helpful. Insulin users should always have a supply nearby as well as some sugar and should carry identification cards or wear bracelets that identify them as insulin-dependent and provide their doctor's phone number.

In type II diabetes, there is often good chance of achieving control by diet and exercise alone, without insulin or diabetes pills. The main goal is usually to lose fat. Many obese diabetics have more insulin than nondiabetics, but their excess fat makes their bodies resistent to insulin. (For tips on losing fat and getting fit, see Section One.) As with type I diabetes, patients should work closely with a qualified nutritionist. For many type II patients weight control is not enough and they require oral hypoglycemic agents (diabetes pills) or insulin.

Diabetics should exercise for the same reasons everyone else should, but particularly for weight control. Therefore, sustained aerobic-type exercises are best. Walking, for example, does more good than weight lifting. In many cases surprisingly small successes lead to big gains. Losing just ten to twenty pounds can significantly improve blood glucose levels and other signs of the disorder. Losing just one pound a week, or even half a pound is cause for celebration (but not with anything edible). However, while exercise takes on added importance for diabetics, avoiding injury from exercise does also. Great care must be taken to avoid stress and trauma injuries to the feet and eyes. In general, walking, bicycling (on a stationary bike unless biking is absolutely safe), and swimming are preferable to running of any kind.

In recent years evidence has accumulated that the risk of diabetic retinopathy, blindness, kidney disease, and other complications can be substantially reduced by rigid control of blood sugar levels, especially in type I diabetes. This may require the use of an insulin pump, careful self-monitoring of glucose levels, or multiple insulin injections. It is also very important to control hypertension in all diabetics.

Hope for the Future. *Beta-cell transplants,* the insertion of healthy insulin-producing cells into the abdominal cavity, is a promising experimental technique. And a variety of drugs are being tested for their ability to prevent nerve damage due to diabetes.

The Recommended Diet

In general, the recommended diet for those with diabetes is the same as for nondiabetics: lots of whole grains, beans, fruits, vegetables, and fish; moderate amounts of poultry and other lean meat and low-fat dairy products. The difference is that diabetics must be more regular in their eating habits and much more careful to avoid binges of excess calories and sugar, as well as chronic, low-level overeating. Also, the saturated fat proscription and the fiber prescription are even more important.

Starchy foods can cause the blood sugar to rise almost as fast as sugar if they are eaten alone. In general, it is best for diabetics to eat high-carbohydrate foods with other foods in order to slow their absorption. A good meal would be a salad, steamed broccoli, rice, and baked fish; a small dessert may be okay as long as the calorie and sugar intake are not excessive.

As we said above, the diabetic's diet should be low in sugar, fat, and cholesterol, moderate in protein, and high in starch and fiber. The reduction of saturated fats and cholesterol is prudent since fats in the bloodstream make the cells less sensitive to insulin, and because diabetics run a very high risk of developing atherosclerosis, which is promoted by high fat and high cholesterol levels. The question of sugar consumption is controversial, but it is clear that the total calorie count is more important.

Sodium intake is also somewhat controversial. Some experts recommend moderate salt restriction for all diabetics on the grounds that it might help prevent or delay hypertension in some of them. It also prepares patients for stricter salt restriction that might be necessary in the future. Since the combination of diabetes and hypertension is so serious, and since the restriction is not a great hardship, moderate sodium restriction for all diabetics seems prudent. It's usually enough to avoid salty snacks like potato chips, and refrain from adding salt to food at the table.

The usual recommendation is that a little more than half of one's calories come from starch, a little less than a third from fats, and a tenth to a fifth from protein. However, there is increasing evidence that consumption of oils from olive, avocadoes, sunflower seeds, and other sources of monosaturated fats in lieu of some of the starch may be beneficial. This means more olive oil–herb sauce on your pasta, but less pasta, and more avocado or almond butter on your sandwich, but less bread. Total calories usually must be restricted and kept nearly the same from day to day as long as exercise levels are constant.

Eating Disorders

The two neurotic eating disorders of serious public health concern are anorexia nervosa and bulimia nervosa. They are similar in some ways, but there are major differences.

Anorexia nervosa is a puzzling and stubborn eating disorder in which normal, successful young people (about 90 percent are women) develop an obsession with their weight, dieting, and often exercise. They frequently use laxatives, diuretics, and enemas to increase their appearance of thinness. They are afraid of food and eating, and become prisoners of eating-related activities and thoughts, compulsive rituals, and endless planning designed to rigidly control and minimize food intake. Many end up looking like starvation victims, and suffer loss of bone mass, thinning of hair, anemia, shrinking of breasts, and loss of menstrual periods, all the while denying that they are unusually thin.

More than 95 percent of anorexics are white North Americans, Western Europeans, or Australians, mostly between ages thirteen and twenty-two, although the condition may begin at practically any age over ten. In women the onset tends to occur around two stressful growing-up milestones: the onset of menses and graduation from high school.

 In the few men who develop the disorder it is usually very severe.

Because of the compulsive rituals (like precisely cutting food into tiny pieces) and the necessity of being in complete control of food preparation and intake, eating becomes a private affair. Social contact is shunned because it tends to encourage eating. So the anorexic becomes reclusive at an age when social contacts and skills are normally expanding and he or she shies away from intimacy. A sense of inferiority and inadequacy is common, and in chronic cases severe depression can be a serious complication, often leading to suicide.

The condition may last for a few months or it may wax and wane for years. Death is a frequent outcome. Estimates range as high as 5,000 a year in the United States. Many survivors suffer years of weakness and sickness due to starvation-induced damage, often to the liver, kidneys, bones, and heart. Diabetics are especially vulnerable to serious harm.

The cause of anorexia nervosa is not clear, but the epidemiology strongly suggests that it is associated with, and perhaps a result of, the cult of thinness that began in the 1960s and is widespread in the United States, Australia, and some Western European countries. Some blame the fashion and advertising industries for perpetuating the problem. In any case, striving for thinness provides the person with an opportunity for precise self-control of his or her behavior as well as extreme achievement. In some cases a young woman may fear her physical maturation and emerging sexuality so much that she starves away her breasts, hips, and menstrual periods. The psychological profile includes insecurity, a sense of powerlessness and inferiority (often in spite of high achievement), a lack of spontaneity, rigidity and extremity in behavior with no appreciation of moderation, and general immaturity.

Bulimia nervosa is a hidden disease—carefully concealed by the victims themselves. People afflicted with this eating disorder indulge in truly enormous binges of overeating (bulimia) and vomiting, almost always very secretly. For most people an average meal is about 1,000 calories. Bulimics consume anywhere from 2,000 to 50,000 calories in one session that may last hours. It may be vomited in several episodes or all at once when the eating binge is over. The amount of food eaten and retained is variable, so bulimics may be emaciated or normal in weight. In most cases weight fluctuates wildly.

The frequent vomiting can cause severe acid burns to the esophagus, gum recession, and dissolution of the enamel of the teeth, leading to rampant tooth decay. It can also cause chloride and potassium deficiencies, heart arrhythmias, heart damage, anemia, and death. Moreover, the problem can become very time consuming and, because of the large quantities of food eaten, very expensive. Shoplifting is often resorted to.

The vomiting habit often starts casually as a diet substitute. If it continues the body's satiety mechanisms become disordered and ever larger meals are required for satisfaction. These lead to more vomiting, and so on. There is a sense of lack of control over eating. Guilt and poor self-esteem follow.

PREVENTION

- **Biology classes** at the intermediate and high-school levels should emphasize human physiology and anatomy, and include discussions of the functions of normal fat. These include keeping the body warm, providing a padding for sitting and lying, and helping keep women fertile by playing a role in estrogen storage and activation. Eating disorders and the dangers of habitual vomiting, fasting, using laxatives, and overexercising should be discussed along with other health problems common to young people, like drug abuse.
- **Good parenting** can help. Firm, intelligent guidance and lots of affection and positive strokes can help children develop a sense of security, self-esteem, and confidence.
- **Some segments of the fashion and advertising industries are starting to use more normal, healthy models** instead of always portraying ultra-thin women as the ideal. A more robust athletic look is more acceptible than it was twenty years ago. If this trend continues we may see a decrease in the incidence of eating disorders.

EARLY DETECTION

Parents of adolescent girls and boys should be able to recognize the early signs of anorexia and bulimia nervosa and quickly take steps, preferably with professional guidance, to meet the problem before it feeds on itself and becomes entrenched. Some signs to watch for are dieting and fasting, excessive concern with bodily appearance and thinness, refusal to eat with the family, social isolation, a sense of inadequacy, and the use of diuretics, laxatives, and emetics. Bulimia may be especially difficult to detect because it is by nature a secret disease and parents don't want to seem nosey or overbearing. Still, be alert for weight fluctuations and unusual or gluttonous eating patterns, especially if accompanied by apparent theft of money, discoloration of teeth, depression, and addictive behavior.

TREATMENT

There are two goals in treating anorexics: first to save their lives; and in the long run to cure them of their delusional afflictions, usually a slow process. This calls for a physician working with a psychotherapist.

Severe cases often require long-term hospitalization. The patient often must be fed through a tube inserted through the nose and into the stomach. In extreme cases total parenteral nutrition may be required to save the patient's life. This involves inserting a tube into a vein in the chest and pumping in nutrients. The psychotherapy can be long and difficult. It is too soon to conclude that a specific approach will or should become standard treatment, but one widely used, often successful method stresses a nurturing, authoritative, nonneutral but friendly posture toward the patient. He or she is repeatedly reminded of the seriousness of the condition and encouraged to face reality and give up the delusions; yet there is always empathy and consideration for the real fears of the anorexic. Strong rapport and trust are developed, hopefully leading to self-trust, self-esteem, growth, and maturity. The barrier and habit of solitude are broken. Group sessions with family members and with other anorexics often help achieve these ends.

Like anorexia nervosa, bulimic disorders generally call for extensive psychotherapy, and sometimes hospitalization with supervision to prevent vomiting. The goals should include interrupting the binge-purge cycle, treating complications that have developed, encouraging acceptance of more body mass and body fat, and fostering self-esteem and healthy relationships.

Epilepsy

People with epilepsy suffer recurrent seizures that resemble electrical storms in the brain, rather than the normal orderly flow of impulses between brain cells. Seizures may be mild and hardly noticeable, perhaps just a blank stare and feelings of detachment; or they may involve convulsions and loss of consciousness. Attacks are often preceded by a peculiar feeling or aura (a premonition that an attack is imminent). The victim may fall, bite the tongue, pass urine, and froth at the mouth. He or she may appear to stop breathing and turn blue before the attack is over. Severe seizures are often followed by sleepiness or confusion.

The electrical storms frequently originate in small, unstable patches of brain matter like scars, which can spread their instability through normal brain tissue. These unstable areas can be created by infections, blows to the head, very high fever, complications during birth, certain drugs and poisons, and tumors. Sometimes there is no obvious cause.

PREVENTION

- **Prevent head injuries.** Wear seat belts in cars and helmets on motorcycles. Young children should be securely strapped into safety seats even for short trips.
- **Prevent toxemia and other complications of pregnancy.** The most important factors here are good nutrition, good prenatal care, avoidance of unnecessary drugs, and delivery in a hospital where facilities are available to deal with complications.

TREATMENT

In an acute attack the head should be positioned for easy breathing. The person should lie on the side, not the back. Tongue biting may be prevented by placing a pad between the teeth. However, you should not put a finger in the mouth of a person experiencing a seizure; a serious bite could result.

Seizures almost always stop by themselves. If they continue one after another without consciousness returning, immediate medical attention is required. Moreover, anyone who has a seizure for the first time should see a physician immediately.

To minimize the risk of seizures occuring those with epilepsy should:

1. Cooperate carefully with the doctor in finding the right drug regimen, and then stick with it. These drugs stabilize the electrical membranes in the brain and prevent the storms from brewing. Report all side effects to your doctor, but never stop taking the drug(s) on your own. Anticonvulsants must be slowly withdrawn, or the risk of seizure will be greatly increased.

2. Maintain a well-balanced diet and don't fast or go on a low calorie diet without a physician's guidance.

3. Avoid alcohol, addicting drugs, psychedelic drugs, and strobe lights.

4. Be active but avoid excessive fatigue or overexcitement and get plenty of rest and sleep.

5. Carry a card or wear a bracelet indicating the problem and how to handle it.

6. Avoid very hazardous occupations and recreations like solitary

 swimming and rock climbing; driving and operating heavy machinery may be restricted by law.

Family understanding and support are very important in helping the person live with epilepsy and lead a normal life. Moreover, by decreasing emotional stress, plenty of love and affection may decrease cerebral excitability and so decrease attacks and help prevent psychological complications as well.

Sometimes epilepsy clears up spontaneously. On the other hand, surgery is sometimes necessary to remove a tumor or a focal area that triggers attacks.

Female Disorders

Cancers, osteoporosis, and sexually transmitted diseases are discussed in detail elsewhere in this section. The following focuses on menstrual and related problems, as well as urinary tract infections. The following disorders are included: **amenorrhea, cervical erosion, CIN (cervical intraepithelial neoplasia), dysmenorrhea, endometrial hyperplasia, endometriosis, fibroid tumors, hypermenorrhea (excess menstrual flow), irregular menses, menopausal symptoms, ovarian cysts, polyps, premenstrual syndrome (PMS), toxic shock syndrome (TSS), and urinary tract infection (UTI).**

THE NORMAL MENSTRUAL CYCLE

When all is normal each month, under the influence of the ovarian hormones estrogen and progesterone the endometrium (uterine lining) thickens, proliferates, and is prepared for the implantation of the fertilized ovum (egg). When fertilization does not occur, the estrogen and progesterone output drops, the endometrium is shed, and a new cycle begins. The cycle is counted from the first day of bleeding to the last day without bleeding. It is normally twenty-one to thirty-five days long, with the flow occurring for one to seven days and requiring one to ten tampons or pads per day.

Amenorrhea

Missing several periods in a row is common and usually normal in girls who have not yet started to ovulate regularly. But if a woman who is normally regular misses her period two months in a row, she should have a physical and gynecological examination. The most likely cause is pregnancy. Malnutrition (caused by fasting, extreme dieting, poor eating habits, anorexia nervosa, or overeating), excessive exercise without an adequate increase in caloric intake, and emotional and physical stress can all cause periods to be missed. Rare disorders of the pituitary gland or ovaries are much less common causes. Amenorrhea due to diet and exercise should not be taken lightly or seen as convenient birth control: It can be associated with the development of osteoporosis, a very serious disorder.

Cervical Erosion

Cervical tissue sometimes erodes because of irritation or trauma from tampon insertion, intercourse, or infection. This may cause pain during tampon insertion and intercourse, and a thick mucus discharge, sometimes containing pus. Cervical erosion makes the cervix more vulnerable to infection, but if no infection develops the symptoms of cervical erosion are often minimal and go unnoticed.

Consult a physician if itching, burning, or other signs of infection occur.

CIN (Cervical Intraepithelial Neoplasia)

In CIN, also called cervical IN, the outer cells of the cervix show abnormalities under a microscrope. These changes sometimes precede cancer and are graded from mild to severe. The latter is also called carcinoma in situ and takes ten years or so to become malignant. CIN causes no symptoms and is detected by a Pap smear.

PREVENTION

The risk of CIN can be minimized by avoiding teenage sexual intercourse, intercourse with many different men, and intercourse with men with genital herpes or genital warts.

Consult a physician: Women should have a Pap smear examination annually from age eighteen or within a year of beginning sexual intercourse.

Dysmenorrhea

In this extremely common condition symptoms are menstrual pain (aching and cramping) in the lower abdomen, sometimes radiating to the back or inner thighs. Nausea, vomiting, diarrhea, headache, dizziness, breast tenderness, fatigue, and muscle pain may also occur. There may be some discomfort a day or two before the period begins, but the most severe pain usually occurs on the first day of menstruation. It may last hours or even days. Dysmenorrhea occurs in all age-groups of menstruating women, but it is more common in the late teens and early twenties and in women who have never given birth. It declines sharply in the mid-twenties.

The usual cause of dysmenorrhea appears to be an excess of prostaglandins, hormones that promote the uterine contractions and blood vessel constrictions that lead to menstrual flow. Excessive amounts cause painful contractions and other symptoms. Other causes of dysmenorrhea are infections, cysts, endometriosis, and intrauterine devices.

SELF-CARE

- **Exercise,** such as swimming, bicycling, walking, or jogging, may help by improving circulation and relaxing muscles. Situps (with knees bent) and leg lifts (one leg at a time) may also help.
- **Sexual orgasm** may help by improving circulation and relieving pelvic congestion. Sexual arousal without orgasm may aggravate discomfort.
- **Heat application** with a hot water bottle, heating pad, or hot bath can help relieve pain.
- **Massage** and deep thumb pressure around the middle of the back on either side of the spine is sometimes good for several hours of pain relief.
- **Aspirin and ibuprofen,** which are prostaglandin antagonists, often help, especially if taken at the first sign of cramps or even before cramps begin. Take two or three regular tablets three or four times each day. Don't use these drugs if you have any stomach acid-related disorders. Stop using them if stools become black or bloody. Acetaminophen does not affect prostaglandins, but it may relieve the pain of cramps and headaches.

Consult a physician if dysmenorrhea is severe or occurs for the first time after age twenty-five.

Endometrial Hyperplasia

This is an excessive build up of the endometrium (lining of the uterus) associated with failure to ovulate. Since the egg is not released, the woman stays in the proliferative (estrogenic) phase of her cycle and her endometrium continues to proliferate. Eventually, frequent or profuse menstrual bleeding occurs. The problem is most common in girls who have just begun puberty and in women around menopause.

Consult a physician if excessive menstrual bleeding occurs.

Endometriosis

Endometriosis is a puzzling disorder in which endometrial tissue (menstrual tissue) appears outside the uterus. One theory is that it backs up and out the Fallopian tubes into the abdominal cavity. It becomes attached to the outside of the Fallopian tubes, ovaries, bladder, and other organs in fibrous, adhesive patches that continue to respond to monthly hormonal cycles. Like normal endometrial tissue, these patches thicken with blood during the latter part of the cycle. Pain, infertility (due to Fallopian tube adhesions), and irregular periods may occur.

SELF-CARE

If a woman with this problem plans to have a child sooner or later, sooner might be better, both to treat the endometriosis by eliminating the monthly cycle and to have the child before the problem causes infertility.

Consult a physician if menstrual pain is severe, intercourse is frequently painful, periods are prolonged and irregular, or chronic pelvic pain occurs.

Fibroid Tumors

Fibroid tumors are noncancerous growths of muscle tissue on or inside the uterus. They are quite common and affect about one in four women, usually in their thirties or forties. Their cause is unknown, but their growth is stimulated by estrogen-containing oral contraceptives; they recede with menopause. Although they sometimes grow very large, they usually are no bigger than a marble, produce no symptoms, and require no treatment. But if a fibroid tumor causes pressure on other organs in the pelvis or if it causes pain or heavy bleeding or contributes to infertility, it can be surgically removed. In some cases this can be done without affecting fertility, but sometimes the uterus must be removed; fibroid tumors are the most common reason for hysterectomy.

 Consult a physician if heavy bleeding or unusual pelvic pain occur.

Hypermenorrhea (Excess Menstrual Flow)

Excessive menstrual bleeding can be inconvenient and even frightening. It should be investigated by a gynecologist because it can lead to iron deficiency anemia and may be a sign of an infection, IUD complications, ectopic (tubal) pregnancy, cancer, hormonal disturbances, or other serious problems. **Consult a physician.**

Irregular Menses

Young women are usually quite irregular in the first one to three years of menstruation because ovulation is often irregular. This is generally nothing to worry about. In more mature women the length of the cycle and of the period and the total blood flow per period are pretty constant, though they may be affected by travel, emotional or physical stress, and illness.

Consult a physician if large, unexplained changes in menstrual patterns occur.

Menopausal Symptoms

In the United States, most women stop menstruating between forty-five and fifty. Ovarian function slows, estrogen levels decrease, and various physiological changes take place. These may include thinning of the vaginal epithelium, decreased lubrication during sexual arousal, painful tetany (spasms) of the uterus during orgasm, and hot flashes due to circulatory instability. Sex drive is usually not affected, but the loss of reproductive capacity may create emotional turmoil. More important are the increased risks of atherosclerosis and osteoporosis.

Consult a physician if you suspect menopause may be starting. Adverse effects can often be prevented or treated with the proper use of estrogens and lubricants.

Ovarian Cysts

These are growths on the ovaries that can cause sharp abdominal pains, sometimes during intercourse, but which sometimes produce no symptoms. Some recede after one menstrual cycle. Others do not recede with the cycle and some of these are malignant. In either case persistant cysts often must be surgically removed to keep them from growing to enormous size.

Consult a physician if unexplained sharp abdominal pains occur.

Polyps

Polyps are benign growths on stalks that develop on the cervix or within the uterus. The cervical type can cause bleeding during intercourse, between periods, and after menopause, or they may cause no symptoms. Uterine polyps can cause excessive menstrual flow, irregular periods, and even infertility. Polyps can be removed if they cause problems.

Consult a physician if unusual or excessive bleeding occurs.

Premenstrual Syndrome (PMS)

About a week to ten days before menstruation many women experience a variety of symptoms such as bloating and weight gain due to water retention, tender or swollen breasts, headaches, backaches, irritability, depression, anxiety, lethargy, joint pain, hives, craving for sweets, and decreased tolerance to alcohol. In most cases the symptoms are short-lived and merely a nuisance, but sometimes they are severe enough to disrupt normal functioning.

The leading theories of the cause of PMS are estrogen excess, progesterone deficiency, and decreased levels of the neurotransmitters (brain chemicals) dopamine and serotonin. These chemical changes are believed to lead to sodium and water retention, low blood sugar, and other consequences that account for the symptoms of PMS. Caffeine may aggravate symptoms in some women.

SELF-CARE

- **Minimize intake of salt** to reduce water retention.
- **Exercise regularly** to improve your general sense of well-being and to decrease water retention.
- **Avoid caffeine,** at least on a trial basis.

Consult a physician if:
- symptoms occur often and are severe;
- bleeding is heavy for several consecutive periods.

Toxic Shock Syndrome (TSS)

In TSS there is sudden sickness with such symptoms as fever, vomiting, and diarrhea. If untreated, blood pressure becomes dangerously low and shock often ensues. Damage to the liver, heart, and kidneys may occur. TSS is caused by a powerful toxin produced by certain strains of *Staphylococcus aureus* bacteria when they proliferate in large colonies.

PREVENTION

"Super-absorbant" tampons have been associated with TSS. Women with a history of TSS should avoid all tampons. Others should use them sparingly—not at night—and change them every four to six hours. Hands should be washed well before inserting tampons. The vaginal area should be kept clean with daily washing. Tampons should *not* be used for nonmenstrual purposes. (Abnormal discharge should be discussed with a physician.)

See a physician immediately. There is no self-care for TSS. Remove any tampon and see a doctor at once if fever plus any of the following occur: diarrhea, vomiting, peeling of hands or feet, a rash, fainting, dizziness, severe headache, sore throat, vaginitis, or red eyes.

Urinary Tract Infection (UTI)

Bacterial infections of the bladder (cystitis) or urethra (urethritis) usually cause painful, difficult, and frequent urination. Typically there is a strong urge to urinate, but only a little comes out and it burns painfully. The urine may have a strong odor. In severe cases there may be fever, chills, abdominal pain, and bloody urine. Sometimes there are few or no symptoms. These urinary tract infections can spread to the kidneys and cause serious damage, so they must be cleared.

The most common cause is *Escherichia coli,* a bacteria normal to the colon. The most common source of infection is contamination of the urinary opening with fecal bacteria. Women are about ten times as likely as men to contract a UTI because of the proximity of the urethal, vaginal, and anal openings and the shortness of their urethras. Chlamydia and gonorrhea bacteria, which cause common sexually transmitted diseases, also cause some UTIs.

Pregnant women are also more susceptible because the bladder is pressured between the uterus and the pubic bone and may not empty completely. The stagnant urine is a good breeding medium for bacteria.

Hormonal changes may also make the urinary tract more susceptible to infection.

In children recurrent UTIs are often associated with anatomic abnormalities, polyps, or stones that obstruct urine flow. As with adults, the residual urine provides a medium for bacterial growth.

PREVENTION

- **Keep the vaginal and anal areas clean.** Women should clean the anal area by wiping away from the vagina; girls should be taught this early.
- **Don't wear tight pants,** noncotton underwear, or anything else that traps heat and moisture in the crotch.
- **Tampons and diaphragms must be used with care:** Don't leave the former in too long, and make sure the latter fit right and are clean.
- **Be careful during lovemaking:** That which touches the anal area should not enter the vagina. The susceptible woman and her partner should bathe thoroughly before making love. Urinating soon after intercourse helps wash out any bacteria that might have been pushed in. Vibrators (and perhaps motorcycles and horse-back riding) may precipitate UTI in some women.
- **Don't use petroleum jelly.** If a lubricant is needed use a sterile, water-soluble product; ask a pharmacist.
- **Do not postpone urination** when the urge occurs. A full bladder accumulates germs, and excessive pressure on the bladder wall may damage it and make it more susceptible to infection.

TREATMENT

Call a doctor right away if urinary symptoms are accompanied by vomiting, fever, chills, bloody urine, or abdominal or back pain. This is very important to prevent kidney infection.

Drink enough fluid to produce lots of very dilute urine. This will probably be at least two liters per day and more in hot weather. This dilutes and flushes out the bacteria.

Cranberry juice is a popular home remedy. It contains organic acids that apparently act as antiseptics. However, it doesn't work very well, and it may make the burning worse so a little baking soda is often added. Others skip the juice and drink water with baking soda (no more than a half teaspoon per cup) to ease the pain of urination. Those on sodium-restricted diets should *not* try this. Vitamin C in large doses is also popular with some, but there is little evidence that it helps. Home remedies should be considered temporary measures to try before a physician can be seen; they should not be used instead of consulting a physician. Delaying proper treatment increases the risk of more serious infection.

UTIs tend to recur, so proper treatment must also include preventive measures.

Gallstones

The gallbladder is a small sac under the liver that stores bile from the liver and releases it into the duodenum where it helps digest fats. The bile contains bile acids, cholesterol, lecithin, calcium, and other substances. Sometimes these become too concentrated, or supersaturated, and stones crystallize in the sac. These may look like pearls, quartz crystals, or mulberries, and may be white, brown, black, yellow or red, depending on the exact composition. There may be a few large stones or a sludge of hundreds of small ones.

If a stone blocks the duct that feeds bile into the intestine, the resulting spasm of the duct and bladder causes severe pain in the pit of the stomach or upper right abdomen, often radiating to the right shoulder. Nausea, vomiting, fever, and jaundice may occur. Severe complications can ensue, and so it must be treated. The problem is extremely common. Almost a million Americans each year are diagnosed with it. Millions more develop gallstones that never cause symptoms and are never treated.

CAUSE

Why does the bile become supersaturated and give rise to stones? Unfortunately, we do not know. Genetics, age, obesity, and pregnancy are predisposing factors. Dietary protein and fat stimulate bile production, and fat stimulates release of the bile into the intestine, but the role of diet in gallstone formation is poorly understood. For unknown reasons obesity and fasting both promote gallstone formation. Birth control pills and other sources of estrogen tend to promote it, as do some cholesterol-lowering drugs.

PREVENTION

Avoid obesity; fat people are much more likely to get gallstones. However, if you are obese don't fast or go on an extreme low-calorie diet and lose weight rapidly. (See **Obesity** for tips on safe methods of losing weight, below.)

Women who have a family history of gallstones, particularly if they are obese, should consider the risk of gallstones in deciding whether to take birth control pills.

Animal experiments suggest that dietary fiber and soy protein may decrease cholesterol concentration in the bile, so a high fiber diet with tofu, tempeh, and other soy products might help prevent gallstone formation.

TREATMENT

It is generally agreed that treatment is necessary if the stones cause symptoms or if the person afflicted is diabetic. Beyond that there is controversy. Some physicians believe stones always call for surgical removal of the gallbladder, even if there are no symptoms. This is because once stones appear they are likely to continue to form, and sooner or later they are bound to cause trouble. Thus, it is argued that it is better to remove the gallbladder when the person is young and healthy than to wait until surgery is riskier. The organ is not essential; if it is removed, bile goes straight from the liver to the intestine.

Others argue that such major surgery should be avoided unless absolutely necessary. Each case must be considered on the basis of the severity of the problem, age, and general health. In recent years drugs that dissolve stones, shock waves that break them up, and other treatments have proved useful in a minority of patients. Unfortunately, such treatments often need repeating. Only surgery solves the problem permanently.

Hearing Loss and Ear Infections

The ear consists of three compartments: the outer ear with the ear canal leading to the tympanic membrane (eardrum); the middle ear with the three bones of hearing that is connected to the throat by the eustachian tube; and the inner ear where mechanical vibrations are converted to nerve impulses. Hearing problems can originate in any of these three parts and can be caused by a variety of factors.

CAUSES AND PREVENTION

Pushing things into the ear is a common cause of outer ear infection. Common objects for children are pebbles, beads, and pencils; adults prefer toothpicks and ear swabs. The ears should be cleaned with a little finger and soapy water. Don't attempt to remove accumulated wax from your ears unless you have been shown how by a nurse or doctor.

Earwax normally works its way out of the ear canal along with dust and bacteria. Occasionally excessive amounts accumulate and interfere with hearing. Ear swabs are more likely to impact the earwax against the eardrum than to clean it out. A physician, nurse, or you can remove it with a warm water ear syringe. Using an earwax softener first may help. The syringe and glycerol are available at most drugstores. Keep in mind, though, that earwax helps waterproof and germ-proof your ear canals, and helps keep them warm. Too little earwax probably causes more problems than too much (see **Surfer's ear,** below).

Middle-ear infection, known as otitis media, can be viral or bacterial. This can be a stubborn and frustrating problem in young children. If a youngster becomes irritable for no apparent reason, and if he or she pulls or rubs on one or both ears, suspect an ear infection. If infection and hearing impairment are chronic, language and learning problems may develop, so effective treatment is important. These infections are usually treated with antibiotics, but these don't always work. In some cases a surgical procedure called myringotomy may be done. A small hole is cut in the eardrum to drain accumulated pus. This relieves pain, provides a specimen of the microbes for culture, and decreases the risk of serious complications due to spread of the infection. Tubes may be inserted into the middle ear to provide continuous drainage. Some believe that much of this surgery is unnecessary, so be sure all other reasonable methods are tried first and get a second opinion about the surgery.

The infection is promoted by inflammation and blockage of the eustachian tubes, which can be caused by allergy. If the culprit is hay fever, prevention is very difficult, though antihistamines and decongestants may help. If the child is allergic to house dust it might help to get rid of all carpets, or at least to have them thoroughly cleaned with a wet or water-filter vacuum cleaner as frequently as practical. Regular vacuuming kicks up the dust and makes matters worse. Another preventive measure is to keep the child away from cigarette smoke and other air pollution which may cause swelling and blockage of the eustachian tubes.

If the culprit is a food allergy the food can be avoided, if you can figure out what food is involved. It appears that in many cases strict avoidance of milk and all other dairy products clears up the problem. If you decide to try this be sure to provide other sources of calcium (see **Food Allergies,** Section One).

Diving (high or deep-water) can cause perforation of the eardrum and infection of the middle ear. If promptly treated, hearing loss can be prevented. Learn to adjust the middle-ear pressure when diving more than about ten feet deep. Many face masks are constructed so that you can hold your nose while blowing out your cheeks with your mouth closed. This forces air into the middle ear to balance the water pressure against the eardrum from the outer ear.

Swimmer's ear, also known as tropical ear or otitis externa, is an inflammation of the skin of the ear canal. The thickened skin narrows the canal, traps water in it, and causes pain, itching, and partial hearing loss. People with this problem should wear earplugs or dry their ear canals with a hair dryer or isopropyl alcohol eardrops after swimming. (**Caution:** If the alcohol irritates, stop using it.)

Surfer's ear is the growth of bony protrusions into the ear canal as a result of irritation by cold. The bony growths can eventually block the canal and cause deafness. They also trap water and promote infection. Untreated, this condition can require expensive surgery. Use of earplugs whenever exposed to water or wind can conserve earwax, keep the canals warm, and prevent the bony growth. Severe cases may even be reversible if the ears are religiously kept warm with earplugs in the water (except when diving below ten feet) and a hat over the ears out of the water, especially when sleeping. Several months may be required. The best earplugs for surfing have tiny holes that allow some sound to enter while keeping water out, and are leashed together to prevent loss during wipeouts. Ask at a sporting goods store or surf shop.

Excessive noise is perhaps the greatest threat to hearing, or at least the most widespread. Repeated and prolonged exposure apparently harms the inner ear's delicate *organ of Corti,* that converts vibrations to nerve impulses. Loud machinery and loud music are common problems; rock musicians and frequent concert goers often suffer impaired hearing. Portable stereo headphones have become a major threat to hearing; some brands reach deafening levels at only half volume.

Alcohol and other drugs can worsen the danger of loud sounds. Many bars and nightclubs play music so loud it can only be tolerated by drinking alcohol. Alcohol and barbiturates have been shown to weaken the ability of the stapedius muscle to contract; marijuana, tranquilizers, and other drugs may do the same. This small muscle in the middle ear is stimulated by loud sounds to contract and reduce sound transmission to the inner ear. When this safety mechanism is compromised by drugs, the ears are more susceptible to noise damage.

If you are regularly exposed to loud noises at home or at work, consider ways you can reduce the danger to your hearing. When purchasing new equipment such as a lawnmower, food processor, vacuum cleaner, or air conditioner, select the quietest product available. When using a chain saw, riding in a noisy subway, or working in a noisy environment use earplugs, like the flexible foam type with a noise-reduction rating of at least 20.

Dietary fat and cholesterol may affect hearing. The inner ear is highly vascular, well supplied with blood, and has a high metabolic rate. Factors that affect this supply of blood and nutrients may affect hearing. Large intake of saturated fats may cause sludging of the blood and atherosclerosis, which slow microcirculation. Restriction of saturated fats and cholesterol have been reported as helpful in some cases. Other factors that can affect hearing by affecting inner ear circulation or nerve activity are cigarette smoking, alcohol, and hypertension.

It is a good idea to have your hearing tested periodically. **See a physician** about any ear problems, infections, discharge, buzzing or ringing, or apparent diminished hearing.

Heart Disease

A variety of anatomical and functional abnormalities cause potentially lethal disorders of the heart. They may be congenital or due to infections, tumors, or problems in other organs—but all other forms of heart disease are dwarfed by *coronary artery disease* (CAD), also redundantly called coronary heart disease (CHD). CAD is the single most common cause of death in the United States. Most CAD is caused by the deposition of atheromas (fatty, mineralized plaque) on the insides of the coronary arteries that feed the heart muscle. The disease is insidious; it develops over decades until the arteries are so clogged that severe symptoms, or even death, occur without warning. CAD is largely preventable (see **Atherosclerosis,** above).

Hepatitis

Hepatitis means inflammation of the liver. There are many causes of hepatitis, including certain poisons and drugs, gallstones, parasites, and bacterial infections, but the term most often refers to viral liver infections, the most common cause. Only these will be discussed here.

There are four known forms of viral hepatitis: type A, type B, delta, and non-A/non-B. The symptoms are similar, but they are caused by distinct viruses and are different diseases. Types A and B are the most common.

Hepatitis A (HAV)

This infection is very contagious and spreads rapidly where people live in close quarters, share a kitchen, or endure poor sanitary conditions. Prisons, mental hospitals, homes for the retarded, military units, and day-care centers are especially at risk. During the incubation and acute periods, enormous quantities of viruses are excreted with the stool, and invisible traces may contaminate food and water supplies and be passed on by close personal contact. Sexual contact (hetero- *or* homosexual) can also spread the virus. The infection is common among promiscuous people.

The **symptoms** begin two to six weeks after exposure. The first ones resemble the flu—muscle aches, headache, eye discomfort in bright light, and low-grade fever. A few days later loss of appetite, malaise, weakness, nausea, and vomiting may occur. At this point the virus is spread throughout the body. Typically, after about a week of this, the virus invades the liver. The urine turns a brownish color while the stools may become pale. Diarrhea sometimes occurs. Jaundice deepens as malaise and weakness worsen. The right upper abdomen may be swollen and sore due to liver inflammation.

Improvement in all symptoms begins one to two weeks after the onset of jaundice. Full recovery can take several months. The liver is a very resilient organ capable of completely repairing itself after even the most severe hepatitis A infection. About 99 percent of previously healthy individuals enjoy complete recovery. Death is very rare. One bout of this illness confers lifelong immunity.

PREVENTION

- **Immune globulin injections** may be in order if you have been or will be exposed to the virus; ask a physician. For example, if a member of the household or a sexual partner comes down with the infection, or if you are going to an area where sanitation is poor and the disease is common, one or more injections could prevent severe illness, even if infection occurs.
- **Avoid contaminated water** for swimming, fishing, and clamming.

Heed the warnings of your local health department. Also, do not eat raw shellfish, which often harbor live viruses. Always obey the local laws and codes on sewage disposal. This is very important in preventing contamination of water supplies.

- **Avoid intimate contact** with people with hepatitis.
- **Infected people should not handle food, water,** or eating and drinking utensils that others use. If possible they should have separate toilet facilities and their clothes should be washed separately. They should keep their hands scrupulously clean, as should those in close contact with them (household members, fellow workers).
- **Food handlers,** especially in institutions and restaurants, should always wash their hands very well before work. If a food handler is diagnosed as having hepatitis A, he or she should be removed from the job until well.

Hope for the Future: A vaccine is being developed.

Day-Care Centers and Hepatitis A

The problem of hepatitis A outbreaks in day-care centers is steadily growing. Because infected children of day-care age usually have no symptoms and still wear diapers that must be frequently changed, the virus is easily spread among the staff and children, and then to all their families. If hepatitis occurs in one of these families all the families should be alerted to the possibility of infection, and the staff should take preventive measures focusing on diapered children.

It is very important that the staff, children, and parents wash their hands thoroughly and often. Soiled diapers must be handled carefully and properly disposed of. Surfaces used for diaper changing should be impermeable and used exclusively for that purpose. They should be cleaned and disinfected with household bleach diluted 1:32 (½ cup per gallon water) prepared daily and sprayed from spray bottles. Accessories used in diaper changing should also be disinfected each day.

Day-care centers with outbreaks usually need not be closed and parents should not transfer their children to other centers. But the acceptance of new admissions should be suspended or required to receive immune globulin. If even one case occurs in a center, immune globulin for all employees, children, and their families should be considered.

TREATMENT

A well-balanced diet with adequate vitamins, minerals, and proteins will promote recovery by providing the nutrients necessary for liver repair. Attractive meals should be served to help stimulate the appetite, which is often poor. There is no proof that any special or extreme diet is helpful, but a moderate to high amount of protein and a moderate to low amount of fat are thought to help.

Absolute bed rest does not seem to speed recovery, but vigorous physical activity should be avoided. The return to normal activities should be gradual.

Alcohol, tobacco, and all other drugs should be completely avoided. Even nonprescription drugs should not be taken without a physician's approval.

Again, some experimental drug treatments are promising.

Hepatitis B (HBV)

This infection is not quite as common (in the United States) as hepatitis A, is usually more severe, and tends to last longer. The initial symptoms are similar, with a flulike illness for a week or so. The disease is sometimes associated with skin rashes, arthritis, and kidney damage. It is not often fatal in the United States, but it can lead to cirrhosis or cancer of the liver.

Like HAV, HBV can be transmitted through blood, saliva, and feces. An invisibly small speck of blood is enough to infect, so medical technicians and researchers must be extremely careful in handling blood and other body fluids. Acupuncture needles can transmit the virus even if they have been soaked in alcohol or ammonium compounds and appear sparkling clean. The sharing of needles by drug users is a common cause of spread of the virus.

A serious problem involving all modes of transmission is that many people, perhaps 1 percent of the United States population, are **lifetime carriers** of the virus without ever getting sick from it. And those who do get sick are "silent" carriers for the six-week or longer incubation period.

While hepatitis B is a relatively small (but growing) problem in the United States, it affects hundreds of millions worldwide. In some countries 20 percent or more of the population are carriers. Some victims never experience illness during years of infection, yet eventually die of liver cancer or cirrhosis. And if they are women, they often pass the infection on to their newborns at birth. In some areas where hepatitis B is common (parts of South America, Western Africa, southern Italy) the newly discovered *delta virus* or *hepatitis D virus* (HDV) works in concert with the HBV to cause acute hepatitis and cirrhosis.

TREATMENT

Treatment is essentially the same as for hepatitis A: rest, good nutrition, and avoidance of alcohol and other drugs. An experimental treatment with interferon may prove effective.

PREVENTION

The First Anticancer Vaccine. The hepatitis B vaccine is one of the most underutilized preventive medicine tools available. It can prevent not only the misery of the disease itself, but the liver cancer the virus may cause years later. Headlines should have trumpeted the first anticancer vaccine and millions of those at risk should have rushed to get it. Instead, only a small percentage of those who should be vaccinated have been. Hepatitis B vaccination, and in some cases immune globulin, should be considered for those belonging to the following groups:

- **health care workers** in frequent contact with blood, including dentists and hygienists;
- **immigrants** from areas where hepatitis B is common, especially China, Southeast Asia, and central Africa;
- **travelers** to areas where hepatitis B is common;
- **clients and staff in institutions** for the mentally retarded;
- **sexual and other close contacts** with hepatitis B carriers;
- **infants born to hepatitis B-carrier mothers** (all pregnant women should be tested for HBV);
- long-term **prison inmates**;
- **promiscuous** homosexual men (homosexual women don't exchange infectious bodily fluids);
- **users of illicit, injectable drugs** (who frequently share needles);
- **victims of human bites** that break the skin;
- **dialysis and hemophilia patients.**

The main problem with the vaccine is its high cost. Government and health officials have softpeddled the vaccine because they know the cost is too high (about $135) to give it to everyone. Even if just everyone at risk demanded it the price would go even higher. Recombinant DNA techniques may bring the cost down and lead to much wider—perhaps universal—use. There is even hope of eradication of the virus, as was accomplished with smallpox.

GENERAL PREVENTIVE MEASURES

- **Don't inject illicit drugs,** especially not with shared needles or syringes.
- **Dispose of all articles contaminated with blood.** It is best not to share razors, toothbrushes, towels, and the like. This is mandatory with infected people and known carriers.
- **Avoid sexual intimacies** with known carriers of hepatitis B, those who inject illicit drugs, and sexually promiscuous people.
- **In institutions and restaurants** heat sterilization of all food handling implements and careful cleaning of all instruments and surfaces are very important.

Non-A/Non-B Viral Hepatitis (NANBH)

Several other viruses can cause hepatitis, and these will be collectively called non-A/non-B until further study clarifies their role. Like types A and B, they are transmitted through the oral route, infected blood, or shared needles, and the infection can be as severe as with the type B virus. A virus that apparently causes most of these cases has recently been identified; it is called hepatitis C virus (HCV). Since most of the hepatitis transmitted by blood transfusion is NANBH, this discovery should lead to a much safer blood supply.

Hypertension

Sustained high blood pressure, the "silent killer," is a major cause of death in the United States. One out of five Americans is affected, but only half of them know it and only half of these are being effectively treated. Much progress has been made in recent years in identifying and treating hypertensives; this is already being reflected in lower stroke and heart disease incidence. But much more remains to be done.

The problem with high blood pressure is that it damages arteries and vital organs like the heart, kidneys, brain, and retina. It is a major factor in about three-fourths of all heart attacks and strokes. The person often feels completely normal until serious harm has been done. Sudden collapse and paralysis due to a stroke (a damaged brain artery) may be the first symptom.

Hypertension is so harmful that, in general, at every age, the higher the blood pressure, the shorter the life expectancy. For example, a thirty-five-year-old man with a moderately elevated pressure of 150/100 is considered to have about a sixteen-year shorter life expectancy than if he had 120/80. The first number, systolic pressure, refers to the pressure (in millimeters of mercury) during heartbeat; the second, diastolic pressure, refers to the pressure between beats.

There is some difference of opinion about the exact definition of high blood pressure. Generally, a diastolic pressure over 90 is cause for concern, especially in younger people. Systolic pressure is also important, but it is more variable; 150 is slightly high for someone over sixty, but very high for a teenager.

Several readings are usually necessary to be sure the high pressure is sustained and not temporary. For some people hospitals, clinics, doctors, nurses, and the measuring procedures themselves all contribute to "white-coat hypertension" that does not need treatment. There are now practical home measuring devices and even ambulatory devices that can be worn away from home. These are especially useful in borderline cases to avoid unnecessary drug use, inconvenience, expense, and higher life insurance premiums, as well as to assure prompt treatment of those who can really benefit.

CAUSES AND RISK FACTORS

In very few cases the cause of hypertension can be traced to a drug, an adrenal tumor or other hormone disorder, a congenital pinching of the aorta (the main artery from the heart), abnormal kidney function, or poor circulation to one or both kidneys. But in at least 90 percent of the cases no definite cause can be determined, and the condition is called essential hypertension. Fortunately, some important predisposing factors are well known, and this knowledge makes control of hypertension and prevention of early disability and death possible.

Obesity and inactivity are major factors in hypertension. It has been estimated that men 30 percent overweight have about a sixfold greater incidence of stroke and sudden death. In many cases of hypertension, weight reduction is all that is needed to reduce pressure to normal. Moreover, regular aerobic activity can help normalize hypertension even without weight loss.

Excess salt is an aggravating factor in about one-third to one-half the cases. Sodium *is* an essential nutrient but adequate amounts are generally available in natural foods without added salt. In studies of primitive people, those who use salt as a food preserver and as a condiment almost always have significant problems with blood pressure. Neighboring tribes who don't use salt don't have the problem. In parts of Japan where the average consumption of salt is about 30 grams per day, mostly from fermented soy products, almost half the population has hypertension.

The intake of salt in the United States is generally 10 to 15 grams per day, about ten times what it needs to be. Much of this is hidden salt, added to almost every kind of processed food on the market. Hypertension experts suggest that reduction of salt intake to 2 grams per day starting in infancy could bring this huge public health problem under control in one generation. However, this is probably an exaggeration since many people with the disorder are not salt sensitive, and do not benefit from salt reduction. Those most likely to be salt sensitive include blacks, the elderly, and those with a family history of salt-sensitive hypertension.

Excessive sugar in the diet may act synergistically with excessive salt in promoting hypertension.

Inadequate potassium is sometimes a factor in hypertension; it seems to provide some protection against excess sodium intake. When consumption of fresh produce is down and consumption of meat and processed foods is up, hypertension is more likely. The main sources of the mineral are fresh fruits and vegetables, especially bananas, oranges, apples, and tomatoes.

Inadequate calcium and magnesium have been implicated, the former more strongly. The mechanism is not understood, but the effect is strong enough to have prompted clinical trials of calcium supplements as a treatment for hypertension.

Smoking is a factor in hypertension. Other things being equal, smokers are much more likely to develop hypertension than nonsmokers and much more likely to develop the malignant phase of the disease and die than those who don't smoke. Moreover, if a cerebral aneurysm (an abnormal ballooning of a blood vessel) is present, the likelihood of rupture is much greater in smokers.

Prolonged stress may contribute to hypertension. Blood pressure normally increases with excitement or alarm, then drops to normal. In some people, each bout of excessive stress pushes blood pressure slightly higher than before, and it eventually remains higher than normal. Some people who lose their jobs experience blood pressure rises that do not drop until they find new work.

Drugs, including estrogens, indomethacin, phenylpropanolamine (the appetite suppressant and decongestant), amphetamines, and cocaine provoke hypertension in some users. More than an ounce of alcohol a day can cause hypertension in many people.

Excessive licorice can cause hypertension.

Genetics plays a major role in hypertension. The risk factors above affect some people more than others.

PREVENTION

About 11 percent of the population between the ages of twelve and twenty-four have hypertension, and may eventually suffer strokes, brain damage, or heart disease. While hypertension usually becomes apparent later in life, it often begins in childhood, so preventive measures should start early and involve whole families.

Until we know exactly what causes essential hypertension, efforts at prevention will focus on reduction of risk factors whenever possible. This means to eat right, keep active and fit, don't get fat, don't smoke, avoid drug abuse, don't drink more than lightly, and get adequate rest and relaxation. Family members can influence each other for better or for worse in all these things.

Some experts think all families should have blood pressure measuring devices, and record each member's daily fluctuations, regardless of the absence of risk factors or signs of high pressure. We think this is going too far. It is fine to have the device and use it periodically, but excessive worry and compulsive record keeping could do more harm than good. Nevertheless, regular monitoring should become a habit if you are obese or sedentary, or have a family history of hypertension, diabetes, or heart disease.

In the near future DNA testing will identify those at high risk for hypertension and lead to early and more effective treatment.

TREATMENT

Drugs have been the main treatment since World War II. They have unquestionably helped reduce disability and death. Some of these drugs affect the kidneys and some the nerves or blood vessels. They are relatively innocuous, but they do pose certain hazards and must be used as prescribed.

Many patients with mild hypertension (diastolic about 85 to 100 mmHg) can improve by reducing risk factors without taking medications. In borderline cases the decision about treating with drugs may depend on other risk factors, such as smoking, high cholesterol levels, and diabetes. Sometimes after a year or so of successful therapy the drugs can be stepped down carefully and perhaps permanently reduced or eliminated. More likely, therapy will be intermittent.

Fat loss in obese hypertensives is often the most effective treatment, better than either salt restriction or drugs (see Section One for tips on exercise and diet).

Exercise can sometimes help reduce blood pressure even if weight does not decrease. Aerobic exercises such as walking, running, swimming, hiking, rowing, and biking are the best for all-around fitness. Most weight training programs, and even hard work involving heavy lifting or pushing, however, should be avoided.

Salt restriction can be effective in some cases but not others. One of the first effective treatments for hypertension was Kempner's low-salt rice diet. Depending on the individual, the restriction may be moderate or strict; the advice of the physician or dietician must be followed. Unfortunately, there is no quick test to determine who is salt sensitive. Long-term trial and error is the only option, but such efforts can be confused by simultaneous institution of other treatments and dietary changes. One may never know whether salt restriction is really helping.

Nevertheless, salt restriction is effective often enough, it is cheap and safe, and it may help in other common disorders, too, like kidney stones and osteoporosis. Therefore, restricting salt and sodium as much as practical and tolerable seems to be prudent, at least until blood pressure is under control. However, an unfortunate complicating factor in all this is that in a few people salt restriction results in an increase of blood pressure. Clearly, careful consultations with a physician and a dietician are essential.

Polyunsaturates in place of saturated fats in the diet seems to help in some cases. In a study of hypertensive teenagers who were not being treated with drugs, the group that went on a diet rich in corn oil with very little animal fats showed a significant drop in blood pressure compared to the controls, who ate the usual portions of butter, bacon, egg yolks, and whole milk.

Dietary fiber, for unknown reasons, seems to affect blood pressure. A low-fiber diet tends to increase pressure, while a high-fiber diet decreases pressure.

Garlic may help reduce blood pressure. The relatively low incidence of hypertension and heart disease in some Mediterranean countries may be linked to the high consumption of garlic (see Section Four for a closer look at the herb).

Stress control often helps. Yoga, meditation, and biofeedback are all techniques to aid deep relaxation, which helps lower blood pressure. The specific method used is not as important as applying it faithfully and achieving a deep relaxation one to four times a day. The pressure reduction is not just for the duration of the session. The person's baseline pressure may be reduced over a period of weeks, and stay reduced as long as the sessions continue. It tends to rise as the practice tapers of.

All the nondrug methods require more willpower than do drug methods. Because of the lack of symptoms, it is often difficult to muster and maintain the willpower to stick to a treatment. Even the drug users have to be reminded and nagged about keeping up the treatment.

If you are determined to use nondrug methods, such as a low-salt, high-fiber diet, exercising, stopping smoking and drinking, eating garlic, and meditation, or some combination of these, should you avoid or quit drugs and rely completely on the other remedies? In borderline and mild cases, this is probably all right. But in more severe cases, such as when diastolic pressure is consistently above 110, drugs are usually preferable. As the other methods take effect, as weight is lost and the blood pressure drops, the drugs can be gradually reduced. Each individual is different, and whatever works best for him or her is the treatment of choice.

Anyone diagnosed as hypertensive should get a device to measure blood pressure and learn to use it. A doctor or nurse can teach you. Self-monitoring is useful because it involves the person in the treatment and provides more accurate readings than the sporadic office readings that are so often affected by psychological stress factors.

Influenza (Flu)

Influenza symptoms such as weakness, loss of appetite, upper respiratory problems, and a feverish feeling often cause it to be confused with the common cold. But it is really a different and much more serious disease. Every winter there are outbreaks, and frequently epidemics, that afflict millions. The vast majority recover fully, but thousands of elderly and chronically ill people die from the infection or its complications, especially bacterial pneumonia. Moreover, there are occasional pandemics, extremely virulent and deadly outbreaks that result in millions of deaths. The Spanish flu of 1918 killed more than five hundred thousand in the United States and perhaps twenty-five million worldwide, more than any other pestilence including the black plague epidemics of the Middle Ages. The other major pandemics of this century were the Asian flu of 1957 and the Hong Kong flu of 1968.

How to Tell a Cold from the Flu

People have widely differing reactions to colds and the flu, and there is no single symptom that distinguishes the two. In general, however, it can be said that colds come on gradually, usually do not cause high fever (except in children), and have localized symptoms like sneezing and a runny nose. Influenza usually begins with a fever, hits suddenly and severely, and often causes muscle pain, chills, headache, sore and red eyes, flushed skin, and a dry hacking cough. If there is a local flu outbreak and these symptoms appear, the ailment is probably influenza.

CAUSE

Influenza is caused by three basic types of virus, A, B, and C. They are spread from person to person and by contact with contaminated objects. Type A causes the seasonal outbreaks as well as major pandemics and type B causes smaller outbreaks. Type C is rarely a serious problem.

Once inside a host cell a flu virus commandeers its biochemical machinery and uses it to reproduce itself by the thousands. These break out and infect other cells. Most people easily develop antibodies that latch onto the invaders and inactivate them so that a given virus can infect them only once. Unfortunately, influenza viruses have an uncanny ability to change from year to year just enough to confound the immune system. These small changes in structure, known as *drift,* are caused by spontaneous mutations. They are responsible for the seasonal outbreaks, which are usually limited because lingering immunity to the old form provides partial protection.

When a virus undergoes a large change that results in a completely different protein on its surface, lingering immunity to previous strains no longer helps, and a pandemic results that can afflict hundreds of millions. Such large changes, known as *shifts,* are believed to result when two strains of virus infect the same cell and shuffle genes. For example, some scientists believe the Hong Kong flu virus arose when a strain of duck flu virus found its way into a human cell already infected with a human strain. The resulting hybrid struck down about fifty million Americans and left about seventy thousand dead in six weeks.

Wild ducks seem to play an important role in the epidemiology of influenza. The viruses grow rapidly in their intestinal tracts without causing illness, are passed from duck to duck in pond water, and are spread around the world in their feces during migration. They can then be acquired by humans, pigs, horses, turkeys, and other animals.

PREVENTION

Avoid close contact with infected people and do not share drinks, foods, or eating implements. Avoiding crowds during the flu season may reduce the chance of infection.

Don't smoke. It increases the likelihood and severity of infection by reducing the effectiveness of the mucus and cilia that normally trap dust and microbes and keep them out of the lungs. Passive exposure to smoke also increases susceptibility, especially in children.

Get vaccinated every year if you are in a high-risk group. This is one of the most underutilized vaccines. Only about 20 percent of those who should get immunized each year do so. Every spring representatives of the U.S. Center for Disease Control, the Food and Drug Administration, and other medical experts meet to determine what flu virus strains to put in the next season's vaccine, based on information from outbreaks all over the world. Many thousands of different flu virus strains are kept on ice in laboratories for this purpose. Those believed to be likely to result in epidemics are inactivated and placed in the vaccine, which then will stimulate the formation of antibodies to the viruses in those innoculated.

Because the vaccine is expensive and is only effective for about a year, immunization of the general population is not feasible. Instead, it is recommended for the following **high-risk groups** (in order of priority):

- adults and children with chronic respiratory or cardiovascular disorders, and those who are HIV positive;

- residents of nursing homes and other chronic-care facilities;
- doctors, nurses, and others who have extensive contact with high-risk groups;
- otherwise healthy people over age sixty-five;
- adults and children with diabetes, kidney problems, or other chronic disorders.

The antiviral drug amantadine is sometimes used to supplement the vaccine.

TREATMENT

Most people stricken by the flu need only to rest and take lots of fluid to fully recover within a week or so. Vitamin and mineral supplements at the RDA level may be advisable if food intake is greatly reduced, but there is no evidence of benefit from megadoses of vitamin C or other nutrients.

Aspirin can help reduce symptoms in adults, but is not recommended for children because of its possible association with the rare but very serious Reye's syndrome which is characterized by vomiting, violent headache, listlessness, irritability, delirium, and disturbed breathing, and can lead to coma and death. If such symptoms are seen in a child with or recently recovered from a flulike illness, a physician should be called immediately. The aspirin substitute acetaminophin is safe and effective for reducing flu symptoms in children.

For people in certain high-risk groups influenza can be very serious, and their physicians should be notified so that complications can be watched for. The groups include the elderly, those with chronic disease, young children and pregnant women. The antiviral drug amantadine can lessen the severity of the illness if given soon enough, but the side effects often outweigh the benefits.

Kidney Disorders

There are many diseases that affect the kidneys and interfere with their filtering, purifying, and regulating functions. Since the kidneys have a large reserve capacity, the symptoms may be mild until large areas of both kidneys are involved. Then waste accumulates in the blood causing severe illness with nausea, vomiting, headaches, and anemia. If infection is present there may be painful, burning urination with bloody, brown, or cloudy urine.

 In chronic renal (kidney) failure, calcium and phosphate metabolism are disturbed causing weak bones susceptible to fractures, and (rarely) deposits of calcium and phosphate in soft tissues such as the lung, blood vessels, joints, and eyes. In severe renal failure, uremia (urea and other toxins accumulating in the blood) may cause convulsions, coma, heart and lung failure, and ultimately death.

CAUSES

Diabetes damages small blood vessels in the kidneys; **high blood pressure** and **atherosclerosis** damage blood vessels in and leading to the kidneys. **Urinary tract infections** can spread to the kidneys and cause serious damage. **Bacterial infections** like tuberculosis directly damage the kidneys, while **streptococcal infections** can stimulate the formation of antibodies than can damage the kidneys. **Preeclampsia** is a complication of pregnancy that includes hypertension and kidney malfunction. **Too much vitamin D** can cause calcium deposits to form in the kidney. **Various prescription drugs** and combinations of drugs can slowly damage the kidneys; quite likely, all manner of **illicit drug use** carries a risk of kidney damage, both from infections in IV drug abuse, and toxic damage from cocaine, amphetamines, and assorted uppers and downers. Similarly, **alcohol** may be harmful to the kidneys. **Heavy metals** such as lead, mercury, gold, and cadmium, as well as insecticides and other chemicals that get into the body through food, water, and air interfere with normal kidney functioning. In many cases of kidney disease the onset is insidious and the cause is not known.

There is a growing suspicion that **excessive dietary protein** may play a role in chronic renal failure. The toxic breakdown products of proteins apparently damage the kidneys as they are concentrated and pumped out. Tiny amounts of damage daily for several decades can add up to significant loss of kidney capacity. It's almost as if excessive protein accelerated the aging of the kidneys. This is still a controversial concept, and no one knows who is most at risk or what amount of protein is dangerous, but some kidney specialists are chalking this up as yet another reason to keep consumption of meats and other concentrated proteins in the low to moderate range. The people most at risk, if the theory is correct, are body builders and other athletes who consume enormous amounts of protein, sometimes hundreds of grams a day, in the erroneous belief that this will increase their muscle mass.

Kidney stones are common and often very painful. They are most often calcium oxalate precipitates, but calcium phosphate and uric acid stones are also common. They may be the size of a grain of sand or a fist, and can cause infection, bloody urine, and vomiting. The problem tends to run in families and is often chronic, with recurrences throughout life. Stones are more common in men than women, and are rare in children and blacks. All these stones are dangerous, but the worst are those that block the ureter and cause urine to back up into the kidneys; they are also the most painful. Diagnosis is by urinalysis and X-ray of the kidneys.

CAUSES

Causes of kidney stones include: genetic predisposition to high concentrations of calcium, oxalate, or uric acid in the urine; excessive intake of vitamin D, milk, calcium antacids, and oxalate-containing foods; low fluid intake; prolonged bed rest or immobilization, causing demineralization of the bones; and poor diet, especially deficiencies of vitamin B-6, thiamine, and magnesium. Foods high in DNA and RNA (mostly animal meats), acidic urine, and low fluid intake promote uric acid stone formation. Fasting, which mobilizes protein for energy and inhibits uric acid excretion, can do the same. Infections and anatomic abnormalities of the kidney increase the risk by providing a focus for stone precipitation.

PREVENTION OF PROGRESSIVE RENAL DISEASE

The best prevention is to prevent and control hypertension, diabetes, atherosclerosis, and urinary tract infections (see separate discussions of each). One of the most important kidney saving measures may turn out to be very early treatment of hypertension in diabetics. This could save (i.e., dramatically prolong and improve the quality of) millions of lives.

Prevent and control strep throat and skin infections. Children in particular should avoid close contact with those with sore throats, boils, or infected cuts or abrasions. If you have a sore throat and relatives or other close contacts have recently had strep throat, or if there is a red skin rash, fever, or pus in the back of the throat, see a physician right away.

Minimize exposure to heavy metals, insecticides, drugs, toxic chemicals, and plant toxins.

PREVENTION OF CALCIUM OXALATE STONES

- **Drink enough fluid** to make very dilute urine. This will usually be about two liters a day, more in hot weather.
- **Eat a well-balanced diet** with adequate amounts of all the essential nutrients. Avoid excessive vitamin D and calcium-containing antacids. For those at risk for calcium oxalate kidney stones, total dietary vitamin D should not exceed about 800 IU per day; even that amount might be hazardous to those who also get lots of vitamin D from exposure to the sun. Total calcium intake should not exceed about one gram, unless the risk for osteoporosis is also high. In that case the relative risks must be discussed with at least one physician and carefully weighed. A registered dietician can help those with both risks to walk the necessary tightrope.
- **Avoid, or eat sparingly, foods rich in oxalates** such as spinach, dandelion greens, rhubarb, parsley, sweet potato leaves, asparagus, cranberries, chocolate, almonds, peanuts, walnuts, black pepper, beets, pecans, colas, and tea. Theoretically, too much vitamin C may increase oxalate precipitation. A gram or so per day is not thought to be risky, but larger amounts might be.
- **In some cases drugs,** including potassium phosphate, potassium citrate, and diuretics can help prevent stone formation.

PREVENTION OF URIC ACID STONES

- **Drink lots of water,** enough to make very dilute urine. This will usually be about two liters a day, more in hot weather.
- **Eat a well-balanced diet** with adequate amounts of all the essential nutrients. Restrict concentrated purines in the diet—anchovies, sardines, brewer's yeast, organ meats, and the like.
- **Keep the urine alkaline.** A low protein diet is helpful. Too much vitamin C will acidify the urine.
- **Some drugs help** prevent stone formation by reducing uric acid production. Others promote the excretion of uric acid through the urine and thereby increase the risk of stone formation.

Kidney Hygiene for Everyone

Public health and education efforts are rarely aimed at preventing kidney disorders. Those at risk fall into such disparate groups that giving advice to the general public might not seem appropriate. There would seem to be little reason to tell everyone how to prevent uric acid stones when only a few people are at risk for them. However, some of the preventive measures are appropriate for several kidney disorders. So many people are at risk for some or another kidney problem that, taken together, these measures amount to good general kidney hygiene and become relevent to the general public. Conscious attention to them can reduce one's risk of kidney diseases and the pain, disability, and early death they bring. Since many of the suggestions are also the factors in other very common and serious disorders, the suggestions amount to good general health advice and reinforce advice in other sections of this book. Our advice is to:

- **Eat a balanced diet** with moderate to low amounts of protein, sodium, saturated fats, and cholesterol. Avoid excesses and deficiencies of vitamins, minerals, and calories. Remember that hard water can make substantial contributions to calcium and sodium intake, both of which should not be excessive. Avoid unnecessary supplements. Don't fast and don't overeat.
- **Drink enough water** to keep your urine reasonably dilute, especially before, during, and after heavy exercise and heat exposure.
- **Prevent** or assure early detection and treatment of **diabetes and hypertension.** If you have close relatives with these disorders *do not smoke!* Keep your weight down and discuss screening tests with your doctor.
- **If a close relative has had kidney failure,** stones, or other kidney disease, including kidney cancer, consult with your doctor about the potential risks to you.
- **Prevent** or assure early detection and treatment of **sexually transmitted diseases and urinary tract infections.**
- **Prevent** or assure early detection and treatment of various **childhood and adult viral and bacterial infections,** including streptococcal throat infections, pneumonias, hepatitis B, influenza, mumps, measles, chickenpox, tuberculosis, and some sexually transmitted diseases, including AIDS.
- **Pay careful attention to skin wounds and infections.** See a physician for severe cuts, punctures, and other skin wounds, as well as boils and other signs of skin infection.
- **Minimize exposure to household and industrial chemicals,** insecticides, heavy metals, and miscellaneous toxins.
- **Avoid unnecessary drug use,** especially IV drug abuse and alcohol abuse.

TREATMENT

Kidney infection must be treated to prevent permanent damage. If it is not completely eradicated it could spread silently, causing severe relapse and even destruction of the kidneys. It is important not to neglect prescribed antibiotics or any follow-up examination because the infection seems to be gone.

In some kidney diseases large amounts of protein are lost in the urine and must be replaced in the diet. In other cases protein, sodium, potassium, magnesium, water, and some other nutrients must be restricted. The therapeutic diet depends on the type and stage of the disease. Quackery can be deadly here. Only physicians and registered dieticians who are trained in kidney disease are qualified to give advice. Expert care is required to lighten the kidneys' load and prevent toxic levels of minerals, protein wastes, and water from accumulating; at the same time, malnutrition and dehydration must be prevented. If protein is restricted, plenty of carbohydrate and fat is recommended to prevent tissue breakdown.

Dialysis (blood filtering by a "kidney machine") and kidney transplant are offered to patients with uremia.

As for the stones, sometimes they are small enough that they can pass spontaneously, though the process can involve one to several hours, or even several days of severe pain. Strong pain killers may be appropriate. There are several methods of breaking up and removing stones that don't come out by themselves, including shock wave devices and surgery. Each method has its risks and benefits for each patient. Whatever method is used, stones should be analyzed so rational measures can be taken, both to eliminate them and to prevent others from forming.

Malaria

Malaria is caused by infection with protozoa called Plasmodia. Infected female Anopheles mosquitoes transmit the parasite to humans when they draw blood. The victim may experience slight sickness for about an hour at this time. The protozoa enter the liver cells where they grow for five to sixteen days, depending on the species. When they are mature, they break out of the liver and enter the blood, causing fever and chills, and find their way into red blood cells. There they grow for two or three days, depending on the species, then break out, again causing fever, and go into more red cells. The infected blood cells become defective and are destroyed when they rupture.

The body fights the infection fairly effectively and death is rarely due directly to infection. Antibodies coat the parasites and prevent their entry into the red cells. Then they are removed from the circulation by special cells in the bone marrow, spleen, and liver. This battle may go on for years. Complications, such as the damaged red cells clogging up the capillaries, can cause severe damage to vital organs, especially the kidneys, and this can cause death.

There are several hundred species of Anopheles mosquitoes that can transmit the infection to humans. There are at least five species of Plasmodia responsible, but *P. falciparium,* and *P. vivax* account for about 90 percent of the cases. Sometimes these parasites are transmitted from cattle, monkeys, or other animals to humans by mosquitoes. Transmission rarely occurs by blood transfusion or by common use of hypodermic syringes among drug addicts.

Two decades ago malaria was on the decline under the onslaught of insecticides, drugs, and other measures. The optimists once spoke of eradication, but malaria has made a comeback and such hopes have faded. Mosquitoes have developed resistance to the insecticides and the parasites have developed resistance to the drugs. Millions of people are now stricken each year, mostly in tropical and subtropical areas of Africa, Asia, South America, and the South Pacific. India and other countries have experienced enormous increases in malaria incidence and deaths over the last twenty years. Worldwide, perhaps five million people a year die from the disease and millions are chronically infected.

In the United States malaria-carrying mosquitoes were eradicated in the 1940s, so the disease is not acquired here. However, each year about a million Americans travel to countries where the disease is endemic and more and more of them are contracting it.

PREVENTION

If you are entering a malarious area, be prepared. Use mosquito netting, screens, insecticides, and repellants to avoid contact with mosquitoes. N, N-diethyltoluamide or DEET is the best repellant; look for products with it. Since mosquitoes can penetrate cloth, clothing should also be sprayed. The female Anopheles mosquito is active only at night, so you should protect yourself between dusk and dawn.

You should probably also take the prescription preventive medication chloroquine starting two weeks before departure and continuing for several weeks, even if you return in a few days. (Chloroquine usually should be taken for a month after leaving a malarious area.) If you are traveling to an area with chloroquine-resistant *P. falciparum,* ask your doctor about Fansidar, which should be taken at the first sign of fever. Unfortunately, many physicians are not well informed about malaria prevention, so make a point to consult a doctor with experience in the health problems of international travelers. You must follow instructions or risk severe illness.

It is important to understand that even if you take all possible precautions you can still acquire malaria and get sick for up to a year after the trip. Therefore, if you develop any febrile illness in the weeks or months after returning you should see a doctor right away. Malaria is easily treated and becomes serious only if treatment is delayed.

PREVENTION ON A COMMUNITY LEVEL

Eradication is no longer spoken of; reasonable control is the only hope. The tools include draining and filling mosquito breeding areas, insecticides, daily drug use by large populations, and screening blood donors who have been to malarious areas. On the bright side, several vaccines are being developed and human trials have started.

TREATMENT

Cinchona bark was used by the Incas for hundreds of years. It contains **quinine,** which is still used today. **Chloroquine,** a close relative, is the drug of choice for most cases as we mentioned above, but specific treatments change frequently as the organisms change and new drugs are developed.

Other drugs are used to prevent relapses due to some surviving plasmodia in the liver and red cells. It is especially important that the drugs be used *exactly as prescribed,* since the treatment is based on knowledge of the behavior of the various types of Plasmodia.

There is no other effective treatment. Bed rest and fluids are important. Aspirin may ease discomfort. All serious complications must be dealt with by a physician.

Measles (Rubeola)

Measles is a virus-type disease that usually strikes before adolescence. The first symptoms are like those of influenza, with fever, a dry cough, drowsiness, and loss of appetite, and with tiny white spots on the inner cheeks. Photophobia (light sensitivity and avoidance) and itchy, red eyes are common. There may also be a sore throat.

The rash usually appears on about the fifth day, first on the face and then spreading downward. It lasts up to about a week. The spots start out pink and blotchy and tend to darken and merge into red patches. Measles is generally more severe in adults than in children. Complications can be serious. Encephalitis is rare but may cause permanent brain or nerve damage, or even death. More common are secondary bacterial infections and pneumonia, the major cause of death in measles. Such complications are much more likely in the malnourished or chronically ill.

Measles is highly contagious. The virus is spread in droplets exhaled or coughed out, and on articles that come in contact with nose or throat secretions.

PREVENTION

Immunize, preferably at nine months of age and again at fifteen months, but later in those who have not had the disease or been vaccinated. If an outbreak occurs in a school or college revaccination is recommended for all students who were vaccinated before 1980. Before then the vaccine sometimes failed to immunize because of poor handling and storage. Later vaccine contained a better stabilizer.

Measles could be eliminated in the United States and possibly the world if people were more diligent about getting their children vaccinated.

TREATMENT

The patient should be isolated from close contact with others, both to avoid spreading the disease and to avoid exposure to bacteria which could cause complications. The room should be well ventilated, but comfortably warm.

Plenty of fluids should be taken. Ibuprofen or acetaminophen and lukewarm sponge baths may ease discomfort.

Reading is not harmful as long as the required light does not cause discomfort.

See a physician immediately if there is vomiting, convulsion, severe lethargy or headache, or bleeding from the nose, mouth, rectum, or into the skin.

Call a physician if there is an earache, sore throat, or rapid breathing.

Mumps

Mumps is a contagious virus disease that attacks the salivary glands (usually one or both parotids in front of the ears), causing them to swell. Pain, malaise, and fever last from five to seven days. Rare complications include encephalitis (infection of the brain), deafness, kidney disease, pancreatitis (infection of the pancreas), and infection of the ovaries or testicles.

One attack almost always confers lifelong immunity. Subclinical infection (exposure and infection without symptoms), which is very common, also confers durable immunity.

Recent outbreaks, mostly in colleges and the workplace, have affected mostly those born between 1967 and 1977. These people were not as likely to have received the vaccine as children born later, or to have been exposed as those born earlier. Therefore, they have neither natural nor induced immunity, and are now at risk for mumps.

PREVENTION

Mumps vaccine is very effective and safe and is routinely given at fifteen months. Adults who are not immune should receive the vaccine, which is very safe, effective, and inexpensive.

Several states do not require mumps immunization for students attending public schools; these states tend to have the highest incidence. These policies appear to be negligent since there is no good reason not to vaccinate.

TREATMENT

Rest in bed until the fever and swelling are gone. Adopt a liquid diet and avoid sour foods, including orange juice. If the testes are affected a cold pack may help.

Acetaminophen, ibuprofen, or codeine may be desirable for severe pain.

See a physician right away if there is lethargy, convulsions, or a stiff neck. **Call a physician** if there is pain or swelling in the testes, abdominal pain and vomiting, dizziness, or difficulty hearing.

Obesity

Overweight people are far more likely than others to get diabetes, hypertension, abnormal blood lipids, coronary artery disease, gallbladder disease, and a variety of cancers. The excessive storage of energy in the form of body fat so strongly predisposes people to serious diseases that it's reasonable to consider obesity a disease in itself, or at least a disorder. Obesity also aggravates backaches, arthritis, and other health problems. The direct cause of obesity is eating more calories than one burns off. The indirect causes are complex and poorly understood. Most obesity is genetically determined and manifested through central nervous system control of metabolic rate, appetite control, and fat cell number and distribution.

Who Needs to Lose Weight?

One measure of obesity is given by the Metropolitan Life Insurance Company height and weight tables for men and women with small, medium, and large frames. These are the weight ranges for those with the lowest death rates. There are several problems with these tables and they should not be taken as gospel. They don't take age into account; the weights of young and old alike at death are all lumped together, which could be misleading. Women and nonwhites are underrepresented because they buy less life insurance. Moreover, practically speaking, frame size is difficult to determine. Perhaps most important, the tables tell you nothing about fat, which is the important variable here. An athletic, muscular man six feet tall with a medium frame and very little body fat weighing 190 pounds is overweight according to the tables.

A somewhat better measure of obesity is the body mass index (BMI). This is the ratio of the weight in kilograms to height in meters squared (BMI = wt/ht × ht). To calculate your BMI, first find your weight in kilograms and your height in meters. One kilogram is 2.2 pounds. One meter is 39.4 inches. Then divide your weight by the square of your height. The result is your BMI. Refer to the table below to see where you stand. A BMI of 30 indicates obesity and is the beginning of the danger zone; 35 is definitely medically significant. Like the height and weight tables, the BMI has shortcomings, but it's easier to use and the classifications of obesity based on BMI are clear and meaningful.

The best measure of obesity is fat as a percentage of body weight. There is some debate on the exact numbers, but men are approaching obesity at 20 percent fat, women at 25 percent fat. It has long been known that body fat is the important factor, not body weight, but determining body fat has always been difficult. Now new technology may solve the problem. The most promising device measures fat by measuring tissue absorption of near-infrared light. The price for the little instruments, which resemble penlights attached to hand calculators, is still high, almost two thousand dollars, so only health professionals and clinics have them. But such devices may eventually make the bathroom scale obsolete.

MEDICAL CLASSIFICATION OF OBESITY USING BMI

% Desirable Weight	Definition	Grade of Obesity	Excess Fat (lb/kg)	BMI (kg/m²)
MEN				
225	Super morbid obesity	6	175/80	≥50
200	Morbid obesity	5	145/66	45
180	Super obesity	4	110/50	40
160	Medically significant obesity	3	80/36	35
135	Obesity	2	50/23	30
110	Overweight	1	15/7	25
100	Desirable weight	0	0	22
70	Medically significant starvation	−3	−15/−7	15
WOMEN				
245	Super morbid obesity	6	155/70	>50
220	Morbid obesity	5	130/59	45
195	Super obesity	4	100/45	40
170	Medically significant obesity	3	75/34	35
145	Obesity	2	50/23	30
120	Overweight	1	25/11	25
100	Desirable weight	0	0	21
75	Medically significant starvation	−3	−20/−9	15

- Medical risk of obesity is further modified by concurrent illness, complicating organ dysfunction, body fat distribution, velocity of weight change, and age. Relative risk varies from 2- to 15-fold.
- Body mass index was developed by the Nutrition/Metabolism Laboratory, Cancer Research Institute, Boston, Massachusetts.

Reproduced with permission from G. Glackburn, B. Kanders: Medical evaluation and treatment of the obese patient with cardiovascular disease. Amer J Cardio 60: October 30, 1987, pp. 55G-58G.

How Fat Are You?

As stated above, the upper limit of healthy fat percentage is about 20 to 25 percent for men and 25 to 30 percent for women. More fat than this is considered unhealthy, and there are good reasons for substantially lower levels, especially in men. Most athletic men are under 15 percent fat; ultramarathoners can be as low as 3 percent fat. Women who get too thin may develop symptoms of estrogen insufficiency like anovulation, amenorrhea, and bone thinning (osteopororis). Such problems seem to start at about 20 percent fat for the most susceptible women, but some women can be 15 percent fat or less and remain fertile and healthy. In this sense, it appears that some women are genetically determined to be, or at least allowed to be, less fat than others.

Fat percentage can be estimated by an experienced person, usually a nutritionist, dietician, or nurse, using calipers to measure the thickness of the fat layer under the skin. In the most accurate tests, measurements are done on the back of the upper arm, the back of the thigh, the abdomen, and the back. The results are meaningless unless done by a trained person using standardized procedures.

Fat content can also be estimated by underwater weighing. The person sits on a chair hung from a scale and is lowered into a large water tank. The more he or she weighs under water, the less fat he or she has. Some weight reducing clinics, research centers, and college athletic departments have underwater weighing facilities.

To get a rough idea of your fat percentage without an underwater scale, consider these estimates:

If in fresh water you float easily, your fat content is greater than 25 percent.

If you float only with your lungs full, you are about 22 percent fat.

If you sink slowly but definitely even with your lungs full, you are less than 20 percent fat.

If in salt water you sink even with your lungs full, you are 13 percent fat or less.

These are rough estimates subject to error due to residual air in the digestive tract and lungs.

Another measure of fatness is the waist to hip ratio. A tape measure is used and the waist size is divided by the hip size. Ratios greater than .85 in women and .95 in men seem to be associated with a higher incidence of hypertension, diabetes, and other obesity-related problems. However, in practice it's hard to know exactly where to measure.

Here's another way to tell if you have a fat problem. Look into a full-length mirror without your clothes on. Most important, look at your abdomen. Do you have a spare tire or potbelly? Can you grab a handful of fat around your waist, where it counts most? A simple tool superior to the scale, and far cheaper than the near-infrared device, is the tape measure. It can help you keep track of changes in fat even if your weight stays the same. For example, if you exercise regularly for several weeks you might lose lots of fat but little weight because of muscle gain. In that case, your waist should reflect the improvement. Not all excessive fat is equally dangerous. It is the fat around the waist that causes the most trouble. Put crudely, a potbelly is more dangerous than a fat butt.

PREVENTION

Prevention should start early. Obese babies don't always end up obese as children or adults, but the longer they stay fat the greater the risk they will always be fat. Some experts believe that bottle-feeding in the first few days and weeks of life may upset the normal appetite control mechanisms, establish a higher calorie requirement for satisfaction, and result in fatter babies. This could result in a lifetime tendency to obesity. More long-term studies are needed to confirm this, but it is probably another plus for breast-feeding at least for the first few weeks.

More tips: If a bottle is used, it should be offered, not pushed. If the baby gets too fat, the formula can be diluted a little, but only by order of a physician. Sugar and honey should *not* be added to formulas. It may also help to avoid giving solids too soon.

Young children should be given every opportunity to run and play. Parents should spend at least a couple hours a week playing with them and getting some exercise themselves. This sets a good example and creates early positive associations between love, fun, and physical activity. As they get older they should be encouraged to be active in hiking, swimming, bicycling, and team sports. Hiking is an excellent way for the whole family to exercise together. Kids should be encouraged to walk as much as possible; parents shouldn't play chauffeur for short distances without good reason.

Excessive television watching is a major factor in childhood obesity and should be prevented. Health and physical education classes should teach the importance of exercise and fitness to general health. Nutrition education, of course, is also important. Children should be taught the importance of a balanced diet and the consequences of overeating and poor eating habits. Junk food snacks, those that provide plenty of calories and little or no other nutrients, should be kept out of the house; lots of fruit and vegetable snacks should be on hand.

TREATMENT

Obesity is one of the most difficult and frustrating challenges patients and health professionals face. The statistics are so discouraging we won't even mention them; suffice it to say that the vast majority of overweight people who succeed in losing weight gain it back within a year or two. Nevertheless, an effort must be made or the person will get even fatter.

Success is most likely with an integrated approach that includes regular exercise and moderate reduction of calories. It is very important to understand that fat reduction is a long-term process—any attempt at a quick fix will surely result in greater problems. Exercise is important because it uses up calories and increases the capacity of the muscles to burn fat. Calorie reduction can help, but if excessive can cause weakness, apathy, a decrease in activity, a lower metabolic rate, less capacity to burn fat, and eventually more weight gain.

Don't Be a Yo-Yo

Failure to understand these points often leads to the dreaded yo-yo syndrome. Drastic calorie reduction inevitably leads to substantial weight loss, much of which is due to loss of water and some to loss of muscle tissue. When the desired weight is reached, the old eating habits are resumed and the weight comes back plus some because the muscles now have less capacity to burn fat than before the diet. The dieter is disappointed, blames the relapse on lack of willpower, and goes on another diet, perhaps more restrictive than the first. Now the vicious cycle of yo-yo dieting is in high gear. The "cure" turns out to be a curse. Every time a radical diet is resorted to, the body gears up to store fat more efficiently. Not only does the person end up fatter, but yo-yo dieting may increase the appetite for fats and thus increase blood lipids and the risk of cardiovascular disease. The lesson is clear: If you want to lose weight, do it right, or you're probably better off staying fat, especially if you hold the line and don't get fatter.

The difficulty of losing fat rapidly and permanently has given rise to an enormous industry based on false promises and deceit. There is no end to the ridiculous and dangerous diet books, phony weight-loss pills and teas, slimming belts, sweatsuits, and hundreds of other worthless gimmicks and gadgets huckstered to the public. These frauds make proper treatment of obesity more difficult because they confuse people and lead them on wild goose chases. Some also contribute to the yo-yo syndrome.

It is important for the obese person to understand that all this nonsense must be avoided. The only hope lies in regular exercise and moderate calorie restriction, which means no less than 1,000 calories a day for most people. The faster the weight loss, the more likely it is to be gained back; weight loss should not exceed 2 pounds per week. Remember, 1 pound per week is 52 pounds in a year (see Section One for more on nutrition and exercise). If you need more specific advice consult a physician or nutritionist.

228 Behavior Modification

Instead of focusing on food, as diets do, the behavior control approach to obesity concentrates on eating habits. A typical method is to keep a detailed diary of absolutely everything eaten, the amounts, and an estimated caloric intake for several weeks. This is very revealing to most people who try it, and by itself can result in a lower food intake.

A more detailed diary includes not only every bit you eat but when you eat it, under what circumstances, and how you feel at the time. This helps you detect bad eating habits and situations in which you unconsciously overeat. Do you snack while reading or watching television? Does tension with your family or housemates send you to the refrigerator for consolation? Do you clean your kids' plates to avoid wasting food? Do you eat when you are disappointed, bored, or angry?

If you are a TV snacker, try knitting, clipping and cleaning your nails, or flossing your teeth instead. If you are a bored or angry eater, find a better way to handle those feelings. Take a walk or bike ride, call a friend, start a new book, take up a challenging hobby; do anything but punish yourself with food you don't need.

It helps to focus fully on eating at mealtime. Don't read, watch TV, or talk business. Concentrate on the sight, smell, texture, and taste of the food and make the meal satisfying. Eat slowly. If you eat too fast, you will likely be starting on your second helping before your brain has time to develop a sense of satisfaction with the first. Chew slowly and put your fork down for a minute or two every few bites. Let ten to twenty minutes pass between courses or servings of a meal. This may not be practical for every meal, but it's worth trying, especially for your largest meal of the day.

Perhaps the most important concept in behavior therapy is to learn to recognize true hunger and eat only in response to that, rather than in response to external cues. The sight, smell, or thought of food doesn't have to trigger false hunger. Learn to pass up food unless you are really hungry. And when you go to a party, don't eat just because the food is there and everyone else is eating.

Here are some other useful suggestions.

- Shop for food only with a list and only when you are not hungry. This helps keep snacks bought on impulse out of the house.
- Keep food out of sight.
- Don't nibble while cooking.
- Don't feel you have to clean your plate. Learn to prepare smaller

portions. Develop a leftover strategy so you won't feel you have to eat it to avoid waste.

Weight Control Groups

Not all commercial weight-loss programs are worthless frauds; some of the weight control groups can be helpful. Compulsive overeating is often an emotional problem, somewhat similar to alcoholism. It is not surprising, then, that therapy groups similar to Alcoholics Anonymous have evolved. Several large nationwide diet clubs and many smaller regional groups have helped thousands of people lose fat and keep it off.

The success of group programs is based on group support, encouragement, and contagious fervor. Healthy competition between members also helps. Most of the groups provide basic nutrition education and reasonable exercise programs. Regular meetings reinforce the concepts and provide opportunities for people with a common problem to discuss it freely and openly with other people with the same problem. Most people in the United States have access to at least one of these groups. There is no way of knowing which group is best for a given person. It is best to attend a meeting or two before committing yourself.

A Plea for Understanding and Fairness

Normal-weight people and society in general tend to be very unfair, even cruel, to overweight people. The obese are discriminated against in the job market, in applying to colleges, in housing, and in the social arena. They are even insulted and taunted by strangers on the street. Most people feel that obesity is a character flaw, a sign of gluttony, greed, and laziness. In fact, it is very often a genetic problem, especially for those who are severely obese. In our evolutionary history humans have often experienced famine, at which time obese people had a survival advantage. They could live longer by living off their fat. They were then more likely to reproduce and pass on their "fat genes."

Genetically overweight people find it extremely difficult to lose fat and keep it off. They often eat less than their slender peers, but because they have lower metabolic rates, they burn even less. Even their infants, long before they have had a chance to become "gluttonous and lazy," have substantially slower metabolisms than infants of the nonobese. This is not because of thyroid problems, as is commonly believed, but it may be related to something called brown fat, a type of fat cell that burns fat rather than just stores it. It seems that people blessed with lots of these cells can eat more without getting fat. In a sense, their brown fat cells exercise for them while fat people have to exercise for themselves and watch their diets much more carefully. Self-righteous slender people should consider this before they feel superior, and they should no more discriminate against the obese than they would against short or tall people.

Osteoporosis

Osteoporosis is one of the most common, disabling, and costly metabolic diseases. It kills about fifty thousand people each year and disables many more. The bones lose mass and become porous, thin, and weak. Vertebrae collapse and fractures occur from simple stresses like sneezing or bumping against a table, or from no apparent stress at all. These breaks are very slow to heal, and the subsequent prolonged bed rest may lead to serious medical problems.

Practically all postmenopausal women, with the notable exception of blacks, are susceptible. There is gradual loss of bone mass starting in the early thirties in both men and women. By age thirty-five up to 15 percent of total bone mass may be lost. In women, menopause accelerates bone loss. Those who live to the age of eighty usually lose one-third to two-thirds of their entire skeletons and up to six inches of their height. Young women who exercise to excess and lose too much fat, to the point of stopping menstruation, may also develop osteoporosis.

Although men also lose bone mass as they age, the rate of loss is much slower than in women, and osteoporosis is rarely a serious problem, though it may occur in men past age seventy. Black men have the densest bones and are the least susceptible.

CAUSES

Bones are metabolically active reservoirs of calcium, which is being constantly removed and replaced depending on the needs of muscles, nerves, and other tissues. The skeleton is constantly undergoing subtle changes to accomodate changes in activities, stresses, and weight distribution, and in response to diet, hormones, and drugs. Several hormones are involved in bone metabolism, and the change in hormone patterns over time, especially the decline of estrogen in women, tend to promote bone thinning and weakening of the bones.

Genetic susceptibility is an important factor in osteoporosis. Whites and Asians who are lean and small are most at risk, particularly if close relatives have the disorder. Whether and when the disorder develops and how bad it becomes depend to a great extent on the other risk factors.

Lack of activity is a major factor in osteoporosis, and sometimes (as in paraplegia and arthritis) it is the only cause. The osteoblasts (bone-forming cells) must bear loads to function properly. A sedentary lifestyle encourages bone demineralization and weakening.

Calcium absorption decreases with age and, especially if combined with reduced calcium intake, this may contribute to demineralization. The development of lactase deficiency (lactose intolerance) may exacerbate the problem.

Cortisone treatment can promote osteoporosis by decreasing calcium absorption and blocking the activity of osteoblasts. After several years of high doses of cortisone, loss of bone mass is commonly 30 to 50 percent.

Smoking seems to promote osteoporosis, possibly by increasing bone acidity and thereby the solubility of the bone minerals, and by hastening menopause. Alcohol and caffeine also promote bone loss. In all of these the strength of the effect and extent of the hazard is not known.

In postmenopausal women, several or all of these factors may be present: genetic susceptibility, decreased estrogen, lack of activity, a diet high in phosphorous and protein and low in calcium, cortisone treatment, and use of tobacco, alcohol, and caffeine.

Osteoporosis can also be caused by various endocrine disorders, inherited diseases, cancers, and organ failures. These cases must be handled in the context of the primary problem. The following discussion does not generally apply to them.

PREVENTION

Girls and women at risk should be identified as early as possible, long before menopause (or removal of ovaries) and the development of the disorder. Family doctors, parents, and perhaps even health and physical education teachers and school nurses should identify adolescents at risk so they can be educated about the impending threat to their health and take preventive measures. Preventing and delaying osteoporosis is very important because reversal of the process and rebuilding the bones is almost impossible. Young women should anticipate the problem far in advance and avoid the risk factors so they can go into the high-risk postmenopausal years with the densest, healthiest bones possible. The following are offered as helpful measures.

Get adequate calcium by eating low-fat dairy products, sardines, salmon, beans, leafy greens, and a variety of vegetables. Lacto-vegetarians generally have strong bones, but vegetarians who avoid dairy products may have inadequate calcium intake (as well as protein and vitamin B-12). Calcium-fortified orange juice is an excellent alternative to dairy products if protein and vitamin B-12 are otherwise provided (see Section One for more on getting enough calcium).

An old adage says that senile osteoporosis is a pediatric disease. That is, the stage is often set for the disease during the teenage years when growth is rapid but calcium intake declines. Mothers can help by education, example, good meal planning and, if necessary, supplementing her milk-hating daughter's diet with calcium-fortified orange juice and powdered calcium carbonate sprinkled into soups and sauces during cooking.

If you do not get adequate calcium in your food, take a supplement, preferably at bedtime since bone decalcification peaks in the early morning before rising. Pure calcium carbonate, like that in popular antacids, is best. Don't overdo supplementation, though; excessive calcium can cause side effects, like constipation and, in susceptible people, kidney stones. Most people should avoid total calcium intake over 2 grams per day, whether at risk for osteoporosis or not. Some people over age sixty have mildly elevated levels of parathyroid hormone that keep their blood calcium too high. Calcium supplements can be harmful in this situation. Older people should check with their doctors before greatly increasing their calcium intake. A simple blood test for the hormone, calcium, and phosphorous levels is all that is needed.

Get adequate vitamin D by being outdoors or taking a supplement of up to 400 units per day. In strong sunlight, about fifteen minutes of head, neck, and arm exposure supplies the RDA. In overcast conditions and less direct exposure, longer or more extensive exposure is required.

Vitamin D supplements can be hazardous, so don't overdo it. Don't take supplements unless you don't eat foods with vitamin D and you aren't regularly exposed to a little sunlight.

Get adequate vitamin C, which appears to promote efficient absorption of calcium. Supplements are not usually necessary; just eat a variety of fruits and vegetables regularly.

Get adequate fluoride, which appears to be as essential for strong bones as it is for strong teeth. If the drinking water in your area does not have fluoride, either naturally or added, try to eat seafood and seaweed three or four times a week.

Get plenty of exercise, but not too much. Even in advanced age increased physical activity can decrease or even stop the slow loss of bone mass. At least some of the exercise should be weight bearing, such as walking, jogging, dancing, or even weight lifting. Swimming and bicycling are not as effective in stimulating bone mineralization. Whatever exercises you do, it's extremely important not to do so much that your periods stop. This can mimic menopause effects on the bones and hasten the ravages of osteoporosis. Underexercise and overexercise in the teen years are believed to be major factors in osteoporosis development. A moderate, sensible level of physical activity is an important osteoporosis prevention measure that parents, teachers, children, and adults at risk should understand.

Watch out for prolonged use of corticosteroids and aluminum-containing antacids. The former promotes bone demineralization and the latter inhibits calcium, phosphorous, and fluoride absorption.

Don't smoke; avoid excessive alcohol and caffeine.

Postmenopausal women (especially slender, caucasian smokers) **should consider estrogen supplements** with their physicians; the hormone can very substantially retard bone loss and effectively prevent osteoporosis or delay its onset. The sooner treatment starts, the better. In properly selected women the risk of adverse effects is very small, and practically zero if the uterus has been removed.

Avoid or minimize prolonged immobilization such as strict bed rest for a back ailment or recuperation from surgery, injury, or illness. Immobility promotes demineralization of bones at a frightening speed. Any more than a week can be significant. The bone loss can persist for months or even years. Avoiding immobility can be a very important preventive measure, even for those not considered to be at high risk, including men.

TREATMENT

After decades of research and clinical trials it appears that a truly effective and safe treatment has emerged. It cannot rebuild bone already lost, so prevention is far preferable, but it can greatly decrease the incidence of fractures and slow further bone loss. The treatment consists of daily estrogen and calcium supplements if dietary intake is not high enough. The evidence for the estrogen is far stronger than that for the calcium, but most experts go along with assuring generous calcium intake.

It has long been know that estrogen is effective in preserving bone, but there has been concern that it might promote cancer of the breast and uterus endometrium, and increase the risk of cardiovascular disease. These fears are unfounded in most cases. There is still concern about a possible link with uterine cancer, but if small doses of progestin are also given the therapy may actually have a protective effect. Each case must be decided individually, with the benefits of the therapy weighed against its risks and those of osteoporosis.

In general, estrogen replacement therapy does not have an adverse effect on blood pressure, body fat, blood fats, or other risk factors in cardiovascular disease. In fact, some studies suggest that estrogen replacement therapy greatly decreases the incidence of heart attack in postmenopausal women, perhaps by increasing HDL-cholesterol levels.

Another hormone that inhibits bone demineralization, calcitonin, is proving useful in those who can't take estrogen. Several other therapies show great promise, and some may become mainstays. These include etidronate, a drug already used successfully in less common bone disorders; thiazide diuretics, which are important hypertension drugs that decrease calcium excretion by the kidneys; and supplements of fluoride that seem to promote bone strength but can cause stomach distress and other side effects.

No matter what therapy a woman is receiving, she should also follow the preventive measures discussed above.

Pneumonia

In a pneumonia the lungs are inflamed and breathing tends to be difficult; there may be fever, chills, chest pain, coughing, and weakness. Pneumonias were once the number one cause of death in the United States. Antibiotics have reduced mortality, but pneumonia is still a major problem. The very young and those over fifty with other health problems are the most susceptible.

CAUSES

There are at least fifty different causes, including chemical irritants and even allergies. By far the most common causes are a couple dozen bacteria, fungi, and viruses. AIDS is an increasingly important cause or facilitator of all these infectious pneumonias.

Organisms that can cause pneumonia are often present in the normal respiratory tract; decreased resistance allows them to grow explosively and become virulent. This poor resistance can result from malnutrition (often associated with drug addiction and alcoholism), colds, influenza, diabetes, chronic bronchitis, emphysema, chronic exposure to dust and fumes, and cigarette smoking.

PREVENTION

Maintain good general health with good nutrition, exercise, and adequate rest.

Avoid chronic exposure to fumes, dust, and smoke. If you are recovering from an illness or surgery, get adequate rest, avoid crowds, and avoid stresses like exercise or getting cold and wet.

Don't smoke; it weakens your defenses against all the pneumonia-causing microbes. **Don't drink excessively;** alcoholism opens the door to various pneumonias.

A pneumonia vaccine against many strains of the pneumonia-causing bacteria is available and is advisable for those over sixty-five, those with lung disease, and those who have had their spleens removed.

Prevent influenza; pneumonia can be a complication. Many who should be vaccinated annually are not (see **Influenza,** above).

Other vaccines, some already developed, are likely to gain wide use sooner or later and have a significant impact on pneumonia incidence. These include vaccines against cytomegalovirus (CMV), various influenza strains, Epstein-Barr virus, chlamydia, tuberculosis, legionella bacteria, and, we all hope, HIV. (See also **AIDS, Tuberculosis, Influenza, Diabetes.**)

TREATMENT

Tests like sputum culture help determine the cause of the pneumonia. Most of the bacterial cases can be helped with antibiotics. Hospitalization may or may not be necessary. Bed rest is very important, and sometimes oxygen is necessary. A liquid diet is preferred at first. In a long illness, or when nutrition status is poor, a high-protein, high-calorie diet with vitamin and mineral supplements is advisable.

Viral pneumonia often develops during what seems to be a bad cold. Many common viruses, including influenzas and CMV, are culprits. Antibiotics don't help. With adequate rest and good nutrition, it usually runs its course in two or three weeks. But **don't ever self-diagnose viral pneumonia** and decide you can treat yourself. Even if your original symptoms were caused by a virus, you could have acquired a secondary bacterial pneumonia, and failure to treat it with antibiotics could be lethal. See a physician if you have severe symptoms.

Rabies

Rabies is one of the most ancient, horrible, and fascinating of all diseases. First mentioned in the twenty-third century B.C. in the pre-Moses Eshnunna Code, rabies is a virus disease that attacks the nervous system of all warm-blooded animals, including humans. Symptoms may vary substantially, but they often conform to the description provided by an Italian physician in 1546:

> Once the disease takes hold the patient can neither stand nor lie down: Like a madman he flings himself hither and thither, tears his flesh with his hands, and feels intolerable thirst. This is the most distressing symptom, for he so shrinks from water and all liquids that he would rather die than drink or be brought near to water; it is then that they bite other persons, foam at the mouth, their eyes look twisted, and finally they are exhausted and painfully breathe their last.

This fear of water gave rise to the term *hydrophobia,* once the common name for rabies.

Rabies is essentially 100 percent incurable and fatal. Only two or three people in the last four thousand years are believed to have survived the devastating infection (once it had established itself), one being a woman saved by injections of interferon. Symptoms may not develop for many months after exposure, but once they appear it is too late for the vaccine to work and there can be very little hope. Thus it is critical that immunological prevention occur as soon as one suspects the infection may have been introduced.

CAUSE

Rabies is caused by a virus that enters the blood and concentrates in the brain. If it simply killed its host quickly, it might perish with its victim instead of being passed on. But the genetic material and protein coat of the virus have evolved a mechanism to ensure that it gets passed on: The virus attacks areas of the brain in a way that makes the animal restless, irritable, and very aggressive. It will then roam for miles, attacking many times without provocation and passing on the virus with its saliva.

The most common sources of human infection are bites and scratches from dogs, cats, rats, bats, squirrels, foxes, raccoons, skunks, mongooses, and various farm animals. There have been a few cases of infection occurring with cornea transplants from people who had undiagnosed rabies at the time of death.

PREVENTION

Only a handful of humans contracts rabies each year in the United States, but the cost of this control is eternal vigilance and a lot of money, especially when people fail to take the primary preventive measures. For example, in Florida a raccoon was taken from the woods and kept as a pet. When it became sick it was taken to a veterinarian, whom it bit. It also bit his assistant. The raccoon was then killed and found to have rabies. The subsequent immunizations, investigations, and counseling cost more than $20,000. In another case, a dog in California bit three people and was killed when it appeared ill. Tissue tests were positive for rabies. The subsequent investigations and immunizations of dozens exposed to the dog cost more than $100,000.

Thousands of people in the United States, and about a million worldwide, receive rabies immunizations each year because of exposure to rabid or possibly rabid animals. The cost of rabies control, the number of people needing the shots, and the risk to people and their pets could be greatly reduced if people would strictly follow these preventive guidelines:

- **Vaccinate pets and livestock against rabies.**
- **Do not take wild carnivorous mammals** (especially skunks, raccoons, bats, and foxes) **for pets,** try to handle or pet them, or

get close enough to be scratched or bitten by them.

- **If you *are* scratched or bitten** by a wild carnivore or an unwanted or stray dog or cat, or even licked on a tiny scratch or abrasion, the wound should be immediately and thoroughly cleaned with soap and water. **Call a physician right away.** If possible without risking further exposure, the animal should be captured or killed for rabies testing.
- **Immunization** will be required if it is determined that you might have been exposed to rabies. This will include one injection of rabies antibody (passive immunization) and four to six injections of rabies vaccine. This prophylaxis (or preventive) regimen is nearly 100 percent effective and very safe, though there are sometimes side effects. The virus may remain latent for hours or many days, depending on the severity of the wound and the amount of virus left in it; the vaccine will be effective as long as it is administered before dissemination and nervous system infection.
- **If you are bitten or scratched by a rodent** (such as a rat, mouse, chipmunk, squirrel, hamster or guinea pig), rabbit, hare, or farm animal, clean the wound thoroughly and call a physician. Regional conditions vary, but the chances are that immunization will not be required.
- **Quarantines must *not* be evaded.** Many islands are completely free of rabies and use quarantine periods of several months for imported dogs, cats, and other susceptible animals to keep the virus out. People who smuggle in animals to avoid the quarantines risk introducing the virus, an irreversible and very costly disaster.
- **Preexposure prophylaxis** is advisable for those at high risk of exposure to rabies. They should receive the vaccine *before* being bitten, scratched, or otherwise exposed. Candidates include veterinarians and their assistants, biologists and lab workers working with susceptible animals or with the virus itself, spelunkers, trappers, animal control officers, and travelers to areas where rabies is common. This is important because exposure can occur without one's knowledge. For example, cave explorers can inhale the virus from infected bats or even be bitten by bats without feeling it.

TREATMENT

Once clinical signs of rabies are evident, the only treatment that offers any hope of survival is interferon injections. However this treatment is extremely costly and not likely to succeed; this is why prevention is so important.

Rubella

Rubella, also called German measles, is a viral infection similar to measles (rubeola), but its duration is shorter and it is milder. There is low fever and malaise, and in about half the cases a fine rash. Sometimes there is pain in the joints or enlarged and tender lymph nodes. The illness itself is rarely more bother than a common cold; almost half the time the infection causes no symptoms at all.

The importance of rubella lies in its potential for causing miscarriage and very serious birth defects—cataracts, nerve deafness, mental retardation, heart problems—if a pregnant woman is infected during the first three months of gestation.

PREVENTION

All children should be vaccinated when they are between one and two years old; the live attenuated virus is very effective and safe. If a woman is to be vaccinated, it must be certain that she is not pregnant and will not be for three months. Prior to a planned pregnancy a woman can be tested for immunity to rubella. Some states require the test prior to marriage.

TREATMENT

Rest, liquid diet, and lukewarm sponge baths are usually sufficient. Those affected should **avoid contact with pregnant women.**

Sexually Transmitted Diseases (STDs)

At least twenty diseases are transmitted by sexual contact, oral and manual as well as regular intercourse. The most important in the United States are, in approximate order of prevalence, venereal warts, chlamydia, gonorrhea, genital herpes, cytomegalovirus (CMV), trichomoniasis, nonspecific bacterial vaginitis, and syphilis. Hepatitis B and AIDS are important STDs discussed separately, above.

Ano-genital venereal warts are caused by human papilloma virus (HPV). They are important because of their increasing incidence and their association with cervical cancer. It has been estimated that 20 percent of all female cancer deaths worldwide are due to HPV. Infected women should be examined for abnormal cervical cells every six months. Penile cancer may also occur, but is not nearly as common. There are not always obvious lesions, but subclinical infection can be detected by applying vinegar, which turns infected areas pale.

Standard wart removing methods are usually successful. Self-treatment should *not* be attempted. Sexual partners should be treated or recurrence is likely. There are about fifty strains of the virus, so development of a vaccine is unlikely.

Chlamydia trachomatis bacteria infections cause nongonococcal urethritis (NGU), which is now even more common than gonorrhea. Nearly 10 percent of all sexually active American women have chlamydial infections. Inner-city clinics report an incidence of nearly 25 percent. The infection can result in ectopic pregnancy, miscarriage, female sterility, and pneumonia and eye infections in the newborn. Men may develop inflammation and pain of the testes, sperm ducts, urethra, and prostate. Symptoms are often mild, just a slight discharge and slight urinary pain. Very often there are no symptoms, especially in women, so screening sexually active young women is of growing importance. All pregnant women should be screened. When found or strongly suspected, treatment is with an antibiotic. Sexual partners should be treated or reinfection is likely. There is growing hope that a vaccine can be developed.

Gonorrhea ("the clap") is caused by *Neisseria gonorrhea* bacteria that infect the mucous membranes of the reproductive organs, urethra, rectum, eyes, and throat. Sterility can result from infection of the prostate or sperm ducts in men, or the Fallopian tubes or ovaries in women. Generalized gonorrhea can cause arthritis, liver disease, and serious skin rashs. Infection of an infant's eyes during birth can cause blindness. This is the reason for the silver nitrate or penicillin eyedrops at birth.

Most women and some men who have the disease show no symptoms in spite of the severe infection that is damaging internal organs and being spread to others. This is why sexually active, nonmonogamous people, especially women, should be tested for gonorrhea once or twice a year. Routine gynecological examinations should include a gonorrhea culture and check for pelvic inflammatory disease (PID).

When symptoms do occur, they may include burning urination, vaginal or penile discharge, irritation of the vulva, pain on defecation, or abnormal anal discharge. Untreated cervical gonorrhea can lead to PID with Fallopian tube infection that can cause fever, nausea, vomiting, burning during urination, heavy vaginal discharge, and severe lower abdominal pains. Any of these symptoms, whether they occur in you or in any of your sexual contacts, should send you running to a clinic or physician. Antibiotics are usually effective. In general, all partners of infected people should be assumed to be infected and should be treated. Because chlamydial infection is so common in those with gonorrhea, there is a trend towards treating gonorrhea patients for chlamydia too.

Genital herpes infections are caused by the Herpes simplex virus-1 (HSV-1) and increasingly by HSV-2, which causes oral herpes (cold sores). The lesions can be quite painful and recur periodically in 5 to 25 percent of the cases. However, contrary to some scare stories, herpes does not destroy sex lives and mental health, and recurrences are generally much less severe than the original outbreak. For the majority of those affected, the affliction is a relatively trivial problem.

Nevertheless, herpes is a growing problem and a serious one because it may promote cervical cancer in women and severe brain damage and death in infants. It sometimes causes serious eye infections and is a major threat to people with compromised immune systems. For these reasons herpes needs to be better controlled. A vaccine may help in the future, but for now the best way to slow down the spread of the virus is for the public to understand it and the disease it causes and to take preventive measures.

Herpes lesions are painful blisters that break and form crusty sores. They shed millions of viruses and are extremely contagious. During a recurrence viruses may be shed before sores appear. There is often tingling, burning, or itching in the affected area, and sometimes general malaise and a feeling of impending illness. This is called the *prodrome.* **The single most important preventive measure** is to recognize the lesions and the prodrome and to strictly avoid sexual contact while they are present. This includes oral-genital contact because the virus that causes cold sores can also cause genital herpes and vice versa.

Acyclovir is an expensive prescription drug that can reduce the severity and frequency of outbreaks. It is not recommended for continuous use unless six or more outbreaks occur each year. No other treatments are effective. Pain may be relieved by keeping the area clean and dry and avoiding tight clothing that irritates the area and traps moisture.

The question of nonsexual transmission of herpes arises because studies have shown that the virus can live for several hours on plastic, glass, clothes, towels, and other surfaces as well as in unchlorinated water. But this survival of the virus does not mean it can infect people. Without mechanical friction infection is highly unlikely to occur, and nonvenereal transmission is very rare. However, until we know more, it is considered prudent for those with herpes sores or the prodrome to use separate towels, silverware (for oral herpes), and the like, and to be careful about sharing objects with infants and young children. Those with the infection should take care not to innoculate other parts of their own bodies, especially their fingers, eyes, and any area where the skin is broken with a scratch or abrasion.

Preventing herpes in the newborn is especially important. This can usually be accomplished by Cesarean section if genital herpes lesions are present at the time of birth. But sometimes the lesions are small and go unnoticed, and sometimes the virus is shed when there are no lesions. Until a more sensitive test for shedding viruses is available, the best tool is careful examination of pregnant women who have had herpes or whose sex partners have had it.

Cytomegalovirus (CMV) is a very common virus in the herpes family that produces symptoms in only a few of those it infects. Most people acquire the infection sometime during their lives; it is the most common known infection of fetuses and the newborn, but disease from the infection is not common. The most severe infection occurs in infants, for whom damage to the liver, bone marrow, or brain is often fatal. The virus crosses the placenta to the fetus if the mother has the infection. She rarely has any symptoms or knowledge that the virus is present. Sometimes symptoms suggesting influenza appear, including sudden onset of fever, malaise, and muscle and joint pain.

The virus can apparently be passed on by any close contact, including sexual intimacy, and by blood transfusions. It has been found in semen, mother's milk, urine, feces, saliva, cervical secretions, and blood. Promiscuous homosexuals have a very high incidence of CMV infection. People with AIDS, those receiving immune suppressing drugs after organ transplant, and those with otherwise compromised immune systems are at high risk for serious disease from CMV. Unfortunately, there is no effective treatment. The best hope for future prevention is a vaccine being developed.

Trichomoniasis is caused by a parasitic flagellate, *Trichomonas vaginalis,* that can survive on wet objects like douching equipment, sponges, and washcloths, but is usually sexually transmitted. The symptoms in women include vaginal itching, bad-smelling yellow-green frothy discharge, burning pain, and a frequent urge to urinate. Men usually have no symptoms in spite of harboring the parasite and passing it on to women.

Treatment is with metronidazole (Flagyl), except in pregnant women, who can get some symptomatic relief from vaginal suppositories, vinegar douches, and other measures. Male sex partners must also be treated. Condoms should be used until both partners are cleared of the infection.

Nonspecific vaginitis, or bacterial vaginitis, is caused by a variety of common bacteria. The symptoms include itching, a fishy-smelling, grayish, flour-pastelike discharge, and sometimes a mild burning sensation. The common infection has been thought to be a relatively minor nuisance, but there is now evidence that it can cause premature labor and infertility. Women who use IUDs have a much higher incidence. Oral contraceptives seem to have a protective effect.

Syphilis is less common but more serious than most other STDs. It is caused by the *Treponema pallidum* bacteria, which can penetrate the thin skin around the genitals, anus, and mouth, spread to the nervous system and heart, and cause brain damage, insanity, paralysis, heart disease, and death. The only symptom in the first stage is a painless sore or ulcer on the genitals, lips, breast, fingers, or around the rectum. It appears one to several weeks after contact. Without treatment the sore disappears, but in most cases a rash appears either all over the body or just on the hands and feet. Wartlike growths may occur around the ano-genital area. There may be fever and swollen lymph nodes. This second stage also clears up and the latent phase with no symptoms begins. It may last from a few weeks to twenty years, with occasional relapses to the second stage. Eventually the third stage begins with the infection of the heart and brain.

Because of the long incubation period, the seemingly minor nature of the initial lesion, and the long latent period, syphilis is often not detected and treated early. It is important for sexually active people, particularly homosexuals, who are the most likely victims, to be aware of the symptoms and see a physician if syphilis is suspected. The blood test is very accurate and should be taken once a year by anyone who has more than one sexual partner. If the test is positive, all partners should be treated.

Treatment is with antibiotics.

PREVENTION OF SEXUALLY TRANSMITTED DISEASES

- **Avoid sexual contact** with anyone with an STD.
- **Avoid multiple contacts.** Know your sex partner(s) well enough to ask about possible STDs.
- **See your physician about treatment** if a partner has an STD.
- **Use condoms.**
- **Use spermicidal foam, cream, or jelly.** Besides killing sperm, they may deactivate germs that cause gonorrhea, syphilis, AIDS, and

possibly chlamydia, venereal warts, and other sexually transmitted diseases.

- **Urinate and wash genitals after intercourse.**

Stomach Acid Related Disorders

The stomach makes a potent acid, hydrochloric acid, to aid in digestion. The digestive tract itself is normally protected from injury by this acid, but sometimes the protection breaks down. The stomach itself and the tissues closest to it, the esophagus just above the stomach and the duodenum just below it, can suffer varying degrees of chemical injury and inflammation, leading to different syndromes.

In **acid-related gastritis** there is inflammation of the entire stomach lining and usually a burning pain or sensation of hunger just below the breast bone. Sometimes there is nausea, vomiting, lightheadedness, and sweating, but there may be no symptoms.

In **peptic ulcer** there is an erosion, a little crater, of the mucosa (interior lining) of the stomach or duodenum (upper intestine). This injury can progress to a perforated ulcer, in which a hole has been burned through the stomach wall. This is, of course, a medical emergency. Severe bleeding and gastrointestinal obstruction are serious complications that may occur.

Esophagitis is injury to and inflammation of the esophagus, usually due to reflux or return of acid stomach contents. A sphincter muscle at the bottom of the esophagus usually keeps stomach contents from rising, but this muscle may be weakened by alcohol, nicotine, and possibly other drugs. The weakness may also be inherited or acquired with aging.

The **causes of acid-related disorders** include inherited susceptibility, and chemical and emotional stimulation of excessive acid production. An inborn lack of protection of the stomach or duodeum from its corrosive juice, or a weakness in the esophageal sphincter muscle, combined with acid stimulation by nicotine, alcohol, caffeine, aspirin, or other drugs, leads to an ulcer. Sustained emotional stress—worry, fear, anger, and the like—can contribute to the acid production, and sometimes is the main factor; even noise can be a problem. A stubborn bacterial infection is often associated with ulcers, but its significance is unclear.

PREVENTION

Avoid or minimize the use of all forms of alcohol; all forms of nicotine, including nicotine gum; aspirin, ibuprofen, and other anti-inflammatory drugs commonly used in arthritis; and all sources of caffeine and relatives such as theophylline. Decaffeinated coffee can be easier on the stomach, but in some it stimulates as much acid flow as regular coffee, either by a conditioned reflex association with the flavor or by the action of oils or other substances in the coffee.

Avoid excessive stress and emotional turmoil.

Eat a balanced diet; make certain you are getting adequate vitamin A. This nutrient is especially important in ulcer prevention because of its role in maintaining the healthy functioning of the mucus-producing cells that line the stomach and protect it from digestion by the powerful acid-pepsin juice. Don't take excessive vitamin A.

SELF-CARE

- **Practice all the preventive measures above.**
- It may be helpful to **eat four or five small meals** rather than two or three big ones. This avoids too much stomach distension, which increases gastric secretion. However, bedtime snacks should be avoided since they often lead to acid secretion while sleeping and pain hours later in the middle of the night.
- **Liquid protein supplements with free amino acids** stimulate gastric secretion and should be avoided. Highly concentrated protein foods like drinks with protein powder, brewer's yeast, and eggs can also promote hyperacidity and ulcers.
- There is no question that **severe or prolonged physical, mental, or emotional stress** can aggravate ulcers. For example, in wartime bombing raids ulcer incidence skyrockets, even among those not hurt. This is an extreme case, but some households are practically war zones. Many people seem to improve upon hospitalization or otherwise changing environments, removing themselves from the sources of tension and frustration. Relaxation techniques such as meditation and biofeedback are sometimes helpful.
- **Reflux esophagitis can be minimized** by avoiding large meals just before lying down (or avoiding lying down after a big meal), elevating the head of the bed, avoiding tight garments, and maintaining normal weight (obesity puts pressure on the stomach,

pushing contents upward).

- **Antacids,** best taken between meals and at bedtime, have long been standard medication. They relieve the burning pain, and recent studies have shown that they speed healing of ulcers. In esophagitis liquid antacid should be sipped. Since antacids can be harmful, they should be used with caution and awareness of their side effects. Don't use them daily for more than two or three weeks without consulting a physician.
- **Simply drinking lots of water** or juice, which dilute the stomach acid, can often relieve the pain.
- **Soothing herbal teas** include camomile, anise, fennel, and flax seed. Some herbs are likely to irritate the stomach lining and should be avoided, including peppermint, spearmint, and such stimulating herbs as gotu kola, guarana, desert tea, yohimbe, mate, and damiana.

See a physician immediately if you have very severe abdominal pain, black or bloody stool, or are vomiting; these may indicate a bleeding ulcer.

Consult a physician if you have repeated attacks of heartburn or indigestion for more than ten days.

TREATMENT

Medical treatment is likely to consist of all or most of the prevention and self-care measures above plus daily doses of very effective and safe drugs that suppress acid production. These drugs prevent perforated ulcers and the necessity of surgery. Some specialists are treating some stubborn ulcers with antibiotics, but this treatment is not widely accepted.

It is important to remember that healing an ulcer does not always mean permanently curing it. Most ulcers tend to recur. Care and watchfulness are required for life if hemorrhage, surgery, and even removal of the stomach are to be avoided.

Stroke

Blockage of or damage to an artery that feeds the brain results in damage to the brain—a stroke. Symptoms such as muscle weakness, numbness, visual distortions, loss of speech, or partial paralysis may occur. In a severe episode, in which a brain artery hemorrhages or is closed by a clot, severe brain damage, paralysis, dementia, and even death may occur.

CAUSES

Atherosclerosis—fatty blockage of the arteries—is an important factor in the vast majority of cases of cerebral vascular disease (CVD). When brain and neck arteries are severely blocked, blood supply is decreased, and tiny clots can do major damage by plugging arteries.

High blood pressure can lead to a stroke by promoting atherosclerosis, weakening the cerebral artery walls, and causing cerebral hemorrhage.

Osteoarthritis of the neck, with degenerative changes in the spine near the vertebral arteries, can cause compression of the arteries and obstruction of brain circulation.

Heart arrhythmias and heart attacks can lead to strokes by promoting the formation of clots in the heart that can then travel to the brain.

Severe anemia (insufficient red blood cells) limits the oxygen-carrying capacity of the blood, **and polycythemia** (too many red cells) can impede normal circulation and contribute to CVD.

Cigarette smoking contributes to stroke by increasing clotting and by accelerating hardening of the arteries and promoting hypertension. Heavy marijuana smoking may have similar effects.

Heavy alcohol consumption while taking anticoagulant medication increases the risk of hemorrhagic stroke in which bleeding into the brain damages the cells.

Oral contraceptives increase the risk of stroke in women who are over thirty-five and who smoke.

Chiropractic manipulation of the neck can cause strokes, even in young people. Since there is little evidence of benefit, they should be avoided.

PREVENTION

Because strokes can be so devastating, prevention is much preferable to even the very best treatment. While they remain a major cause of death and disability, the mortality from strokes has steadily declined for almost two decades, apparently because of better treatment and widespread attention to some of the major risk factors.

Hypertension, high blood cholesterol, and diabetes are all risk factors that must be prevented or detected and treated. Proper eating habits are important in both prevention and treatment of these disorders, and therefore in the prevention of stroke. Some simple dietary changes can have dramatic effects on the risk of stroke. For example, potassium is so important that the risk of having a stroke is much lower for those who consume generous amounts of fruits and vegetables than for those who eat very little. Other dietary measures can reduce your risk further. (See separate discussions of the three major disorders associated with stroke, **Hypertension, Atherosclerosis,** and **Diabetes.**)

Migraine headaches may be a sign of dangerous spasms of cerebral arteries that can lead to strokes. Anyone who gets migraines should consult a physician about stroke risk as well as head pain.

Don't smoke tobacco, take cocaine, or take amphetamines. Stopping smoking, no matter how long one has smoked, can greatly decrease the risk of stroke. The benefit seems to become significant about a year after stopping and grows to an enormous 50 percent reduction of risk after five years.

If you are considered at high risk for a stroke **there is no harm in eating fish and garlic** every other day or so, but do not attempt to treat yourself with such things as fish oil pills, aspirin, and large amounts of garlic. These might turn out to be useful but they could also result in excessive anticlotting activity in the blood, and an increased risk of a hemorrhagic stroke. Therefore, it is important to discuss with your doctor any use of aspirin, fish oil, or concentrated garlic.

When consulting with a physician about using birth control pills, be sure he or she knows all about your alcohol, tobacco, and other drug use, migraine headaches if any, and your family history of circulatory disorders, early strokes, and heart attacks.

Avoid chiropractic manipulation of the neck.

EARLY WARNING SIGNS

In many cases there is a history of transient ischemic attacks (TIAs), in which the blood supply to a brain area is cut off for a few seconds, minutes, or hours. Symptoms may include transient partial paralysis or numbness on one side of the body, or visual or speaking difficulties. These episodes can be confused with certain forms of epilepsy or migraine and must be thoroughly evaluated, no matter how brief; proper treatment could prevent a stroke.

Stroke-preventing Surgery? Carotid endarterectomy, an operation designed to prevent strokes by cutting open the carotid artery and clearing out the atherosclerotic plaques that impede blood flow to the brain, makes good theoretical sense. Unfortunately, however, the surgery itself may precipitate a stroke, and it is steadily losing popularity. It is appropriate in some cases, and is done tens of thousands of times each year, but it remains controversial. Proponents say it could prevent strokes in even more patients; critics say it is done unnecessarily and inappropriately far too often. You probably shouldn't have it done without consulting at least two physicians.

Consult a physician if you have unexplained symptoms resembling a TIA (see above). Depending on the severity of the TIA(s), age, blood pressure, and other factors, you may need treatment to prevent a stroke. The most effective medicine so far is aspirin in small daily doses. It helps prevent clots from forming by reducing platelet aggregation. In severe cases surgery may be required to unblock an artery.

Call a physician immediately if someone experiences symptoms which may indicate a stroke (listed above). Emergency treatment of a stroke victim depends on the area of the brain affected. Various drugs can help dissolve clots if given right away.

TREATMENT

Rehabilitation programs (mostly various exercises) can bring gratifying development of remaining functions to compensate for those lost. Success depends mostly on the extent of the damage but partly on emotional factors that determine the patient's enthusiasm and effort. Adequate nutrition must be provided; protein and calories are especially important because of protein breakdown and tissue wasting.

250 Tick-Borne Diseases

Of all the pesky little parasites and miscellaneous biters and stingers in North America, ticks pose the greatest threat to the general public. Of course, more people get bitten by mosquitoes, but they don't carry malaria, yellow fever, or other serious diseases here. Severe allergic reactions do occasionally lead to death after bites and stings from ants, bees, and the like, but the number is small compared to the several thousand each year who get seriously sick after tick bites.

The many kinds of ticks carry a wide variety of disease-causing bacteria, protozoa, and viruses. They cause such diseases as Lyme disease, Rocky Mountain spotted fever (RMSF), Ehrlichiosis, Colorado tick fever, Q fever, relapsing fever, tularemia, and babesiosis. Each is caused by a different microbe that is generally carried by a different tick, though some ticks carry more than one infectious agent and some microbes like more than one kind of tick. To complicate matters, most ticks are happy with any number of mammalian hosts, as well as birds and even armadillos, and many animals can host several different varieties of ticks. Most of them can occur almost anywhere in the country, but there are some regional patterns.

As tick populations ebb and flow around the country and human exposure to ticks changes, the patterns of the diseases change. The most important tick-borne disease in recent years has been Lyme disease, which is caused by a spirochete, an organism similar to the one that causes syphilis. It can cause a mild illness with low-grade fever and a rash, which is sometimes followed weeks later by severe headaches, poor concentration and memory, and other signs of encephalitis. Cardiac symptoms, like fainting, palpitations, and shortness of breath may also occur. Months or years later recurrent attacks of arthritis may occur. Sometimes the nervous system involvement is also chronic or recurrent. Severe headaches and even psychotic behavior may occur years after the bite. (You think the "Twinkie defense" was interesting? Wait until you hear, "Your Honor, the tick made me do it.")

Most tick-borne illnesses involve a rash, fever, headache, and muscle pain, or some combination of these. Without treatment progression of the disease may include pneumonia, anemia, kidney failure, and nerve damage. It's not important for you to know what animals carry what ticks that carry what diseases in what part of the country. Just remember that *all* ticks, whether you get them from contact with animals or from the woods, bushes, grassy plains, or your own lawn, carry a risk of serious disease. Early diagnosis and treatment are very important, sometimes life saving. Prevention, of course, is even better.

PREVENTION

Keep ticks off of you and keep from being bit. If walking in heavily infested areas, cover all your skin except your hands, neck, and face. Tuck your pants into your socks, and your shirt into your pants. You may want to fasten flea collars around your ankles. Light colored clothing is preferable because you can see the ticks more easily. Insect repellants with DEET can be sprayed on your skin, your shoes, and your clothing.

Remember, many people get tick bites without knowing it. Some of the most dangerous ticks are the smallest and hardest to see, so be alert and look carefully. If you may have been exposed, examine yourself, your hair, clothing, and bedding before going to bed. All family members and pets should be examined up to several times a day depending on season, location, and activities. The most important time not to get bit is while sleeping because the longer the bloodsucker is attached, the more likely it is to transfer whatever dangerous germs it might be carrying. Hikers, campers, rural residents, and all who work with animals, take note: Don't go to bed with ticks in your bedding, sleeping bags, or underwear. If there are ticks in your area don't sleep with your pets.

If you are bit remove the tick as quickly and carefully as possible. Whether you should then consult a physician depends on duration of the bite, subsequent signs and symptoms, and your general health. Healthy people with tick bites that lasted only a couple of hours or so and cause no symptoms will probably be okay. Diabetics, pregnant women, and HIV positive people, on the other hand, should report any tick bite to their doctors. In some cases preventive antibiotics will be advisable. In any case, all tick bites should be noted and considered later, should mysterious symptoms develop in future months.

Strangely enough, tick-borne diseases are not always transmitted by tick bites. It appears that the urine and blood of infected animals can transmit some of the diseases if they come into contact with a person's eyes or mouth or a scratch or abrasion. Farm workers, horse caretakers, slaughterhouse workers, cat owners, and veterinarians should take note. Removing and especially squashing a tick puts you at risk. Even airborne transmission may occur in some cases. Q fever, for example, can be transmitted to someone who cleans up after a cat gives birth, handles cat litter, or is just around an infected cat a lot. Bites from infected animals might transmit infection, but this has not been proved.

HOW TO REMOVE A TICK

Grab the bugger as close to its mouth as possible and pull steadily. Use tweezers, forceps, or your fingers protected by rubber gloves or a tissue. You can also sterilize a needle with a lighted match, insert it just under the tick's head, and gently lift it out. *Don't squash it.* Either flush it down a drain or stick it to a piece of cellophane tape to perhaps show a physician later. Wash the area and your hands. Deeply imbedded ticks that can't be removed so easily might weaken their hold if sprayed with ethyl chloride, a cooling product, or perhaps even cooled with ice.

HOW NOT TO REMOVE A TICK

Don't twist, jerk, or squash the tick. Don't apply petroleum jelly, nail polish, alcohol, or other chemicals, or flame.

Hope for the Future: A vaccine against Lyme disease is in the works, but development of vaccines against all tick-borne diseases is unlikely. The preventive measures above will always be important.

TREATMENT

Early diagnosis and prompt treatment is important in tick-borne diseases because they can be very serious, even lethal, but they respond well to antibiotics. Therefore, if you develop any sickness after exposure or possible exposure to ticks, consult a physician. Even if you don't remember a tick bite, if you were around ticks and get sick soon after, or develop mysterious symptoms weeks later, you should talk to a doctor.

Tuberculosis

Tuberculosis (TB) is a growing problem in the United States. At least ten million people are now affected. Most cases are in urban pockets of poverty, malnutrition, and close quarters with poor ventilation. Contact with immigrants from areas of high incidence is often a factor. Outbreaks have occurred in shelters for the homeless. As many as 50 percent of all the homeless people in the United States may be infected. Infection is also very common in those with AIDS.

The tubercle bacillus, *Mycobacterium tuberculosis,* can infect the bones, joints, skin, gastrointestinal system, and other organs, but it most often involves only the lungs. The bacteria invade the tissue and cause abscesses, bleeding, and tissue death. The early symptoms are usually mild—fatigue, loss of appetite, and low fever. Gradually, serious symptoms like bloody sputum and high fever develop.

Infection via raw milk is common in some areas, but in Western countries where milk is pasteurized the bacteria are almost always contracted by inhalation of infective droplets suspended in the air. People with active lung infections leave a mist of infective droplets suspended in the air when they cough. Crowded, poorly ventilated living quarters promote the spread of the bacteria. Most of those exposed develop strong immunity right away and never get sick; in others the infection gains a foothold but is walled off, and they don't get sick until months or years later when resistance is low. Malnourished and otherwise weakened people are more likely to get sick soon after exposure.

PREVENTION

Those who are infected, as determined by a skin test, but not yet sick can usually benefit from preventive therapy with an antibiotic called isoniazid. Those who should be tested include people who have been in close contact with those known to be infected; are HIV positive (infected with the AIDS virus); are entering nursing homes; are Asian immigrants; work as food preparers or handlers; are chronically malnourished; are infants born to infected parents; are schoolchildren in communities with high TB incidence; are homeless; or are intravenous drug abusers. Certain health care workers should also be tested.

Isolation and treatment of those with active TB are important preventive measures. Those in contact with contagious patients should wear masks and have regular skin tests or chest X-rays. The patient must cough and spit in ways that do not spread infection.

The BCG vaccine, a freeze-dried preparation of a strain of TB bacteria, is of limited value, but is widely used in newborns in developing countries. It has the disadvantage of converting negative skin test reactors to positive reactors by tricking the immune system into acting as though infection has occurred. This prevents early detection by skin test and treatment with isoniazid.

Good nutrition, especially adequate protein, calories, and vitamins A and C, is important in tuberculosis prevention. Malnourished children are very vulnerable during growth spurts.

Given the growing incidence of drug-resistant infection and the lack of a truly effective vaccine, it is likely that eradication of tuberculosis must await eradication of poverty, overcrowding, and malnutrition. However, there is some hope that an effective vaccine will be developed.

TREATMENT

Contagious patients should be isolated and treated in a hospital for a couple weeks, or at home if infection of others can be prevented there. Good nutrition and bed rest in a cheerful, comfortable environment are important.

Drugs are usually very effective. Isoniazid and other antibiotics are usually given in various combinations for several months. Side effects must be monitored and the drugs adjusted accordingly.

Vision Loss

Worldwide, the most important causes of vision loss, partial or total, are malnutrition (especially vitamin A deficiency), glaucoma, and infections—particularly trachoma, a chronic inflammation due to a strain of *Trachomatis chlamydia.* (Close relatives of this organism cause the common sexually transmitted disease known as chlamydia.) However, in the United States, the most common causes are cataracts, glaucoma, diabetes, and accidents. Improper use of extended-wear contact lenses is a growing menace.

Cataracts

The lens of the eye is unique—a crystal-clear living tissue floating freely in a fluid (the aqueous humor) without blood or nerve supply. In cataract development the lens gradually (sometimes rapidly) clouds over and vision gets dimmer until it is essentially lost. There is no pain or inflammation, just blurring and dimness. Cataracts usually develop in both eyes simultaneously or nearly so. They can happen at any age, but are much more common in older people. There are many causes and types of cataracts, including senile, diabetic, drug-induced, metabolic, and radiation-induced.

Senile cataract is by far the most common. Almost everyone's lenses get a little hazy with age. As the lens metabolism becomes less efficient waste builds up and cloudiness develops. Overall nutrition seems to be much more important than any specific nutrient. In animal studies various combinations of vitamin and amino acid deficiencies lead to cataracts. In malnutrition due to poverty and war, cataracts develop at a younger age. Deficiencies of protein, vitamins A and C, and the B vitamins are especially conducive to early cataract formation. Diabetes, like malnutrition, encourages early development of senile cataract.

Prevention of Senile Cataract

Assure adequate nutrition throughout life, especially in later years when activity and nutrient intake tend to decrease.

Wear good sunglasses. Senile cataract formation is promoted by exposure to ultraviolet radiation. Ophthalmologists recommend sunglasses for all those with high exposure to the sun including farmers, sailors, lifeguards, beach lovers, and construction workers. Use only those that are guaranteed (on the label) to stop 100 percent of the ultraviolet (UV) radiation. If you wear eyeglasses an optician can apply UV blocker as a clear coating. Protecting your eyes from UV radiation can also prevent the formation of a pterygium, a little growth that forms on the cornea and can distort and blur vision. Protection from UV radiation is growing in importance as the ozone layer thins and develops holes.

Drug-induced cataracts are most often caused by long-term use of moderate to high doses of corticosteroids (cortisone-type drugs). The phenothiazines, used to treat serious psychiatric disorders, can also cause cataracts. Always be aware of the hazards of the drugs you use, and use the lowest effective doses. Have your eyes checked frequently if you are taking corticosteroids or phenothiazines for months or years.

Metabolic cataracts are rare. Probably the most common are those that develop in children with galactosemia, a hereditary lack of an enzyme necessary for the metabolism of galactose from milk sugar. The consequent accumulation of galactose-one-phosphate damages various tissues, including the lens. Strict avoidance of milk, milk products, and all other sources of lactose and galactose is necessary.

Rubella (German measles) during the first three months of pregnancy can cause congenital cataracts. It can be prevented by vaccination before pregnancy.

Radiation-induced cataract is not common except for the accelerated development of senile cataract caused by sunlight. However, it is theorized that accumulated exposure to excessive X-rays, color television, radar, microwaves, and other radiation may be a factor in some cases.

Treatment of Cataracts

When vision in the better of the two eyes is so poor that daily activities are interfered with, surgical removal of the lens is recommended.

 In most cases, a permanent plastic lens is then implanted in the eye. It is imperceptible and usually restores vision to near normal.

Glaucoma

The front chamber of the eye is filled with a clear fluid, the aqueous humor, which is constantly secreted into the eye by fluid-producing cells and drained out through tiny canals. In glaucoma the drainage is defective, so fluid accumulates and pressure in the eye builds up. This decreases blood supply to the optic nerve fibers, which are slowly destroyed, resulting in loss of vision starting at the periphery. Sight lost this way can never be recovered, so early detection and treatment are very important.

The most common type of glaucoma is the insidious chronic type that usually begins after age thirty-five and tends to run in families. Signs of early chronic glaucoma include loss of peripheral vision, recurrent blurred or foggy vision, morning headaches, pain around the eyes, and halos around lights. Unfortunately, **there are usually no symptoms** and no apparent visual defects until damage has been done. This is why regular checks for glaucoma are important.

Acute glaucoma is only about a tenth as common as chronic, but is a significant cause of blindness. About 1 percent of people over thirty-five have a narrow space between the iris (the colored diaphragm) and the cornea, which predisposes them to acute glaucoma in which the iris balloons forward and blocks the drainage canal. The rapid buildup of pressure causes blurred or cloudy vision and severe pain. The eye is usually red and there may be nausea, vomiting, and severe headache. **See a physician immediately if** these symptoms occur. Vision will be lost completely and permanently in a day or two without treatment.

In susceptible people, this sudden canal blockage can be precipitated by anything that dilates the pupils, including prolonged sitting in the dark with open eyes as when watching a movie or television, careless use of eyedrops or internal medicines that dilate the pupils, and blows to the head.

Prevention of Blindness Due to Glaucoma

Have your eyeball pressure checked. Early detection is the best defense against chronic glaucoma. The simple, painless examination of intraocular pressure should be done about every three years after age thirty-five, and earlier and more often if there is a family history of glaucoma. You don't necessarily have to go to an ophthalmologist for this test; your family physician may be able to do it.

Blacks are far more susceptible to the disorder. About 15 percent of all blacks in the U.S. will eventually get glaucoma. This is almost three times the national average. Blacks with a family history of glaucoma, diabetes, or hypertension should be tested annually from age twenty.

If glaucoma is discovered, it is extremely important to follow the ophthalmologist's instructions. Eyedrops are usually used to control the pressure, mostly by increasing the fluid drainage. The drops must be taken as ordered and the eyes should be examined regularly. Other drugs and eyedrops should be avoided without a doctor's approval. When drops are not effective, pills are usually prescribed. In the rare cases where medical therapy is not effective, laser or other surgery may be necessary to reduce the pressure and prevent blindness.

In acute glaucoma, creation of a passage through the iris allows proper drainage to resume and prevents blindness. This is done with a laser beam or simple, quick surgery. Probably the most important measure to prevent acute glaucoma in those predisposed is examination of the anterior chamber angle before instilling drugs into the eyes.

Infant glaucoma can be caused by rubella infection during the first trimester of pregnancy. This is yet another reason for rubella prevention by vaccination.

Marijuana and alcohol both reduce intraocular pressure for several hours, but they are impractical as glaucoma treatments because adequate doses would mean round-the-clock intoxication.

Prevention of Vision Loss Due to Accidents

Suffice it to say that special care, including the use of safety goggles when appropriate, should be taken by carpenters, construction workers, chemists and other lab workers, and those who play tennis, handball, and racketball.

Prevention of Vision Loss Due to Diabetes

Diabetics run a high risk of vision loss due to cataract, glaucoma, and diabetic retinopathy. The risk can be decreased by good nutrition and careful control of blood sugar (see **Diabetes,** above). All diabetics should see an ophthalmologist at least once each year.

Proper Use of Extended-wear Contact Lenses

Millions of Americans are now using contact lenses that don't have to be removed every day; they can be worn for up to a week. Some ophthalmologists consider them corneal time bombs and do not recommend their use. The danger is that infections, abrasions, scarring, and ulcers may develop on the corneas. Severe and permanent visual impairment can result. The risk is much higher than with regular contacts. In order to minimize the danger the following precautions should be strictly adhered to:

- **Never wear the lenses longer than one week.**
- **Sleep without the lenses** at least once a week.
- **Remove and clean the lenses** whenever it seems necessary. Always wash your hands before handling the lenses.
- **Use the lubricating drops and cleaning solutions exactly as prescribed.** Don't change products without consulting your ophthalmologist. Don't make your own solutions.
- **Never put your lenses in your mouth** or moisten them with saliva.
- **Remove your contacts for swimming;** this reduces the risk of bacterial contamination under the lenses.
- **Avoid accidentally drying out the eye** with a hair dryer, clothes dryer, or oven.
- **If exposed to an open car window,** a strong fan, or a nearby air conditioner or heating vent, protect your eyes from the wind.
- **When flying in aircraft** with very dry air use more lubricating drops.

Even if you do everything right you can still have problems. If an eye becomes irritated, uncomfortable, or red remove the lens immediately and consult your ophthalmologist. Don't take chances!

Are Nonprescription Reading Glasses OK?

Reading glasses can now be legally sold at retail outlets without an eye examination or prescription. Like prescription glasses, they compensate for the normal loss of focusing ability that usually starts at about age forty. They are priced at about $10 to $20, compared to $25 to $100 for prescription glasses plus the cost of the optometrist's examination and prescription. The only potential problem with the products is that they may cause eyestrain in the form of fatigue of the eye muscles in some cases. This is because the pupillary distance, the distance from the center of one lens to the center of the other, is uniform. But the pupillary distance of human eyes varies from person to person. Prescription lenses, on the other hand, are made to meet individual needs. However, this is usually not a problem with nonprescription glasses.

WHAT ABOUT RADIAL KERATOTOMY?

Radial keratotomy (RK) is surgery performed on the cornea for the purpose of correcting slight to moderate nearsightedness without the inconvenience of wearing glasses and contact lenses. The procedure has been performed in the United States since about 1980, and its effectiveness has been recognized by the American Academy of Ophthalmology. At least 80 percent of the time it works well and patients are satisfied. The problem is that nearly 10 percent of patients are very dissatisfied because of a variety of side effects including overcorrection leading to farsightedness, reduced twilight vision, worsened astigmatisms, corneal erosion leading to pain and blurred vision, and fluctuation of vision requiring the use of several sets of glasses through the day. This is a high rate of unhappiness for elective surgery on young, healthy people.

If you are considering RK ask the eye surgeon what the rate of satisfaction has been with his or her procedures. Weigh the risks against the benefits you expect. More precise corneal shaping with fewer side effects can apparently be done with lasers. This could turn out to be a big improvement over RK and a major development in eye care, so be patient, don't rush into the usual RK surgery, and keep in touch with a good ophthalmologist.

OZONE DEPLETION THREATENS YOUR VISION

Ultraviolet radiation from the sun promotes not only cataracts, but damage to the retina. Excessive exposure burns the retina, diminishes visual acuity, creates little islands of blindness, and may generally speed up the aging of the retina. The problem is not very common, but the danger is growing as more people are enjoying the outdoors while the ozone layer above the earth is thinned and develops holes. Just as the skin cancer rate doubled during the 1980s, the incidence of solar retinopathy, snow blindness, and macular degeneration (damage to the retina with central-vision loss) may greatly increase in the 1990s. As with cataracts, the best preventive is to wear good sunglasses when you must be exposed to bright sunlight. The thickness of the ozone layer above a given area can change dramatically, like the weather. Reports of UV levels along with the weather will probably become common in the near future.

Section Three

SELF-CARE AND RATIONAL USE OF THE HEALTH CARE SYSTEM

Self-Care and Rational Use of the Health Care System

Recommended Examinations by Age

Common Emergencies

Symptoms: When to Self-Treat and When to Consult a Physician (symptoms are listed alphabetically)

Medical care professionals and facilities are both overused and underused. That is, people often go to an emergency room when they should go to a doctor's office, and to a doctor's office when home treatment would suffice. They ignore symptoms that should be medically evaluated, and they fail to get checkups and vaccinations indicated for risk groups they belong to. This chapter is a guide to self-care and the rational use of professional care.

Recommended Examinations by Age

All ages: Regular dental checkup and cleaning every six months to about age 12 and at least every year after that. We all need various vaccines at different ages. (See **Vaccines** in Section Four for details.)

Ages 7 to 11: Screen for coronary artery disease (CAD) risk factors including blood pressure, cholesterol levels, fitness, and family history of CAD, diabetes, and smoking. Screen for scoliosis at least once a year from about age 9 to 14. Check vision and hearing.

Ages 17 to 25: At least one complete medical history and physical examination including blood pressure and cholesterol checks, electrocardiogram, eating habits and nutrition status, and tests for sexually transmitted diseases if sexually active. Men should learn to check their testes for signs of cancer and do the check every month for life. Women should have a Pap test at age 18 or within a year of beginning sexual intercourse, and annually thereafter. Everyone should have at least one examination for glaucoma before age twenty-five, more if there is a family history of the problem.

 All adults: Blood pressure check annually. Blood cholesterol check every year or two or as advised by physician. Glaucoma check every three years or as advised by physician.

Ages 30 to 35: Complete physical and medical history. Women should learn to do a breast self-exam (see below) and do the check every month for life.

Ages 40 to 60: Electrocardiogram (ECG) at age 40 for all. Periodic check for prostate cancer in men. Complete physical, including checks for colo-rectal cancer, and medical history every two to five years for men and women. Colo-rectal tests more often for those at high risk. Annual breast exam by physician for all women.

Ages 60 to 75: Complete physical exam and medical history every year or two.

Ages 75 and over: Complete physical exam and medical history every year.

All women should have a baseline mammogram some time after age 30, depending on breast cancer risk. In most cases mammography is advisable every year or two after age 40. Postmenopausal women at high risk for osteoporosis should consult a physician about possible estrogen replacement.

Pregnant women should have a battery of tests and examinations. Good prenatal care from the first weeks in the pregnancy is important to the health of the mother and the baby. (See **Birth Defects and Sickness in the Newborn,** Section Two.)

Genetic Screening Is Coming!

Actually, it's already here. DNA and chromosome tests have been developed for fifty-odd familial diseases that affect about seven hundred thousand Americans. But this is peanuts. In the 1990s genetic tests will probably be made available for hypertension, atherosclerosis, Alzheimer's disease, dyslexia, various cancers, common psychoses, and several other common diseases that now affect about seventy million Americans. The importance of genetic testing could increase one hundred-fold by the turn of the century. Theoretically, early detection should lead to the golden age of preventive medicine. Whether this actually happens depends a great deal on the will of individuals and the nation. It's a question of philosophy, psychology, economics, and politics.

Common Emergencies

In some situations medical care is needed right away and the people present must think straight and act quickly. They must decide whether to call an ambulance, drive the patient, or call a cab, and whether the patient should go to a hospital or doctor's office. Generally speaking, if the patient has a personal physician who can be quickly reached by phone, he or she should be consulted before making a move. If a decision must be made without a physician, keep in mind that ambulances are expensive and often not as fast as a car that is already on the scene, but they come with experienced medics and drivers. A car is usually the fastest way to get a patient to a doctor, but should not be used if movement might cause further harm, if the available car is unsafe, or if the available driver is intoxicated. Taxicabs should also be considered if they are readily available.

An ambulance should be called when there is a severe back or neck injury or compound fracture (with a bone protruding from the skin) that could be aggravated by inexperienced hands. In such injuries time is not as important as careful handling. An ambulance should also be called if resuscitation, say from drowning or smoke inhalation, is required. An ambulance should also be called in any of the emergencies below if other safe and fast transportation is not available.

Bleeding that is severe and cannot be stopped by direct pressure must be dealt with quickly. The patient should be driven to a doctor's office if one is nearby or to an emergency room.

Breathing trouble that is severe even at rest requires immediate medical attention. The person's physician should be called. If he or she cannot be reached the patient should be driven to a hospital.

 Broken bones and knocked-out teeth usually require medical attention. In the case of a simple fracture of anything but the back or neck, the patient should be driven to a hospital. The injury can be splinted with almost any straight piece of wood or plastic or just heavily taped, but this is unnecessary if medical care is minutes away. If an adult tooth is broken or knocked out, it should be wrapped in a clean cloth and taken immediately to a dentist.

Burns that are obviously severe, especially on the hands or face, require immediate medical attention. The patient should be driven to a hospital and his or her physician should be called.

Choking on food or any other item can lead to suffocation and death. If medical personnel are more than a minute or so away, the abdominal thrust (Heimlich maneuver) should be applied. Stand behind the person and bring your hands together at the base of the sternum (just under the diaphragm). Give a sharp thrust in and up; the idea is to force the diaphragm up to force air out of the lungs, which propels the object out of the windpipe. If another person is present, he or she should try to contact a physician in case the object won't come out.

If an infant or small child is choking, place it across your lap with head and arms hanging down. Using the heel of your hand, give several thumps between the shoulder blades.

Labor in a pregnant woman at an unexpected time is an emergency. Her physician should be called and she should be driven to a hospital.

Near-drowning, like choking, can be treated with the abdominal thrust, which expels water, vomitus, and other foreign matter from the lungs, and serves as a form of artificial respiration. Place the person in the supine position (lying on the back) with his or her head turned to one side. Place your hands, one on top of the other, at the base of the sternum. Give a sharp thrust in and up. Repeat intermittently until all water is expelled. If the victim does not start breathing, try mouth-to-mouth respiration. While you are doing this someone should be calling an ambulance or physician.

Shock is a serious disturbance of blood circulation that can occur subsequent to injury, hemorrhage, poisoning, adverse drug reaction, heart attack, and other conditions. The skin is pale, the pulse and breathing are rapid and weak, blood pressure is very low, and thirst may be extreme.

The patient should be kept warm and lying down with the head slightly lower than the body. He or she should be driven to a hospital.

Stupor or disorientation, as indicated by extreme confusion, drowsiness, or near-unconsciousness, requires immediate medical attention. The person should be driven to a hospital right away.

Unconsciousness requires immediate medical attention. The patient should be driven to a hospital right away.

Symptoms: When to Self-Treat and When to Consult a Physician

Self-care is natural and inevitable. We all treat ourselves, and sometimes friends and family members, for a wide variety of symptoms, ailments, and injuries. If this were not so doctors would have to work twenty-four hours a day and our medical bills would bankrupt us. It is important, though, to know when to get professional help. In the following pages signs, symptoms, and conditions are presented alphabetically for easy reference.

See a physician immediately means the patient should be driven to a doctor right away, preferably the person's own physician who is more likely to be familiar with the patient's problems. If possible, the doctor should be called first to avoid a trip to a hospital when the doctor's office would suffice or to the office when hospital care is needed.

Consult a physician means to call and discuss the problem with a physician or his or her trained assistant (often a nurse), and possibly to make an appointment for that day or later, depending on the nature and severity of the symptoms.

Abdominal Pain

Abdominal pain is most often caused by gas, hyperacidity, and mild intestinal viral infections, but it can also be caused by bacterial food poisoning, appendicitis, diverticulitis ("left side appendicitis"—actually inflammation of little abnormal pouches ballooning out from the intestine), ectopic pregnancy, tumors, and other serious problems. If you are unsure of the source or cause of the pain, avoid all food, sip water, relax, and see what direction the symptoms take.

See a physician immediately if:
- the pain is very severe or associated with vaginal discharge or bleeding;
- any stool or vomitus is very dark or bloody.

Consult a physician if:
- you are pregnant or possibly pregnant;
- there is nausea, vomiting, diarrhea, constipation, painful urination, or fever.

Abrasions

See **Cuts, Abrasions, Punctures, and Animal Bites.**

Acne

In this skin disorder, which affects mostly teenagers, the openings of the sebaceous (oil-producing) glands become plugged with enlarged dead cells. This traps the normal skin oil, which accumulates under the plug and pushes it toward the skin surface. This whitehead, which becomes a blackhead from exposure to the air, is called a *comedo*. It cannot be washed off since it is slightly below the surface. Bacteria then break down the oil into free fatty acids that irritate the tissue and cause inflammation. This pimple is usually resolved by the body's defenses, or it drains and heals. But sometimes it grows, damages surrounding tissue, and results in permanent scarring. Surging hormones, especially testosterone and progesterone, trigger acne development. It cannot be cured but it can be controlled.

SELF-CARE

Keep your face clean with two or three gentle washings a day using mild soap and warm water. Vigorous scrubbing can aggravate acne by injuring and plugging the drainage canals of the sebaceous glands. Soaking the face with a hot clean washcloth or steaming it with a pot of boiling water before washing may help. *Don't* squeeze comedos. This can injure the skin and cause blemishes and scars. Pimples that have come to a head can be gently pressed after a hot compress.

Keep oily hair away from acne-prone skin. Cutting or restyling may be necessary. Greasy hair itself does not cause or aggravate acne, but the oil can be transferred to the face. Avoid touching the affected areas, especially after eating oily foods. Habitual touching, rubbing, or resting the face on the hands can aggravate acne. Avoid oily cosmetics, lotions, creams, and hair products. They can promote plugging of the openings. It has been estimated that half of all cosmetics are capable of provoking acne. Avoid harsh shampoos and keep all hair products away from the face.

Acne Medicines. Try a product with *benzoyl peroxide,* which helps dry and peel the skin and decrease the population of the responsible bacteria. Follow directions carefully. Products containing *resorcinol* with sulfur can help, but they should be avoided by blacks since the chemical can discolor their skin.

Consult a physician if the self-care remedies don't help and the acne is severe, causing scars, harming self-esteem, or discouraging normal social interactions.

A Note on Prescription Acne Medicines. If your doctor prescribes an acne medicine, it will most likely be an antibiotic or a vitamin A derivative, either tretinoin for topical use or isotretinoin for internal use. It is extremely important that you follow directions exactly and read the patient package-inserts that come with the medicine.

Animal Bites

See **Cuts, Abrasions, Punctures, and Animal Bites; Insect, Spider, and Jellyfish Stings and Bites; Tick-Borne Diseases** (Section Two).

Anxiety Disorders

Anxiety is a normal short-term reaction to stressful situations; we all experience it from time to time. Anxiety disorders, however, are chronic irrational reactions that can have profound effects on one's work and social life. There are several types and, taken together, they constitute the most common psychiatric disorder in the United States. In **panic**

 disorder there are sudden attacks of intense fear with an overwhelming sense of doom and fear of dying or going insane. The fear is accompanied by such physical symptoms as trembling, palpitations, excessive sweating, dizziness, gasping for breath, nausea, and a sensation of choking.

In **generalized anxiety disorder** there is excessive and unrealistic worry for many months about two or more life circumstances, like the safety of one's children and the security of one's job. The anxiety is accompanied by such physical symptoms as restlessness, shortness of breath, hyperventilation (overbreathing), dry mouth, muscle tension, and trembling. The other important anxiety disorders are **agoraphobia** (fear of being in public places), **obsessive-compulsive disorder** (persistant repugnant ideas and ritualistic, stereotyped behaviors), and **posttraumatic stress disorder** (following fires, earthquakes, battles, etc.).

Symptoms resembling those of anxiety disorders can be caused by caffeine, nicotine, cocaine, marijuana, antidepressants, antihistamines, and many other drugs, and by withdrawal of narcotics and sedatives. They can also be caused by peptic ulcer, heart disease, and other disorders. These must be considered before an anxiety disorder is diagnosed.

Consult a physician if you repeatedly experience panic attacks, anxiety, obsessions, compulsions, or the physical symptoms described above, and they are not relieved by stopping all self-medication and recreational drug use.

Back Pain

The most common type of back pain is an ache in the lower back that can usually be prevented or treated with simple measures (see **Backaches** in Section Two). Sometimes, however, back pain is a symptom of kidney disease, pelvic infections, tumors, osteoporosis, or other serious problems.

See a physician immediately if there is also:

- very dark or bloody stools or vomitus,
- severe abdominal pain.

Consult a physician if:

- back pain is very severe;
- there is also urinary difficulty, fever, or sore throat;
- there is also severe menstrual pain or heavy vaginal bleeding.

Blood in the Semen

Bloody semen is fairly common. It may be due to a broken blood vessel or inflammation of the seminal vesicles, the tubes that carry the semen. Neither is serious. However, the symptom can also be caused by a diseased prostate gland, and therefore should be evaluated. Consult a urologist if blood appears in the semen.

Blood in the Urine

This is often due to overexercise. However, it may also be due to infection, inflammation, kidney stone, or even bladder cancer. Consult a physician.

Boils and Similar Infections

A boil, or furuncle, is a localized bacterial (usually staphylococcal) abscess of the skin and underlying tissue, which usually starts at the base of a hair follicle. Most boils come to a head and drain spontaneously, but sometimes the infection spreads under the skin and into deeper tissue, forming several interconnected boils. This is called a *carbuncle.* Boils can be very serious because the bacteria may enter the blood and go on to infect the heart, bones, joints, and other tissue. Infections similar to boils often arise at the site of skin injury.

PREVENTION

Clean all cuts, scratches, and abrasions as thoroughly as possible. Use mild soap and warm water. Remove every particle of dirt, sand, or coral. Antiseptics can be painful and are rarely necessary. Shaving the underarms promotes boils in some, apparently by leaving the hair follicle open to bacteria in the warm, moist environment subject to much friction.

SELF-CARE

The area should be kept clean with several washes a day; injury and irritation should be avoided. To reduce pain and stimulate head formation and drainage, apply very warm salt-water compresses several times a day. *Do not* squeeze or press a boil or attempt to open it. This could cause the infection to spread under the skin and delay healing. Draining boils are highly contaminated and should be covered with sterile gauze to prevent spreading the bacteria. Hands should be washed before and after dressing the wound.

See a physician immediately if there are streaks leading from the infection, or if you experience fever, dizziness, or vomiting.

See a physician today if you have a boil on your face, or if you have more than one boil.

Consult a physician soon if you frequently get boils and other skin infections.

Bone and Connective Tissue Injuries

Sprains, strains, and other injuries due to stresses and trauma common in sports are discussed in Section One. These injuries also occur in a wide variety of accidents such as falling off ladders and down steps, or slipping on wet sidewalks and in bathtubs. In most cases the self-care measures discussed in Section One are sufficient, but sometimes a physician should be consulted.

See a physician immediately if:

- a fracture is obvious or likely and involves the thigh, pelvis, back, or neck (call an ambulance in cases of the latter two);
- a limb is crooked, cold, numb, or blue;
- a suspected fracture is accompanied by heavy sweating, dizziness, or other severe symptoms;
- a joint (knee, ankle, wrist, elbow, or shoulder) is deformed, moving abnormally, or in severe pain.

Consult a physician if:

- an injury involves severe bruising and pain, but a fracture is uncertain;
- pain from an injury lasts more than a few days and severely limits use of the affected part.

Breast Lumps (Fibrocystic Breast Changes)

See also **Cancer—Early Warning Signs.**

Nearly half the women in the United States will have lumps in their breasts sometime in their lives (usually between ages eighteen and fifty), while their ovaries are functioning. The lumps are either long fibers that form a solid, scarlike mass or small pockets filled with fluid or semisolid material. The breasts may become heavy, painful, and tender. The pain and discomfort may be continuous, but is often most severe during the week or so before the menstrual period. Some believe that dietary fat, caffeine, and nicotine might promote the fibrocystic changes, but the evidence is weak.

SELF-CARE

Some relief can be obtained by wearing a supporting bra. Try avoiding or cutting back on fatty foods, coffee, colas, and smoking.

Consult a physician if breast lumps occur. They must be evaluated.

Breathing Problems, Chest Pains, and Palpitations

Breathing problems and chest pains are often due to anxiety, abdominal gas, and colds, but they can also be indications of a wide variety of serious health problems including asthma, emphysema, bronchitis, and heart disease. Smokers can often get rid of these symptoms by quitting.

Palpitations (racing, pounding heart) not associated with other symptoms are not necessarily abnormal and are usually not an emergency. If they happen often try avoiding coffee, tea, and all other sources of caffeine and related stimulants.

See a physician immediately if:

- breathing difficulties occur in an infant;
- the symptoms are associated with an insect sting or any drug use;
- severe chest pain or a sensation of crushing pressure occurs around the breastbone, either arm, or the jaw;
- breathing difficulties, except controllable asthma, occur at rest or in association with chest pain, severe fatigue, or palpitations

(resting pulse over 120 beats per minute);

- irregular pulse, dizziness, or profuse sweating occur.

Note: In this set of symptoms delay can be deadly; prompt medical care can be lifesaving. The latter three may be signs of a heart attack, which can be aborted with clot-dissolving drugs if they are given within two or three hours.

Consult a physician if:

- known asthma is unusually active and difficult to control;
- breathing difficulties occur after slight exertion or while sleeping;
- chest pain or palpitations (resting pulse over 120 beats per minute) occur repeatedly for several days.

Burns

First degree burns are superficial and minor. A moderate sunburn and a tongue burn from hot food or drink are examples. **Second degree burns,** like a severe sunburn or a burn from a motorcycle muffler or stove, cause blistering, splitting, and peeling of the skin. **Third degree burns** char and destroy the skin, including the nerves (so pain is minimal), and can lead to severe fluid loss, infection, and scarring. First and second degree burns should be immediately immersed in cool water (not ice) to minimize tissue injury. However, excessive cooling can further damage tissue, so cold applications should not exceed a couple of minutes unless a physician is consulted.

See a physician immediately if a burn is:

- obviously very severe, yet relatively painless (third degree);
- very painful and extensive, with blistering or splitting of the skin (second degree);
- very painful and on the hands, feet, eyes, ears, or face.

Consult a physician if:

- a burn or severe sunburn does not heal in a few days or has pus;
- you suffer a second degree burn and your tetanus immunization is not current or is uncertain.

Cancer—Early Warning Signs

We should all be familiar with the early warning signs of cancer, as well as the self-examinations and screening tests relevent to us.

Consult a physician if:

- there is unusual vaginal bleeding or discharge between periods or after menopause;
- the monthly breast self-examination shows unusual signs (see below);
- a cough or hoarseness lasts more than about ten days or blood is coughed up;
- there is rectal bleeding or large changes in bowel habits unexplained by dietary changes;
- urinary difficulties in a man are persistant or associated with pain in the pelvis or back;
- a monthly testicular self-examination reveals a lump or enlargement;
- there is persistant difficulty swallowing or a lump in the throat;
- stomach pains or digestive difficulties last more than a couple weeks;
- swollen lymph glands last more than three weeks;
- persistant fatigue, weight loss, mild fever, nausea, or repeated infections occur;
- a lump, white spot, or red or scaly area persists on the lip or in the mouth;
- there is a persistant, unusual skin lesion like an open sore that lasts three weeks or more, a white or yellow area that resembles scar tissue, or a mole or wart that bleeds or changes in color or shape.

More on Early Cancer Detection

Breast self-examinations should not be considered a substitute for an annual breast examination by a physician, which is recommended for all women over forty. Careful palpation by an experienced physician is a very sensitive detection method. These examinations should start much earlier in women whose sister or mother has had breast cancer.

A breast self-examination once a month should become a lifetime habit for women, starting at about age thirty, earlier in women with a strong family history of the disease. You should actually do three exams: one in the shower, one before a mirror and one lying down.

 They should be done about one week after the menstrual period when temporary hormonally induced changes will be minimal.

In the shower use flat fingers over every part of each breast to check for any lump or thickening. Use the right hand for the left breast and vice versa.

Before a mirror look for changes in the contour of each breast such as swelling, dimpling, puckering, skin irritation; or changes in the nipples such as whitish scale or distorted shape. Do this with arms at your sides, then with arms raised high overhead, then with hands on hips and pressing down firmly to flex your chest muscles. Finally, gently squeeze each nipple; report any discharge to your physician.

Lying on your back put a pillow or folded towel under your right shoulder and your right hand behind your head. With flat fingers of the left hand, press gently in small circular motions, systematically covering every part of your breast, including the nipple. Repeat for the left breast. Report any lump you discover to your physician.

Mammography, a safe and painless low-dose x-ray of the breasts, is perhaps the most important tool we have for saving lives by early cancer detection. Unfortunately, there is no consensus on how early and how often it should be done: Some experts believe they should be done starting at age 40; others say to wait until age 50. If the screening starts too early the net cost of finding each cancer is very high. Moreover, false positives result in unnecessary anxiety and further testing. Clearly, though, women at high risk should have mammographies done early and often. Some experts recommend the first mammography at age 30 for women whose mother or sister has had breast cancer and age 40 for the rest; others say age 40 for high-risk women and 50 for the rest. Nonetheless, it is agreed that mammography should be done every year or two for all women from age 50 to about 75.

Breast implants, usually made of silicon and inserted for cosmetic purposes, might make early detection of cancer more difficult. This should be considered, especially if a woman's relatives have had breast cancer.

Men also get breast cancer. It is not nearly as common as in women, but it tends to be deadlier. Men should see a physician about any lumps or unusual changes around their nipples.

Screening for Cervical Cancer. Pap tests are recommended for all women from age 18 or within a year of starting sexual intercourse. After three annual, negative Pap tests, testing every other year or so may be adequate depending on risk factors.

Screening for Colo-Rectal Cancer. Annual rectal examinations are recommended for people over 40, and annual fecal occult blood tests for those over 50. After 40 a proctoscopic examination should be done every 3 to 5 years. People who have had ulcerative colitis or rectal polyps, or a strong family history of bowel cancer, are at high risk for colon cancer and should discuss more frequent tests with their physician.

A testicular lump or enlargement should be reported to a physician. Monthly self-examination can save lives because these cancers spread rapidly. After a warm shower or bath, examine each testicle between the thumb and fingers and feel for hard lumps, slight enlargement, or a change in the consistency. Testicular cancer is primarily a young man's disease. Self-examination is especially important between the ages of fifteen and thirty-five and should be taught in high-school health and physical education classes. Undescended testes have a very high risk of developing cancer. Parents should have their infant sons checked for this.

Stomach pain or digestive discomfort that continues for two weeks or more should be discussed with a physician. People with pernicious anemia or lack of hydrochloric acid are at higher risk for stomach cancer and should have regular checkups.

Moles, freckles, or warts that have changed in color or shape or that bleed should be examined by a dermatologist. So should a brownish or blackish band running up and down a fingernail or toenail. People who have had skin cancer, especially melanoma, which can recur many years later, should have regular examinations for life. Some experts believe that all moles present at birth should be removed. This is controversial, but all such moles should certainly be examined and watched. If you have more than twenty moles, even if they all appear normal, you should ask a dermatologist to examine them.

A persistant lump, white spot, red area, or scaly area on the lip or in the mouth should be seen by a physician. Tobacco smokers and chewers should regularly and thoroughly examine the mouth area for signs of cancer. With your fingers feel the sides of your neck and under your jaw. Look at and feel the lip area, inside and outside the mouth, for color changes and lumps. Look and feel for white scaly areas and lumps all over the inside of the mouth, including the gums, cheeks, roof, and floor. Pull the tongue out and hold it to the right and then left to look for lumps and growths. Use a good light for this examination and do it at least once a month so you know your mouth well and will quickly notice any changes.

Chest Pains

See **Breathing Problems, Chest Pains, and Palpitations.**

Common Cold

Consult a physician for coldlike symptoms if:

- sore throat is severe,
- fever is high,
- breathing is difficult,
- thick greenish or yellowish phlegm is coughed up,
- you are HIV positive or have diabetes or other chronic disease.

Constipation

Experiencing difficult bowel movements with dry, hard stools is a common complaint from people with poor diets. It should be dealt with to prevent hemorrhoids and diverticular disease. One bowel movement a day is normal and most common, but more or less is not necessarily abnormal. The need to strain while defecating is probably the best criterion of constipation.

SELF-CARE

Constipation can usually be prevented or cured with proper diet, adequate fluid intake, and exercise. Try eating more fruits, vegetables, and whole grains and drinking more water. Prunes and prune juice are especially helpful. Psyllium seed laxatives are helpful but expensive. Exercise regularly; even a casual walk can help. If you must use aluminum-containing antacids, use the type that also contain magnesium. Avoid using stimulant laxatives and enemas.

Consult a physician if:

- stools are consistently pencil-thin;
- defecation is painful or accompanied by bleeding.

Convulsions, Seizures

In a severe seizure consciousness is lost, the body goes rigid, and the limbs and head jerk rhythmically. During a seizure the head should be positioned for easy breathing. The person should lie on his or her side, not the back. Don't put your finger into the mouth lest a serious bite result. Seizures usually stop within seconds and the person regains consciousness.

Call a physician immediately if:

- seizures continue one after another;
- the patient is an infant;
- the seizure is the patient's first ever. Any witness to the seizure should try to remember exactly what happened and describe it to the physician.

Consult a physician if a seizure occurs.

Note: Epilepsy is a neurological disorder in which the person suffers recurrent seizures due to abnormal electrical discharges in the brain (see Section Two for details).

Cough and Hoarseness

Most coughs are caused by smoking and common viral infections. A productive cough due to a respiratory infection should not be treated. It is better to expel the excess mucus. A dry cough can be treated with any nonprescription medicine containing dextromethorphan.

See a physician immediately if:

- coughing starts suddenly in a child due to choking on a piece of food or other small object and you cannot remove it using the abdominal thrust (see **Common Emergencies,** above);
- there is also excessive drooling or difficulty breathing in a young child.

Consult a physician if:

- coughing occurs in an infant less than three months old;
- a cough in an infant or young child sounds like a seal's bark or is associated with rapid or difficult breathing (this may be a sign of severe croup, a respiratory viral infection common in young children);

- a cough produces thick, foul-smelling mucus or blood;
- a cough lasts more than a week or is associated with a fever for five days;
- hoarseness lasts a week in a child or a month in an adult.

Cuts, Abrasions, Punctures, and Animal Bites

Minor wounds can be treated by thoroughly cleaning with soap and water. Simple puncture wounds, like a needle prick to the finger or stepping on a tack, should be allowed to bleed freely to clean them. All wounds should be kept scrupulously clean until they are completely healed. Bandages can hold the edges of a wound together, help keep dirt out, hasten healing, and minimize scarring.

See a physician immediately if the wound:

- is very severe with bleeding that cannot be stopped with pressure, edges that cannot be held together by a bandage, or the possibility of nerve damage (as indicated by numbness or inability to move the affected part normally);
- is difficult to clean or you cannot remove the glass, metal, or other culprit;
- is a deep puncture;
- is a puncture of the eyes or genitals.

Consult a physician if:

- the wound develops pronounced inflammation (redness and swelling), pain, or pus;
- you have not had a tetanus shot in the last ten years or are not sure;
- you are bitten or scratched by any wild mammal or domestic mammal of uncertain rabies vaccination status.

Dandruff

Dandruff is skin flaking off the scalp. A certain amount is normal and adequately controlled by washing with a mild shampoo. Aggravating factors include strong or concentrated shampoos, rough treatment of the scalp during washing and drying, hot water, saltwater, scratching the scalp with a hairbrush, and excessive washing and brushing.

SELF-CARE

Avoid aggravating factors. Use dandruff shampoos with zinc pyrithione or selenium sulfide and use them in the lowest effective amounts. The effectiveness of these products tends to wear off. It might help to switch between the two types and even rotate in regular shampoo frequently to reduce tolerance to dandruff shampoos.

Consult a physician if self-care measures don't help and dandruff is severe with large flakes, very oily scalp, crusting, hair loss, or other scalp abnormalities.

Delusions

See **Hallucinations and Delusions.**

Dementia

Consult a physician if a middle-aged or elderly relative shows obvious signs of reduced mental capacity such as inability to recall recent events or do simple arithmetic, poor judgment, or getting lost (see **Dementia and Alzheimer's Disease,** Section Two).

Depression and Mania

Depression is characterized by sadness, low energy, a sluggish feeling, inability to experience pleasure, difficulty sleeping, and appetite changes. The cause is poorly understood, but some cases appear to be associated with low levels of certain brain neurotransmitters. Manic depression, or bipolar depression, is characterized by mood swings. In the manic or "high" phase the patient is energetic and euphoric with increased libido, appetite, and confidence. This gives way to depression with lethargy, apathy, and a feeling of hopelessness.

SELF-CARE

Lean a little on family and friends in times of need. Don't hide disappointment, grief, or anger. Get out of any job or business that makes every day a miserable chore to live. Get adequate rest, eat right, and exercise some every day.

Consult a physician if you experience suicidal urges or several weeks of unexplained fatigue, sadness, insomnia, or loss of libido.

Diarrhea and Vomiting

Acute diarrhea and vomiting, which may occur together or alone, can be caused by a wide variety of bacteria, virus, and protozoa that infect or poison the stomach, small intestine, and colon. Chronic diarrhea (lasting more than two months) is sometimes caused by microorganisms, but it is more often caused by irritable bowel syndrome, inflammatory bowel disease (like ulcerative colitis and Chron's disease), and other noninfectious and nontoxic factors. Acute diarrhea can often be prevented by careful attention to the factors discussed in Section One related to food poisoning. Travelers to developing countries must avoid raw foods and tap water. In day-care centers special precautions are necessary: Children with diarrhea must be excluded. Staff and children must keep their hands clean. Toys and other shared objects and surfaces should be cleaned *daily* since microbes can live on them for days, even weeks.

Simple diarrhea, whatever its cause, is almost always self-limiting. It subsides in a day or two without treatment. The simplest remedy is to avoid any foods or drinks suspected of causing or aggravating the problem, drugs not recommended or prescribed by a physician, and most dairy products since the lactose aggravates diarrhea even for those who are not normally lactose intolerant. Water should also be taken to replace lost fluid. Fruit juices may aggravate the problem due to their sorbitol content. All caffeinated and very sweet beverages should be avoided. If diarrhea lasts more than a day, make a mixture of half a teaspoon of salt, half a teaspoon of baking soda, and four tablespoons of sugar in a liter of water. Drink it when thirsty to prevent dehydration. Avoid alcohol; it promotes urination, diarrhea, and dehydration.

SELF-CARE

Sip water, soup, vegetable juice, or the solution described above. Avoid fruit juices and other very sweet liquids, sorbitol-containing products, dairy products, magnesium-containing antacids and dietary supplements, caffeine, and fatty foods. For chronic diarrhea one or more of these proscriptions may become permanent. For example, you may turn out to be lactose intolerant (most black and Asian adults are to some extent) and will have to avoid milk unless the enzyme lactase has been added. Or you may be sensitive to sorbitol. If you have irritable bowel syndrome, which is characterized by long-standing chronic diarrhea, cramping, and gas with no known cause, you may have to avoid all the culprits above plus increase your dietary fiber and perhaps take a commercial fiber supplement, preferably one with psyllium seed. All chronic diarrhea should be evaluated by a physician.

See a physician immediately if:

- stool or vomitus is very dark or bloody;
- there is also severe abdominal pain, stiff neck, or headache;
- there is also confusion or extreme lethargy in a young child.

Consult a physician if:

- medication is being taken—it may be the cause or it may be rendered ineffective by the symptoms;
- there are signs of dehydration (thirst, intensely yellow urine, dry mouth, inelastic skin), diabetes, pregnancy, urinary problems, or a recent head injury;
- there is no improvement within three days.

Dizziness and Blacking Out

There are several innocuous reasons for faintness or vertigo (dizziness, visual field spinning, or lurching). Sometimes one need only recover from the flu, a cold, or alcohol or other drug intoxication, or not stand up too quickly in order to recover from the symptoms. Avoiding cigarette smoke and excessive caffeine may help. Sometimes medical attention is required (see also **Motion Sickness** and **Anxiety Disorders**).

See a physician immediately if:

- unexplained loss of consciousness occurs;
- the symptoms are associated with hives (a severe allergic reaction may be in progress).

Consult a physician if:

- severe vertigo unrelated to a cold or flu occurs;
- the symptoms are related to drug use (medicines, alcohol, cocaine, or any other).

Ear and Hearing Problems

Common causes of ear pain, stuffiness, itching, and hearing problems are allergies, colds, swimmer's ear, surfer's ear, and unusual wax accumulation. The problems can usually be cleared up with simple home treatments, but sometimes medical care is necessary.

Consult a physician if:

- there is hearing loss or ear pain unexplained by excessive wax accumulation, a cold, or allergy;
- there is itching, pain, or redness of the ear opening and canal lasting more than five days;
- there is ear pain followed by a white or yellowish discharge;
- there are signs of ear or hearing problems in an infant or child, like the child rubbing and pulling an ear and trying to scratch the ear canal, a lack of reaction to sounds, or slower than expected language development.

Eye and Vision Problems

Except for minor allergic itching and easily removable foreign objects, most eye and vision problems should be evaluated and treated by a family physician, ophthalmologist, or optometrist.

See a physician immediately if there is:

- an injury to the eye, such as a cut or puncture, or a blow that affects vision or causes severe pain;
- something in the eye that remains after flushing the eye with water;
- a solvent, acid, or other chemical that gets into the eye and causes pain or severe irritation that persists after copious flushing with water;
- sudden vision loss in one or both eyes or the appearance of halos around lights;
- inflammation of an eye that occurs while a cold sore or genital herpes is present;
- pain involving contact lenses;
- unusual sensitivity to light;
- any unusual or alarming symptom or visual change.

Consult an ophthalmologist if there is:

- eye pain, itching, dryness, redness, or discharge that is severe or persists longer than two days;

- visual loss or visual defects that seem to be progressively worse;
- a discharge that resembles pus;
- inflammation of the tear ducts.

Fainting

See **Dizziness and Blacking Out.**

Fatigue and Weakness

Excessive fatigue is most commonly caused by insufficient rest, lack of exercise, too much exercise, boredom, depression, and abuse of alcohol, marijuana, caffeine, and other psychoactive drugs. Attention to these factors often brings relief. However, fatigue and weakness can also be signs of illness or malnutrition requiring medical attention.

Consult a physician soon if unusual or unexplained fatigue persists for several days.

Chronic Fatigue Syndrome (CFS)

CFS is characterized by fatigue, general weakness, headache, sore throat, mild fever, muscle and joint aches, insomnia, depression, painful lymph nodes, and abdominal pains. It may last for months or even years. In a very similar condition called *fibromyalgia* (or fibrositis), soft tissue aches and pains predominate, but many of the symptoms are the same as in CFS; some experts suspect the two will prove to be the same disease.

Some physicians believe that CFS is due to chronic infection with one or another common virus. They advocate extensive and frequent testing, sometimes for years. Since there is essentially no treatment, the purpose of all this expensive care is apparently to assure the patient that he or she has a "real" disease and is not a hypochondriac.

It may be true that chronic fatigue is caused by one or more viruses, but no one knows which one(s). Suspects include Epstein–Barr virus (EBV, which really does cause the acute flulike illness mononucleosis), coxsackievirus B, cytomegalovirus (CMV), and several others. Perhaps an undiscovered virus or even a cumulative effect of two or more viruses is the culprit. Until we have more definitive diagnostic methods and effective treatments, extensive testing for possible virus infections seems pointless and wasteful.

Patients should understand that they may very well have a chronic virus infection of some kind. But the only treatment that is reasonable and often effective is proper rest, exercise, nutrition, and, in some cases, antidepressant medication. A prescription for the latter does not mean the doctor thinks the problem is "all in your head." For all we know, these drugs may counter the effects of some virus(es). None of the herbal remedies, vitamins, or bizarre diets promoted in "health food" stores are effective.

Fear, Irrational

See **Anxiety Disorders.**

Fertility Problems

Ten to fifteen percent of all young couples in the United States have some problem with fertility. About half of these can be traced to the woman, a third to the man, and the rest to incompatibility between his sperm and her fluids and tissues. When we consider the complexity of the events that lead to fertilization, implantation, gestation, and birth, it is not surprising that things can go wrong. Fertility specialists can often find the cause of the trouble and prescribe effective therapy. However, the examinations can be time consuming, inconvenient, unpleasant, and expensive, so couples should consider a number of simple remedies before seeking help unless, of course, there is an obvious or suspected problem like infection or lack of ovulation and periods.

General Measures and Remedies Worth Trying

Men should avoid exposure to pesticides, alcohol, marijuana, tobacco, and other unnecessary drugs, as well as jockstraps, tight pants, frequent prolonged baths, and other causes of overheated testes. If they work in a hot kitchen or factory they should wear the coolest possible clothes. They might increase their intake of vitamin C foods or even take supplements up to 500 milligrams per day for a couple weeks; the vitamin seems to decrease sperm agglutination (clumping). This is not likely to help men who have adequate vitamin C in their blood, but may help those who have had low intakes for months or years.

Women should, of course, be having periods. Even then they should confirm that they are ovulating. They should faithfully record their basal temperature every morning for several months (before rising or being active). If it does not increase by ½ to 1°F for several days in about the third week of the cycle, ovulation may not be occuring. They should also note the length of the second half of the cycle. If the temperature increases at the normal time, but the period starts within a week instead of two weeks of ovulation, it may be reasonably suspected that the corpeus luteum (a part of the ovary) is not producing enough hormones. Making these observations before seeing a specialist can save time and money.

Women should maintain good general health, avoid exposure to chemicals and drugs, and make sure they are not exercising or dieting so much that periods stop. Caffeine intake should be minimized; as little as a cup of coffee each day reduces the likelihood of pregnancy in some women. They should not use lubricating jelly before intercourse and should stay in bed for up to a half hour after intercourse. They should avoid douching other than to try a mild baking soda douche (one or two tablespoons per quart of water) before intercourse to counter semen that is possibly too acidic.

Couples should have intercourse several times a month on various days during the menstrual cycle for at least a year. Most women are fertile around midcycle, i.e. about fourteen days from the first day of each period. A day before ovulation is probably the best time for intercourse. Couples should make sure ejaculation occurs deep in the vagina, which usually means he should be on top of her. They can try abstinence for four to seven days or for the first half of her cycle in order to increase his sperm concentration.

Seeking professional help. If a solid year of effort and home remedies do not bring results, couples should carefully select a fertility specialist, based on advice from their family physician, her obstetrician, and friends who have been successfully treated. If possible, consult a physician who is certified by the American Board of Obstetrics and Gynecology as a specialist in fertility. Expect lots of questions, discussions, tests, and examinations. The purpose is to detect any hormonal or anatomical abnormalities, or infections that might affect fertility.

If the problem lies with the woman possible treatments include antibiotics to clear up any chronic infection, hormones to stimulate ovulation, and surgery to remove scarring, adhesions, tumors, and other growths that interfere with the functions of the tubes, ovaries, or vagina.

If the man is the source of the problem, it is usually because of defective sperm or low concentration of sperm in his semen. Sometimes diabetes, varicose testicular veins, or bacterial infections can be found and treated.

Other options include artificial insemination, either with the partner's sperm or an anonymous donor's, and *in vitro* fertilization, in which an egg from the woman is fertilized with sperm in a laboratory and then reimplanted into her uterus.

Fever

The normal resting body temperature is about 98.6°F (37°C), but it can be almost a Fahrenheit degree lower or higher without being a sign of illness. Eating and excitement can raise the temperature, and exercise can increase it to about 103°F. (A higher temperature associated with exercise may be a sign of impending heat stroke.) A fever is a resting temperature above 100°F, except in ovulating women.

The most common causes of fever are viral and bacterial infections such as measles, chickenpox, flu, and strep throat. Temperatures under 104°F are not usually dangerous. A fever is part of the body's attempt to fight off the infection, so unless it causes significant discomfort or is over 104°F there is no reason to treat it.

SELF-CARE

If relief is needed, a lukewarm sponge bath and aspirin, acetaminophen, or ibuprofen are usually effective. Don't give aspirin to children who may have chickenpox or influenza. Water and at least a little food or juice should be taken. Cotton clothing and bedding are preferable because they absorb perspiration.

See a physician immediately if the fever is not obviously caused by a minor illness or if the temperature is above:

- 104°F,
- 100°F in an infant younger than four months of age,
- 100°F and there is also a stiff neck, seizures, rapid breathing, confusion, or other alarming symptom(s).

Consult a physician if a fever:

- persists for more than three days;
- persists for more than one day in an infant between four and twelve months of age;
- is associated with a rash or hives;
- is associated with drug use (licit or illicit).

Frostbite

Frostnip is mild and superficial frostbite. The skin may be numb or mildly painful, blanch with pressure, and have a waxy appearance. True frostbite causes severe pain, blisters, and bluish skin. Underlying tissues are frozen hard and do not give when the area is gently pressed.

SELF-CARE

Frostnip can be treated with general warming and warm water (not more than 108°F) or gentle pressure with warm hands. Do not rub, expose to high temperature (like an oven or open fire), or apply ointments, lotions, or medicines of any kind. Avoid drinking alcohol and using tobacco.

See a physician immediately if pain is severe, the skin is blistered or bluish, or the tissue is frozen hard. Wrap the affected area in a blanket to protect it from bruising, keep it elevated if possible, and get to a hospital.

Consult a physician if mild frostbite becomes painful, blue, or swollen as the area warms up.

Fungus Infections

Various fungal infections of the skin occur on the scalp, head, trunk, genitals, nails, hands, and feet. Reddish or greyish patches with itching, stinging, and scaling are the usual symptoms. On the trunk and scalp the lesions can appear ringlike and sometimes cause the hair to fall out. Several fungi produce this type of infection, which is spread by contact with infected people or their clothing or from infected pets, especially cats. In the case of athlete's foot, moist areas in showers and around swimming pools can harbor and spread the fungi. These fungi are very widespread, possibly even present on most people's feet most of the time. Some people are much more susceptible than others, for unknown reasons.

PREVENTION AND SELF-CARE

Avoid sharing towels, clothing, hairbrushes, and the like. Avoid scratching, rubbing, or even touching an affected area. Keep the skin, especially the feet, clean, cool, and dry. It may be necessary to decrease activity in order to decrease heat and moisture. Stimulants like coffee, tea, and colas may increase perspiration. Wear clean, dry, loose clothing and shoes. For athlete's foot, wash between the toes and dry well twice a day. A drying agent like calamine or talcum powder will help keep the area dry. Whenever possible go barefoot or wear sandals to allow maximum ventilation.

Nonprescription products with tolnaftate or miconazole are often very effective. However, it is important to use them only if necessary because allergic reaction and irritation are common. Those with allergies should test the medicine on a small area of skin before using. It is important not to overtreat if irritation and dermatitis are to be avoided.

Consult a physician if self-care measures don't work. In very stubborn cases, a physician may prescribe a drug that gets into the skin via the blood and kills the fungi. It is particularly effective when the face, neck, trunk, and nails are affected.

Hair Loss

Many men and some women lose substantial amounts of hair as they age. This is usually caused by genes and hormones and there is *no cure,* the sensational claims for quack remedies notwithstanding.

In alopecia areata, hair is completely lost in a limited, usually small, area. The scalp is normal and there is no known cause. The hair usually regrows within a year. The problem often recurs within a few years but eventually resolves itself.

SELF-CARE

If baldness runs in your family and you start to lose your hair without scalp abnormalities, you'll probably have to learn to live with it. A prescription drug, minoxidil, is heavily promoted as a baldness remedy, but it is expensive, it must be used indefinitely, and its effects are impressive in only a small minority of patients. If apparent alopecia areata occurs keep an eye on the affected area for scalp abnormalities. Make sure your hair loss is not caused by tight braids or ponytails, or by habitual hair pulling.

Consult a physician if hair loss is associated with scalp redness, scaling, oozing, or other abnormality, or if hair is present but fails to grow normally or breaks easily. A fungus infection may be the cause.

Hallucinations and Delusions

These are serious symptoms that can be caused by drug abuse, drug withdrawal, or psychosis. In any case, a physician should be seen right away.

Hand and Wrist Pain

See also **Joint Inflammation and Pain.**

The most common cause of pain, numbness, tingling and weakness in the fingers, hand, and wrist is carpal tunnel syndrome (CTS). In this condition the median nerve is compressed in the narrow passage through the wrist. Many conditions predispose one to CTS, including arthritis, gout, diabetes, pregnancy, and thyroid problems. However, the most important cause is probably occupational trauma. Workers commonly at risk are word processors, assembly-line workers, meat packers, deboners, those who use vibrating tools, truck loaders, piano players, and others whose hands and wrists are repeatedly stressed or flexed. CTS is a serious occupational hazard that employers should protect their workers from. If you suspect your job is responsible for your symptoms, discuss the problem with your boss, your union representative, or OSHA (Occupational Safety and Health Administration). Sleeping with the wrists sharply flexed or with the head resting on a hand can aggravate the problem.

Consult a physician if simple measures such as rest, stretching, and padding vibrating tools don't work.

Headaches

Possibly the most common of human pains, headaches arise from the arteries or muscles of the head and neck or from abnormal neurotransmitter activity in the brain.

Tension headaches or muscle contraction headaches are the most common. The pain, usually tightness and pressure without exact location, comes from sustained constriction of scalp, neck, and face muscles. Poor posture on the job (at a desk, cash register, or assembly line) with prolonged flexion (bending) of the neck can trigger such a headache. Depression, fatigue, and emotional stress can also be factors.

Self-care: Remedies include rest, quiet, warm bath, gentle massage, aspirin and other pain relievers, and meditation and relaxation exercises. The frequent victim may benefit from more rest and relaxation, and less emotional and mental stress.

Migraine headaches are often preceded or accompanied by visual and psychological changes and sometimes nausea and vomiting. The pain, which is usually limited to one side, is pounding and often incapacitating. Migraines are fairly common, especially among young women; they affect perhaps 8 percent of the United States population and tend to run in families.

Suspected precipitating factors include certain foods (strong cheeses, red wines, chocolate, pickles, cured meats, and foods with MSG or nitrates), niacin in large doses (which can dilate the blood vessels), alcohol, caffeine, nicotine, estrogen (naturally during the menstrual cycle or from oral contraceptives or estrogen replacement therapy), excessive sun, and chemicals (fumes and vapors), including perfumes. Sometimes very common foods, such as milk, wheat, corn, eggs, soybeans, and peanuts, cause migraines. Detection of the culprit(s) in these cases requires an elimination diet (also called an allergy diet), followed by challenges with suspected foods. If you suspect a food is causing headaches don't try a radical diet without consulting a physician or registered dietician.

Self-care: Treatment includes relaxation, certain drugs, and biofeedback. At the first sign of an attack it is important to sit or lie in a quiet, dark room. Two to four aspirin or the prescribed dose of migraine medication, taken right away, may abort the attack. It is very important not to take aspirin or any other pain killer too often; this will aggravate the problem. If you find yourself taking drugs on more than two days a week, ask a physician about nondrug remedies. Biofeedback can be especially helpful. And consider the herb *feverfew*. Chewing one or two fresh leaves each day may reduce the frequency and severity of migraines.

Cluster headaches, like migraines, may be associated with changes in the blood vessels of the neck and head; some specialists consider them migraine variants. They are distinguished from typical migraines by a knifelike piercing pain around and behind one eye, tearing, and nasal congestion. The pain is very severe but nonthrobbing, and the onset and cessation are sudden. The headaches tend to occur in clusters of several a day with recurrences every few weeks or more often. Cluster headaches are much less common than migraines, do not run in families, and affect men much more often than women. Simply stopping smoking often provides dramatic relief from recurrent attacks.

Sinus headaches can be brought on by sinusitis, colds, or hay fever. In sinusitis, the sinuses—cavities in the facial bones that normally drain through small openings into the nasal passages—become congested and inflamed due to bacterial infection. The pressure build-up from the trapped mucus and pus causes facial pain, headache, and sometimes tooth pain. Sinus infections can be very serious. If you suspect this is the cause of your headache, **consult a physician** right away.

Prevention and self-care: Treat colds properly. Drink plenty of fluids and get lots of rest. Avoid cigarette and other smoke to prevent irritation, inflammation, and obstruction of the sinuses. Do not abuse decongestant sprays; the resulting chronic congestion could aggravate sinusitis. These products should not be used for more than three days. Blow your nose gently and without pressing hard to avoid forcing infected mucus further into the sinuses. Be alert for irritation from swimming in chlorinated or salt water. Use a nose clip if necessary.

Drug headaches are caused by alcohol, tobacco, cocaine, and marijuana, either simultaneously with intoxication or as an aftereffect or hangover.

Toxic headaches can be caused by exposure to chemicals such as benzene, gasoline, paints, formaldehyde, and glue.

Caffeine-withdrawal headaches are fairly common in those who normally drink coffee, tea, or colas every day, and then suddenly stop. Taking caffeine after the headache starts is often not effective, but aspirin may help. Ease off caffeine rather than quitting "cold turkey."

Hypertension headaches occur in about 10 percent of those with hypertension. They usually occur in the morning. They may be very severe and resemble a migraine, but migraine medicines should not be used. Antihypertensive drug therapy is usually necessary.

Bruxism headaches can be caused by excessive clenching and grinding of the teeth or excessive gum chewing. Learn to relax and decrease emotional tension.

TMJ headaches. Abnormal temporomandibular joints (where the jaw meets the skull) can cause headaches, neck and shoulder pain, and other symptoms. The joint dysfunction may be due to arthritis, injury, habitually clenching the teeth, biting on hard objects, excessive gum chewing or other overuse, or malocclusion (bad bite). TMJ should be considered a possible cause of the symptoms if there is pain or clicking noises when the jaw is moved, if the jaw seems to lock, dislocate, or has limited movement, or if the teeth are sore or excessively worn.

Self-care: When symptoms flare up eat soft food; alternate ice and heat application; don't chew gum or clench a pipe or cigar between the teeth; sleep with a single flat pillow; don't sleep on your stomach; and develop jaw awareness to avoid clenching or grinding teeth when awake.

Many dentists are trained to detect and treat TMJ syndromes. A removable plastic biteplate fitted to the upper teeth and worn for about four months (except when eating or brushing the teeth) often solves the problem. Other remedies include fixing bad teeth, replacing missing teeth, spot grinding of high spots in the bite, braces, and surgical repair of the joints. Symptoms often clear up without treatment in a few weeks, so don't rush into radical or expensive treatment.

Carbon monoxide poisoning often causes headaches and dizziness in those who use gas kitchen stoves for supplemental heat. Poor ventilation and smoking increase the likelihoood of carbon monoxide poisoning.

Dehydration and heat stress can cause headaches. Drink lots of water before and during prolonged exercise or exposure to the sun or heat, including sauna baths.

IMPORTANT

Rarely a headache is a sign of a tumor, meningitis, stroke, glaucoma, diabetes, or other serious problems. Anyone with a severe headache of unknown origin, a headache associated with nausea, fever, or other symptoms, or a headache associated with head injury, even days after the injury, should see a physician.

See a physician immediately if:

- a headache is associated with a head injury;
- there is also fever, stiff neck, or visual problems;
- a severe headache comes on suddenly and is unlike any previous one.

Consult a physician if:

- headaches have persisted for three days or longer;
- frequent headaches are worse in the morning.

Head Injuries

Head injuries that involve or put pressure on the brain or cranial nerves require immediate medical attention.

See a physician immediately if there is:

- unconsciousness, seizure, stupor, visual changes, or lack of memory of the injury;
- vomiting;
- irregular breathing or heartbeat;
- bleeding or other fluid from the nose, eyes, ears, or mouth;
- blackness around the eyes or ears;
- any other suspicious or serious symptoms.

Heartburn and Hyperacidity

Excessive acid production and inadequate protection by the gastric lining are the most common causes of a burning sensation in the stomach and beneath the breastbone. Stomach acid refluxing into the esophagus can also be the culprit. (See **Stomach Acid Related Disorders,** Section Two.)

It is important not to ignore these symptoms because the problem can result in serious tissue injury. Very effective prescription drugs are available to deal with acid-related problems.

SELF-CARE

Don't lie down after eating, avoid tight clothing, drink generous amounts of water, take antacids (occasionally), and avoid alcohol, cigarettes, aspirin, ibuprofen, and caffeine. Eat small frequent meals.

See a physician immediately if there is very dark or bloody stool or vomitus.

Consult a physician if:

- pain is severe and seems to involve the back;

- pain lasts more than three days;
- pain is not easily controlled with antacids.

Heatstroke

Heatstroke is most likely to occur with overexercise in a hot environment when water intake has been inadequate. A body temperature above 104° F and climbing is dangerous and must be treated to prevent convulsions, brain damage, and death. The patient should be immersed in cool water or wrapped in wet cloth until he or she can be taken to a hospital.

See a physician immediately if heavy exercise or work is associated with extreme fatigue, confusion, headache, dizziness, racing pulse, and hot, dry skin.

Hemorrhoids

A hemorrhoid is a mass of dilated, tortuous veins in the anorectal area. Hemorrhoids usually result from habitual straining during defecation, often associated with small stools and constipation. They can cause severe itching, bleeding, and pain, and sometimes require medical treatment.

PREVENTION AND SELF-CARE

Eat generous amounts of whole grains, vegetables, beans, and fruits. Drink lots of water. Exercise regularly; walking is especially good for those prone to hemorrhoids. Be gentle when wiping yourself. If you neglect these things and do develop hemorrhoids, get back on track right away. For symptomatic relief try petroleum jelly or zinc oxide; they are soothing and prevent irritation.

Consult a physician if:

- hemorrhoid symptoms are severe and not relieved by the above simple measures;
- hemorrhoids are bleeding (check the toilet paper) or causing stools to be pencil-thin.

Hiccups

A hiccup is a spasm of the diaphragm. A stubborn attack of hiccups can be very annoying, even exhausting. Here are three home remedies worth trying:

(1) Eat two teaspoons of plain, dry, white granulated sugar.
(2) Breathe into a paper bag for several minutes.
(3) Lie on your back on a bed with your shoulders extending several inches beyond the edge. Stretch your arms beyond your head, take a deep breath, and hold it as long as you can. Repeat if necessary.

Consult a physician if hiccups last more than a couple hours, or if you get them every day. Hiccups are rarely caused by a serious disorder.

Hoarseness

See **Cough and Hoarseness.**

Hyperventilation Syndrome

Stress and anxiety frequently cause a person to unconsciously hyperventilate or overbreathe. There is often a sense of needing to yawn, and one may try to have a good satisfying yawn. This lowers carbon dioxide in the blood, which causes tingling of the extremities, lightheadedness, tightness in the chest, palpitations, and blurred vision. Other symptoms, such as nightmares, tremors, weakness, and fatigue, may also occur. The fear caused by the symptoms leads to further hyperventilation, and so on. Episodes may last for minutes or hours. They may become so frequent that the syndrome is nearly continuous, though varying in intensity.

SELF-CARE

When you feel an attack starting take a brisk walk or do some other moderate to vigorous exercise, or get busy with some chore, hobby, or game. Sometimes the problem is aggravated by excessive attention to one's breathing. Vigorous activity or absorption in something that takes your mind off your breathing may help. Don't drink coffee or take other stimulants.

You may be advised to lie down in a quiet place, relax, and stop taking deep breaths and sighing. Or hold your breath for brief periods, or breathe into a paper bag for a few minutes to get your carbon dioxide level back to normal. The theory is good and it may help some people. The problem is that these techniques increase attention to breathing and if you can nip the problem in the bud by a little exercise, you won't develop low carbon dioxide levels.

See a physician immediately unless the symptoms are familiar to you and have been evaluated by your doctor.

Consult a physician if the above symptoms occur often and are not helped by self-care measures.

Infertility

See **Fertility Problems.**

Insect, Spider, and Jellyfish Stings and Bites

Most of these can be treated by removing any remaining stinger(s) and applying ice. See also **Tick-Borne Diseases** in Section Two.

See a physician immediately if:

- this or a previous sting has led to signs of allergic response such as difficulty in breathing, fainting, abdominal pain, hives, or a rash;
- the culprit was, or might have been, a black widow or brown recluse spider.

Consult a physician if the wound is very inflamed and painful, pus develops, or there is fever or other unusual symptoms.

Jaundice

Jaundice, a yellowing of the whites of the eyes, is caused by an accumulation of bilirubin (a product of normal red blood cell breakdown) in the blood. It can be a sign of hepatitis, cancer, blood disease, or other serious problems.

Consult a physician if you notice changes in the color of the eyes, skin, or perspiration.

Joint Inflammation and Pain

The most common types of arthritis are gout, osteoarthritis, and rheumatoid arthritis. In gout, there is crystalization of uric acid in joints or tendons. In osteoarthritis, joints gradually become inflamed, painful, and stiff with aging and wear and tear. In rheumatoid arthritis, besides joint inflammation and pain, there is often systemic illness (involving the whole body). Specific prescription medicines are used for each type of arthritis.

Consult a physician if:

- there is severe pain, swelling, or inability to use a joint;
- joint pain is accompanied by fever;
- the problem is chronic or sometimes associated with a general feeling of sickness or weakness.

Lumpy Breasts (Fibrocystic Breast Changes)

See **Cancer—Early Warning Signs; Breast Lumps (Fibrocystic Breast Changes).**

Lice

Head and pubic lice are common, the former mostly in children and the latter mostly in adults. These insects are very small and hard to find without a magnifying glass. Their egg clusters, called nits, are little white lumps stuck to hair strands. Lice bites cause intense itching. Head lice are commonly spread between children during play. Pubic lice, also called "crabs," can spread during sexual contact. Both types can also be spread by infected linen, clothing, and furniture.

SELF-CARE

Use a nonprescription product from a drugstore along with a fine-tooth comb to remove the nits. Wash bedding and clothing at the same time. Close friends of children and sexual partners of adults should be inspected and treated if necessary.

Consult a physician if self-care fails, or if severe infestation and scratching has led to skin irritation, bleeding, or scabbing.

Mania

See **Depression and Mania.**

Menstrual and Related Problems

See **Female Disorders** in Section Two. Here is a summary of indications that one should see a physician.

See a physician immediately if:
- symptoms of toxic shock syndrome occur. There is no self-care for TSS. Remove any tampon and see a doctor now if fever plus any of the following occur: diarrhea, vomiting, peeling of hands or feet, a rash, dizziness, fainting, sore throat, vaginitis, red eyes, or severe headache.
- symptoms of ectopic pregnancy occur—i.e., you are or may be pregnant, and you experience severe abdominal pains and abnormal bleeding.

Consult a physician if:
- you miss your period two months in a row;
- itching, burning, or other signs of vaginal infection occur;
- menstrual pain is severe or occurs for the first time after age twenty-five;
- excessive menstrual bleeding occurs;
- menstrual pain is severe, intercourse is frequently painful, periods are prolonged and irregular, or chronic pelvic pain occurs;
- heavy bleeding or unusual pelvic pain occurs;
- large unexplained changes in menstrual patterns occur;
- you suspect menopause may be starting. Adverse effects can often be prevented or treated with the proper use of estrogens and lubricants;
- unexplained sharp abdominal pains occur;
- unusual or excessive bleeding occurs;

- premenstrual symptoms, like bloating, irritability, and headaches, occur often and are severe;
- bleeding is heavy for several consecutive periods;
- premenstrual syndrome includes severe depression, anxiety, or suicidal impulses;
- any other unusual symptoms occur.

Mental and Emotional Problems

Minor mental and emotional problems are best dealt with with the help of family and friends, but sometimes professional attention is required.

Consult your doctor, who may refer you to a psychiatrist or clinical psychologist if you or a loved one experience:

- suicidal or homicidal urges;
- unexplained fatigue associated with sadness, headaches, decreased libido, or insomnia;
- extreme anxiety, phobias, hallucinations, delusions, confusion, or temper tantrums;
- symptoms of an eating disorder, such as being repulsed by food or eating compulsively.

Motion Sickness

Motion sickness, or seasickness, consists of nausea, cold sweats, pallor, fatigue, and sometimes vomiting provoked by the motion of a boat, car, or other conveyance. It is apparently triggered by conflicting information from our eyes and the balance organs of our inner ears. For example, if you read in a car that's going around curves and up and down hills, your eyes detect little or no motion, but your inner ear senses a roller-coaster ride.

SELF-CARE

If you're on a boat, try to be active rather than sit still. Help with the fishing or steer the boat. Don't go below deck except to sleep. If you must just sit, look at the waves or the horizon; anticipate the motion and "ride" the waves. If you're in a car, focus your gaze outside. Children should have a good view out a window. If you decide to use a nonprescription drug like atropine or cyclizine to combat motion sickness, remember to take it well before the trip starts or it will have little effect.

See a physician if you anticipate severe motion sickness. A prescription antihistamine works well and has few side effects.

Mouth Sores

There are several kinds of sores than can occur in and around the mouth. The most common are canker sores and oral herpes. Canker sores are painful little ulcers with a yellowish border surrounded by a red zone. The cause is unknown, but they may be precipitated, or at least aggravated, by some toothpastes and foods. They usually last a few days to a week. Herpes infections usually do not require immediate medical attention, but consulting a physician may be useful for the consideration of treatment with acyclovir (an antiviral drug) and for counseling on symptomatic treatment and avoiding the spread of the virus. Avoid touching the sore since you could spread the virus. Be especially careful about touching infants and sharing objects with them.

Consult a physician if:

- you have painful, recurrent, or persistant mouth sores;
- you have white patches on the roof of your mouth;
- you developed mouth sores after starting a medication;
- you have a persistant, painless sore or lump anywhere in or around the mouth.

Nasal Discharges and Bleeding

Nasal discharges are almost always due to colds or allergies and can be treated with simple home remedies and nonprescription drugs (see Section Four). Nosebleeds are usually due to excessive nose blowing, trauma to the nose, and habitual nose picking (especially in children). Nosebleeds almost always stop by themselves, but may require ten to fifteen minutes of pressure on the nose. The person should sit upright. Applying ice may help.

Consult a physician if:

- the discharge is thick and foul-smelling;
- the discharge is clear or bloody and began after a head injury;

- nosebleeds are frequent and unexplained;
- nosebleeds are caused by snorting drugs.

Nausea

See **Diarrhea and Vomiting; Motion Sickness; Anxiety Disorders.**

Night Sweats

Heavy sweating unrelated to ambient temperature and humidity can have several possible causes. If it comes on gradually it may be due to obesity or smoking: Overweight people tend to perspire more to keep cool; smoking damages the lungs and makes them less efficient at releasing moisture, and sweating compensates for this. Losing weight and quitting smoking are obvious remedies.

Consult a physician if heavy night sweating is not due to a cold or other apparent infection, or if night sweating lasts for more than two weeks.

Palpitations

See **Breathing Problems, Chest Pains, and Palpitations; Anxiety Disorders.**

Panic

See **Anxiety Disorders.**

Pinworms

These intestinal parasites are extremely common, especially in children. They cause intense itching around the anus, where the females go to lay their eggs. Restless sleep and scratching are common signs of infection. The worms occasionally migrate into the vagina or urethra. Scratching leads to contamination of eating utensils, doorknobs, and other objects with the eggs, which can be swallowed by others. Shaking contaminated bedding and clothing can release eggs into the air. These can be inhaled and swallowed by others, who then become infected.

Consult a physician if you suspect pinworm infection. The nonprescription drug pyrantel pamoate works well and may have to be taken by the entire family. Children's fingernails should be kept short. Hands should be washed frequently, especially after bowel movements. Clothing and bedding should be washed, but not shaken. Bedrooms should be vacuumed frequently.

Poisoning

In any case of suspected poisoning **a physician should be called or seen immediately.** If one cannot be reached, call the local poison control center.

If the ingested substance is known to be a drug or poisonous plant (for example, aspirin, iron, apricot kernels, toxic mushroom, or oleander), induce vomiting with a finger down the throat or warm salty water (about one-half teaspoon per cup). Be prepared to give syrup of ipecac or activated charcoal if so advised by a doctor or poison control center.

If the material is a caustic substance such as battery acid, bleach, drain cleaner, furniture polish, or gasoline, do *not* induce vomiting—give activated charcoal or milk.

PREVENTING POISONINGS

Keep all drugs, nutritional supplements, skin and hair products, and household chemicals out of the reach of young children. Keep only those household chemicals you really need and use, and get rid of old containers. Use all dangerous chemicals with proper protective clothing, safety glasses, and the utmost care. Keep syrup of ipecac and activated charcoal on hand.

Punctures

See **Cuts, Abrasions, Punctures, and Animal Bites.**

Rash

See also **Shingles.**

See a physician immediately if:

- hives or itching are associated with rapid or difficult breathing or dizziness, or occur subsequent to drug use;

- a rash suspected of being measles, rubella, or chickenpox is associated with rapid or difficult breathing, stiff neck, severe lethargy, headaches, convulsions, vomiting, or bleeding from the mouth, nose, rectum, or under the skin;
- a fine, rough rash occurs on the trunk and extremities, and there is a fever (this could be scarlet fever, a strep infection that can cause heart and kidney problems).

Consult a physician if you develop a rash unfamiliar to you.

Rectal Bleeding

See a physician immediately if blood is black or burgundy and appears to be mixed into the stool itself.

Consult a physician if blood is bright red and appears on toilet paper. (See **Hemorrhoids,** above.)

Rectal Pain or Itching

See **Hemorrhoids; Pinworms.**

Scabies

This is skin irritation caused by infection with a tiny mite that burrows under the skin, usually between the fingers, under the arms, at the elbow crease, or behind the knees. Intense itching leads to scratching, which can predispose the skin to bacterial infection. Inflammation and blistering often obscure the telltale burrows. Infection spreads easily by personal contact, and contaminated clothing and bedding.

SELF-CARE

Use the nonprescription drug benzyl benzoate (25 percent), applying it all over the body except the face and close to the vaginal or penile opening. Leave it on for twenty-four hours.

Consult a physician if you cannot find benzyl benzoate, or if inflammation is very severe and affected areas develop pus.

308 Scoliosis

Scoliosis is a lateral (sideways) curvature of the spine, which appears S-shaped from the back. Mild curvature causes little or no problems, but if allowed to progress it can cause degenerative arthritis of the spine, disk disease, severe back pain, sciatica, narrowing of the chest cavity, and difficult breathing. It usually appears between ages ten and fifteen and can rapidly worsen during the growth-spurt years. It is often overlooked, though, until it is severe. While equally common in boys and girls, it tends to be more serious in girls. The cause is unknown, but the disorder tends to run in families. It is not caused by and should not be confused with poor posture.

Early detection and treatment are important to prevent the disorder from becoming severe. A brace along with an exercise program can correct the curvature enough to prevent complications. Exercises alone are of little or no benefit. In a few very severe cases surgery is required, followed by a cast for several months.

Some mild curvatures get worse and require treatment; some do not. It is important that all cases be watched carefully through the adolescent years so treatment can be started as soon as it becomes necessary. Despite claims to the contrary, there is no evidence that chiropractic manipulations are an effective and safe treatment for scoliosis. Delay in getting proper treatment can lead to long-term problems.

Early Warning Signs

Parents, physicians, teachers, and school nurses should be alert to the following signs in adolescents.

Consult a physician if:

- one shoulder is higher than the other, one arm hangs lower, or one shoulder blade is more prominent;
- hips are tilted or the waistline is more indented on one side;
- a pronounced curve is seen when tracing the backbone with a finger;
- one side of the back is higher than the other when bending forward;
- hemline or pants legs are uneven;
- leaning to one side.

Seizures

See **Convulsions, Seizures.**

Sexual Dysfunctions

Anorgasmia

Some women have never experienced orgasm. Sexual excitement occurs, but it only goes so far.

Self-care: Avoid deceiving your partner, by faking an orgasm, for example. Communicate your needs and desires. Avoid scheduled sex and demands for performance placed on either partner. The focus should be on prolonged pleasure and affection as goals in themselves, not as means to the goal of intercourse and satisfaction. Become aware of your own body by self-exploration to orgasm if possible. Learn what you like, then guide your partner.

Consult a sex therapist if these measures don't work.

Erective Impotence, Primary

In this condition, a man has never attained an erection sufficient for vaginal penetration while with a woman. The cause is usually psychological.

Consult a sex therapist if you know you are heterosexual, but have never been able to attain or keep an erection while with a woman.

Erective Impotence, Secondary

This is a repeated lack of erection after previous successes. The cause may be psychological or it may be physical, such as diabetes, atherosclerosis, or drug use. If erections do occur in dreaming or fantasizing, the lack of response with a partner is very likely psychological. But if erections never occur, the cause is probably physical.

Fear is the most common psychological factor in secondary impotence. Fear and sexual arousal are not compatible. The fear can be caused by a single past failure, perhaps due to excess alcohol, marijuana, cocaine, or other drugs. Memories of the failure induce fear of failure the next time. Subsequent efforts are more difficult as the fear of failure grows with each failure.

Self-care: Stop using all alcohol, marijuana, cocaine, tobacco, amphetamines, and other unnecessary drugs. If you are taking a medicine you suspect is interfering with your sex life, discuss the problem with your doctor. Antihypertensive drugs are the most common culprits. Antihistamines and decongestants, including nasal sprays, should also be suspected. In relaxed sessions with your partner, focus on total enjoyment, not performance and not erection. If you do experience an erection, don't rush to intercourse; let the erection come and go in several sessions. This should firmly associate your partner with pleasure while reducing pressure to perform.

Consult a physician if self-care measures don't help.

Painful Intercourse

Common causes include vaginal and cervical infections, endometriosis (see **Female Disorders,** Section Two), complications of surgery, tears in vaginal ligaments, an IUD, and rashes from douches, diaphragms, and contraceptive creams and foams. However, the most common cause is probably inadequate lubrication due to inadequate sexual arousal. Estrogen deficiency after menopause or removal of the ovaries will also cause vaginal dryness and fragility. A water-soluble lubricant can be used, but *not* petroleum jelly.

Consult a physician if you experience persistant pain during intercourse.

Premature Ejaculation

This is the most common sexual dysfunction in men. When a man ejaculates within a few minutes of sex play and cannot delay long enough to satisfy his partner, tension and frustration for both can result. There is no clear definition of "premature," but if a man consistently ejaculates within a few seconds of insertion, or even before insertion, he clearly has a problem.

Self-care: Try the squeeze technique, which often works very well. It's best done with the woman on top. She manually stimulates him just to the point of inevitable ejaculation. To stop it, she presses her thumb against the frenulum (the skin fold on the underside of the penis, just behind the opening) with her first two fingers opposite the thumb, above and below the coronal ridge. Then she resumes stimulation, again just to the point of inevitability before applying the squeeze. This is practiced for several sessions without intercourse or ejaculation until the couple is confident of control. Then she stimulates him as before, applies the squeeze, and inserts his penis, though it may be only semi-erect after the squeeze. They remain still at first, then begin slow pelvic thrusting. If ejaculation seems to be coming, she pulls away and applies the squeeze before reinserting the penis. This is repeated until control during intercourse is established. Patience and care usually bring success.

It might help to use condoms to reduce sensitivity. There are also nonprescription ointments for this purpose. However, they sometimes produce irritation or a rash, in which case their use should be stopped.

Consult a sex therapist if the squeeze technique doesn't work.

Priapism

This is a continuous, painful erection, sustained without erotic stimulation or desire for erection. It usually involves a serious dysfunction of erective mechanisms and may be a symptom of serious disease or a side effect of drugs or hormones. It can cause permanent damage and impotence. Amputation of the penis may be required.

See a physician immediately if priapism occurs.

Vaginismus

During sexual excitement the vagina normally expands to easily accept even the largest penis, but involuntary tightening of the paravaginal muscles can prevent penetration by even the smallest penis. The tightening may also occur during pelvic examination or tampon or diaphragm insertion.

Self-care: The woman and her partner must recognize the problem as a reflex response, not a conscious process. The goal is to desensitize the woman to vaginal insertion. Using a lubricant if necessary, the woman first inserts one finger. When that can be done comfortably, she inserts two, then three, then four. Then her partner inserts a finger, and works up to four. When this is comfortable, he inserts his penis. The process may require great patience and understanding. Recriminations and blaming can retard the process.

Choosing a Sex Therapist

If simple measures taken on your own do not solve your problem, you may benefit from the guidance of a sex counselor. A family physician, gynecologist, psychiatrist, nurse, social worker, or clergyman may be able to recommend a good therapist, or may *be* one. Most urologists are trained to evaluate and treat sexual dysfunctions or refer the patient to an appropriate therapist, preferably a certified sex therapist.

In some cases, it may be better to seek psychotherapy rather than sexual therapy as such. For example, in severe depression sexual dysfunction is just one of several depressed functions, and it would be fruitless to attempt a cure of one symptom. Similarly, if an individual or couple has severe emotional conflicts, the relatively simple techniques of the sex counselor are not likely to improve their sex lives, which cannot be isolated from their relationship as a whole.

Sexually Transmitted Diseases

Most STDs can be prevented by simple measures (see Section Two), but once one is contracted it must be medically evaluated.

Consult a physician if:

- you had sexual contact with a person with a suspected STD;
- you have a sore or wart on your genitals;
- there is a thick discharge from the penis or pain and swelling of the testicles;
- there is unusual vaginal discharge;
- vaginal discharge occurs in a girl before puberty;
- any other unusual genital symptoms occur.

Shingles

Shingles, also called herpes zoster, is a rash with intense burning pain and sometimes a fever. Any part of the body may be affected, but the trunk and face are the most common sites. Only one side of the body is involved. The rash usually clears up in a week or two but may last longer. Nerve damage may occur and cause pain for months, even years.

Shingles is caused by reactivated chickenpox viruses from a previous infection, usually decades earlier.

PREVENTION

A vaccine has been developed that prevents both chickenpox and shingles (in those who have never had chickenpox); it may come into wide use.

SELF-CARE

Keep the hands and nails clean and avoid scratching; this helps prevent infection. Colloidal oatmeal baths (ask a pharmacist) may help relieve itching. Aspirin helps, but in most cases prescription painkillers may be required.

Consult an ophthalmologist immediately if the rash is on the face or an eye is affected. Prompt treatment and close follow-up are essential to prevent serious damage and possible blindness.

Consult a physician if:

- shingles is suspected; prompt treatment can reduce the severity and pain;
- a rash or skin irritation is very severe, widespread, persistent, or shows signs of infection such as weeping and crusting;
- an infant rash has blisters, is more severe in skin creases, or occurs outside the diaper-covered area.

Sleep Disorders

Insomnia can usually be alleviated by regular exercise; avoiding tobacco; avoiding alcohol and caffeine in the evening; and making your bed and bedroom as quiet and comfortable as possible. Reserve the bedroom for sleeping and sex; work should be done elsewhere. Wind down the evening slowly; don't work up until bedtime. Don't go to bed hungry or overly full. Go to bed and get up at the same time everyday. If you can't sleep don't lie there trying or fretting about it; get up and do something else. If these measures don't help and your lack of sleep results in fatigue and sleepiness during the day, consult a physician.

Narcolepsy is an incurable inherited disorder characterized by sudden intense sleep attacks that last from five to ten minutes. Cataplexy is also common in the disorder. This is the sudden loss of muscle tone and physical collapse precipitated by laughter, anger, fear, and other strong emotions. Another common symptom is sleep paralysis, in which the person awakens before muscle tone returns and cannot move, speak, or even open his or her eyes for up to several minutes. Hypnagogic hallucinations may also occur either during wakefulness or suddenly at sleep onset. These are vivid dreams or visions, often of human or animal faces, or an illusion that someone else is in the room. Consult a physician if these symptoms occur.

Nightmares are frightening, vivid dreams in which the dreamer's life is in imminent danger. They may be reactions to recent stress; most people experience them occasionally. If you experience a recurrent nightmare try this: Before going to sleep resolve that if the nightmare occurs you will fight back and attack your tormenter. Success in manipulating the dream this way often ends the recurrence. You should also avoid all mind-altering drugs, especially stimulants. If the nightmares still occur, consult a physician.

Night terrors are as frightening as nightmares, but rather than a vivid dream there is just a sense of terror. Sleepwalking and sleeptalking may also occur. Sleepwalkers should be protected from hazards like open windows and objects that might cause tripping. Regular sleep habits and avoidance of caffeine, alcohol, tobacco, and other mind-altering drugs may help. Children usually just need comforting and support. If the terrors occur at the same time every night, simply waking the child a few minutes before they are "scheduled" and keeping him or her up for five minutes often ends the problem within a week. Adults with recurring night terrors should consult a physician.

Restless legs is a symptom that usually occurs when one is lying down and about to sleep. The legs, especially the lower legs, develop a peculiar discomfort that imparts an urge to kick or shake the legs. The cause is unknown, but caffeine, alcohol, tobacco, and other drugs are suspects. It probably helps to exercise during the day, but exercising when the symptom occurs can either lessen or aggravate restless legs. Applications of heat or cold may help.

Sleep apnea is the recurring cessation of breathing for ten seconds or more, or sometimes for a full minute, during sleep. There is usually loud snoring and thrashing about in bed. Morning headaches, daytime sleepiness, poor memory and concentration, irritability, and loss of sex drive frequently occur. The problem is most common in middle-aged obese men, but it also occurs in the elderly. Self-care consists of losing weight, avoiding alcohol and sleeping pills, and sleeping on your side rather than your back. Since this condition may be associated with several serious health problems and an increased risk of automobile and other accidents, **a physician should be consulted.**

Snoring is more than a nuisance to one's spouse. It may be a sign of sleep apnea (see above). Simple snoring without associated cessation of breathing may be relieved by losing weight and sleeping on one's side.

Sore Throat

Most sore throats are caused by minor viral infections that can be treated with simple home measures like warm salt-water gargles. Sometimes, however, they are caused by bacteria and may require treatment with antibiotics.

Strep throat, or infection with streptococcal bacteria, is much more common in children than adults. It causes throat pain, fever, chills, muscle aches, swollen lymph glands in the neck, and headache. The infection can be diagnosed using a throat culture. (Such cultures are becoming available to the public without a visit to a physician.) Strep throat is a serious problem that requires treatment because it can lead to kidney disease (glomerulonephritis) or rheumatic fever, a complex disease with skin rashes, joint inflammation, and damage to the heart valves. The incidence of rheumatic fever has been increasing lately, so diagnosis and treatment of strep throat are extremely important. If an antibiotic is prescribed, be sure to follow instructions exactly.

See a physician immediately if there is:

- severe difficulty swallowing or breathing,
- excessive drooling in a child or infant.

Consult a physician if:

- there is fever, rash, or pus in the throat;
- a sore throat follows exposure to someone known to have strep throat;
- a sore throat occurs without nasal symptoms or a cough.

Sprains and Strains

See **Bone and Connective Tissue Injuries.**

Stings

See **Insect, Spider, and Jellyfish Stings and Bites.**

Swollen Lymph or Salivary Glands

Swelling of the lymph glands is usually a sign of a localized infection, such as a boil, infected wound, ear infection, or sore throat. More general viral and bacterial illness may also cause swollen lymph glands. Swelling of the salivary glands (below and in front of the ears) is often caused by mumps, for which home treatment is usually adequate (see Section Two).

Consult a physician if:

- a head or face infection is present;
- lymph glands are tender or inflamed;
- swelling lasts more than one week.

Tooth and Gum Problems

Toothaches and bleeding gums can be prevented by proper oral hygiene and nutrition, including fluoride (see **Dental and Gum Disease,** Section Two). When they do occur they should be treated by a dentist.

Consult a dentist regularly and if:

- a toothache occurs;
- gum bleeding occurs, unless it is slight and occasional;
- injury to a tooth occurs; if a mature, healthy tooth is knocked out, rinse it well and reinsert it—or wrap it in a clean cloth—and go to a dentist immediately.

Urinary Problems

Pain and other symptoms associated with urination can be signs of serious problems.

See a physician within a few hours if there is also:
- fever, vomiting, back pain, or bloody urine,
- an unusual vaginal discharge and abdominal pain,
- an unusual penile discharge or genital sore,
- pregnancy or possible pregnancy.

Consult a physician if there is:
- pain during urination,
- unusually frequent urination,
- dribbling or weak urination.

Vaginal Discharge or Bleeding

Vaginal discharges and bleeding are usually normal, but there can be signs of a variety of problems that require medical treatment (see **Female Disorders,** Section Two).

See a physician immediately if heavy bleeding and pain occur during pregnancy or possible pregnancy.

Consult a physician if:
- a discharge is associated with abdominal pain;
- a discharge is associated with vaginitis (see below) and persists longer than about two weeks;
- a discharge occurs in a pre-pubertal girl;
- a sexually transmitted disease is suspected;
- heavy bleeding occurs between periods;
- bleeding frequently occurs between periods;
- bleeding occurs after menopause;
- any unusual discharge or genital symptoms occur.

Vaginitis

Vaginitis, or inflammation of the vagina with itching, burning, and pain during intercourse, can be caused by infection by, or overgrowth of a variety of organisms. Also suspected are excessive douching, using so-called feminine hygiene sprays, and wearing tight pants or underwear and wet swim suits.

PREVENTION AND SELF-CARE

Practice safe sex (see **Sexually Transmitted Diseases** in Section Two). Keep the vaginal area dry; wipe after urination. Wear cotton underwear. Don't wear panties to bed. Avoid "feminine hygiene sprays" and excessive douching. If you are taking antibiotics, report any sign of vaginitis to your physician. If you use a diaphragm, be sure it is clean.

Consult a physician if:

- vaginal itching and pain occur for the first time;
- familiar symptoms of vaginitis last more than two weeks.

Varicose Veins

Normally, valves in the veins close and open with the ebb and flow of the blood, and prevent blood from backing down the legs. But in many women and some men the valves are defective and the blood seeps down through them and pools in the veins. These become distended, push toward the surface, and appear as swollen, stretched, bluish bulges just under the skin. In the vast majority of cases the problem is cosmetic, not medical. Sometimes, though, there are serious complications, such as inflammation, pain, blood clots, or hemorrhage. The valve defects are apparently genetically determined, but the problem is aggravated by obesity, pregnancy, being sedentary, standing for long periods, wearing tight clothes, and constipation. The latter leads to straining while defecating and long sessions on the toilet, which can cause excessive pressure to build up in the leg veins.

SELF-CARE

If you are obese, lose weight. Exercise regularly; walking, swimming, and bicycling are especially good. Try to prevent constipation. Don't wear tight clothes, boots, girdles, or other garments that tend to impede blood flow. If you have a sedentary or stand-still job, find a way to move and flex your legs at least once every hour. Elevate your legs above your heart whenever possible. Wear elastic support stockings during pregnancy or long periods of standing, but avoid those that are tight below the knees. Do not scratch varicose veins.

Consult a physician if a sore, ulcer, rash, bleeding, or pain occurs near a varicose vein.

Vision Problems

See **Eye and Vision Problems.**

Vomiting

See **Diarrhea and Vomiting.**

Weakness

See **Fatigue and Weakness.**

Warts

Warts are slow-growing little bumps than can occur anywhere on the skin. They are caused by viruses and usually disappear within a year or two but may recur or spread to other areas. Most warts are a cosmetic rather than a health problem, but those on the soles of the feet, on the genitals or anus, or on other areas where pain or irritation can occur usually require treatment. Ano-genital warts can be transmitted by sexual contact and apparently cause or promote cancer of the cervix.

SELF-CARE

The immune system controls warts quite well in most people, so treatment is usually not necessary. In fact, rushing to remove warts may deprive your body of a chance to develop immunity. If you lose your patience, though, try a nonprescription product with salicylic acid. Follow directions carefully.

Consult a physician if:

- you have a wart on the sole of your foot or near your eyes;
- you have a wart on or around your genitals or anus (your sex partner should also consult a physician);
- a wart is troublesome because of its size or location.

Section Four

DRUGS AND HEALTH

Drugs and Health

Nonprescription Drugs

- Allergy Products
- Antacids
- Asthma Medicines
- Cold and Cough Medicines
- Diarrhea Remedies
- Diet Aids
- Homeopathic Products
- Laxatives
- Pain-Fever-Inflammation Drugs
- Sleep Aids
- Skin and Other Topical Products

Herbal Drugs and Herbalism

- Herbs That Are Probably Useful
- Herbs Probably Not Effective but Safe in Moderation
- Toxic Herbs That Should *Not* Be Taken Internally

Addicting and Recreational Drugs

- Alcohol
- Amphetamine Group
- Caffeine Group
- Cocaine
- Heroin and Other Opiates
- Marijuana
- Nitrous Oxide
- PCP
- Psychedelic Drugs
- Tobacco

Prescription Drugs and Vaccines

Nonprescription Drugs

As we enter the 1990s the American public spends over ten billion dollars annually on more than a quarter million nonprescription drug products or "OTCs" (over-the-counter drugs). Medical experts and consumer advocates have long maintained that a great deal of this is unnecessary, and we agree. About 700 active ingredients go into the hundreds of thousands of proprietary products on the market. Of these, only about 250 have been found to be safe and effective by FDA (Food and Drug Administration) panels of experts, and many of these are related or redundant. You generally need just one sunscreen, one antacid, one headache OTC, and so on. So ultimately, most people have real need for only about ten to fifteen OTCs during their lifetime.

Unfortunately, the FDA, which is under more pressure from drug companies than from consumers, has been slow to implement the findings of its experts and force the removal of worthless products from the market. While we are fairly well protected from unsafe OTCs, it seems clear that ineffective drugs, irrational combinations, and misleading advertising will be with us for years to come. Add to this the recent enormous growth of the herbal and homeopathic drug industries, which are almost completely unregulated, and the net result is a setback for consumers.

The FDA's rationale for its permissive approach is that the products are widely sold and accepted by the consumers. In other words, they are big business. If the FDA were to go after all the worthless OTCs and irrational combinations, it could put half the industry out of business. Creating unemployment is not part of its mandate, so the Great Medicine Show goes on unabated. It's up to you to educate and protect yourself.

- **Don't use a drug unless you really need it.** In many cases non-drug remedies are safer and more effective.
- **When you do need a drug, take a single-ingredient product.** Combinations of active ingredients usually increase the cost and the risk without increasing the benefit, and don't allow independent variation of the doses. (You may not always need an antihistimine *and* a cough suppressant.)
- **Learn to read labels and ignore advertisements.** Difficult as the task may appear at first, consumers should learn the generic names of the products they use, and learn about their effects, hazards, and proper uses.
- **Always heed precautions** and use the drugs according to the instructions on the label or those provided by your physician.
- **Consult your doctor before taking an OTC** if you are under a physician's care for any chronic health problem or are taking a prescription drug.

In general, with very few exceptions, OTCs should *not* be used for **weight problems, constipation** (except bulk remedies), **nausea, vomiting, "over-indulgence," insomnia, simple nervous tension,** or **hemorrhoids** (except petrolatum and zinc oxide).

It would be impractical to review even a fraction of the proprietary products available. There are not only too many of them, but new ones are often introduced, and old ones keep their names while their ingredients are changed. Therefore, we focus on basic principles in the use of the most important **generic drugs,** the active ingredients that are put into the thousands of products. This information, combined with careful reading of labels, should make OTC drug use as rational as possible.

The following categories of OTCs are reviewed below: **allergy products, antacids, asthma medicines, cold and cough medicines, diarrhea remedies, diet aids, homeopathic products, laxatives, pain-fever-inflammation drugs, sleep aids, and skin and other topical products.**

Allergy Products

Nonprescription products for allergy relief are mostly for the treatment of allergic rhinitis (hay fever), the runny nose, sneezing, itchy and watery eyes, throat irritation, and cough due to contact with pollens and other allergens. (Products for asthma are discussed separately.)

The effective OTCs for allergic rhinitis are **antihistamines,** such as pheniramine, brompheniramine, and chlorpheniramine (note the common suffix *pheniramine*). They counter the effects of histamine in affected tissue, which is responsible for the symptoms. Their most common side effect is drowsiness, which varies widely among people and products. They may also cause dry mouth, difficulty urinating, and occasionally blurred vision. Try different products until you find one that works and has weak side effects. When using these drugs, do not drive or operate dangerous machinery until you know how you are affected.

Antacids

Those under a physician's care for gastritis, ulcers, or other acid-related problems should use antacids only as directed by their doctors. Antacids are also appropriate for *occasional* use to relieve the burning sensation of hyperacidity, commonly called acid indigestion or sour stomach, and for heartburn, the burning sensation caused by the acidic contents of the stomach rising into the esophagus. Thick liquid antacids are best for the latter because they coat the esophagus. No one should use an antacid regularly or frequently without consulting a physician. Unfortunately the tiny warnings on the labels often have less impact than the commercial hype, and some people develop problems from these drugs.

Hundreds of antacid products are on the market, but there are only a few active ingredients. They are all effective and safe for occasional use, but some are preferable to others in some circumstances.

- **Aluminum** is usually constipating, though less so if combined with magnesium.
- **Calcium carbonate** may be constipating, so a little extra fiber, water, or prune juice may be in order. Those prone to calcium-containing kidney stones should avoid these antacids.
- **Magnesium** tends to cause diarrhea, though less so if combined with aluminum.
- **Sodium bicarbonate** products are effective, but hazardous to those who must restrict sodium intake. Plain baking soda is generally cheaper than tablets with sodium bicarbonate.
- **Combination products** usually contain aluminum and magnesium, which counter each other's side effects. The balance is not always right for an individual, however, and either constipation or diarrhea may occur.

- **Simethicone,** which makes a few big bubbles out of many small ones, supposedly making it easier to pass the gas, is a questionable ingredient in many antacid products because there is no evidence that it is effective in treating abdominal discomfort after eating. The amount of gas in your gastrointestinal tract is not associated with the symptoms and expelling the gas will not relieve them. Moreover, simethicone cannot decrease the total amount of gas present.

Asthma Medicines

Asthma should not be treated with drugs, even OTC's, without consulting a physician. Prescription drugs are often more effective and sometimes safer.

Theophylline and **ephedrine** are the main ingredients in asthma tablets and elixirs. Theophylline is sometimes the drug of choice for asthma, but blood levels must be closely monitored, so self-treatment (without consulting a physician) is not recommended. Ephedrine is an effective but questionable ingredient because it has many side effects including nervousness, loss of appetite, and insomnia. Eventually theophylline may be designated a prescription-only drug, and ephedrine may be phased out for asthma because there are better products. OTC asthma remedies may become a thing of the past.

OTC inhalers for asthma all contain **epinephrine** (adrenaline), which opens the airways to allow breathing. It is generally safe and effective, but short-acting and subject to tolerance. If not used sparingly it may cause nervousness, rapid heartbeat, and other side effects.

Cold and Cough Medicines

There are hundreds of pills and potions marketed as cold remedies, but none can cure a cold. Much of this drug use is unnecessary and undesirable. The heavily advertised multisymptom remedies are particularly irrational. More and more drugs are included in each pill, which always allegedly treats more symptoms than the competition. We've seen up to about twelve symptoms that can all allegedly be treated by one pill.

In truth, few people suffer more than one or two symptoms worth taking a drug for. The shotgun approach exposes the users to unnecessary risks and expense for little more than a placebo benefit. If you are going to use drugs to treat colds, it is best to treat individual symptoms with single-ingredient products. This will expose you to only one or two drugs at rational doses rather than several drugs in a fixed ratio.

The drug industry also does a disservice with its commercials that encourage cold sufferers to take their products in order to keep going (to school, work, shopping) rather than to rest. This delays recovery and increases the exposure of others to the viruses.

Stuffy nose can be treated with nose drops or sprays containing **ephedrine, racephedrine, naphazoline, oxymetazoline, xylometazoline,** or **phenylephrine.** Inhalers with **propylhexedrine** or **desoxyephedrine** are also effective. Sprays with antihistamines (like pheniramine) are questionable remedies for treating colds since histamine is not responsible for the symptoms. There is no need for menthol, eucalyptus, or other aromatic substances that may add to the cost without increasing effectiveness.

Decongestant sprays should not be used for more than three days because severe rebound stuffiness can occur. That is, when the drug wears off the stuffiness is worse than before its use; more is taken, it wears off, and so on. Moreover, regular use for many months or years may be a factor in some cases of impotence, which is not surprising since the drugs are potent vasoconstrictors and can probably cause constriction of the arteries of the penis.

Related drugs are available in pill form, but the topical products are generally preferable because they give high concentrations of the drugs where you want them and less in your blood. However, if relief is still needed after two or three days, you should switch to an oral product (pill or liquid). Look for pseudophedrine or phenylephrine. Phenylpropanolamine is less safe and eventually may be withdrawn from the market. These drugs are all stimulants and should not be taken at night.

Runny nose should not be treated with drugs since it helps the body shed the offending virus and correct inflammation. Be careful, though, not to blow your nose hard since this can spread viruses and bacteria throughout the sinuses and into the eustachian tubes leading to the middle ears.

Productive cough, a cough that brings up mucus, should not be suppressed with drugs since it helps clear the lungs. The mucus can be thinned by drinking plenty of water and spicy chicken soup. Only one OTC, **guaifenesin,** appears to be of some value as an expectorant. It seems to thin the phlegm and sputum and make it somewhat easier to expel.

Dry cough, a cough that does not bring up mucus, can be treated with **dextromethorphan,** which suppresses the cough center of the brain and has few side effects. Look for a product with no other active ingredients. The antihistamines, chlorpheniramine and diphenhydramine, are the active ingredients in some cough medicines, but because of their strong sedative effects they should be used only at night. Antihistamines should be avoided during a cold if they seem to dry or thicken the mucus.

Sore throat due to the common cold can be treated with **aspirin, ibuprofen,** or **acetaminophen.** These should be swallowed whole, not crushed or chewed in gum because they can irritate the throat and do not provide pain relief by contact with the affected tissue. Some sore throat lozenges may sooth and provide temporary relief. Look for **benzocaine, phenol, menthol** or **hexylresorcinol** in the ingredients. Avoid alcohol-based mouthwashes, which do not affect the cold viruses and can irritate sensitive throat tissue.

Fever, headache, and **aching muscles** are unusual in the common cold. They may indicate flu or something else. If very bothersome they can be treated with aspirin, ibuprofen, or acetaminophen, but if they are severe or persistent, consult your physician.

In conclusion, the vast majority of colds can be endured with simple measures (mainly rest and fluids) and, if necessary, simple drugs. Few people need more than a single-ingredient nasal spray for stuffy nose. For a sore throat, a throat lozenge, aspirin, ibuprofen, or acetaminophen may help. If a dry cough develops, a medicine with dextromethorphan and preferably no other active ingredients can be used.

Diarrhea Remedies

Chronic diarrhea can be caused by many things, including irritable bowel syndrome and lactose intolerance. These must be treated with medical guidance according to their causes, as must any diarrhea that lasts more than a couple days or is associated with a fever. OTC antidiarrheals are intended for use in *acute diarrhea* (as opposed to chronic diarrhea) due to viral infections of the gastrointestinal tract, overconsumption of laxative foods and drinks, food poisoning, or reactions to medicines. They should not be used for more than two or three days without consulting a physician.

Activated charcoal, taken in capsules, often relieves diarrhea, gas, and cramping. It absorbs gases and irritating substances and holds them until excretion in the feces.

Aluminum-containing antacids without magnesium are not marketed as antidiarrheals, but many people find them effective as such. This is not surprising since constipation is a frequent side effect of their use for stomach-acid-related problems.

Polycarbophil is a bulk-forming laxative that is supposedly also effective in consolidating stools and making diarrhea less uncomfortable. It is generally safe since it does not slow down the expulsion of infectious agents and toxins, as truly effective antidiarrheals (like opiates) can do by practically stopping bowel activity. But it is apparently only marginally effective and actually has little to recommend it.

Bismuth subsalicylate reduces cramping and frequency of bowel movements in traveler's diarrhea, but large doses are required and aspirinlike side effects may occur in some people. There is considerable controversy about whether it is effective in other types of diarrhea, but it does seem to help in some viral cases. Bismuth is a heavy metal and potentially toxic. Heavy or prolonged use can cause severe nerve toxicity that can take months to recover from. The subsalicylate is hazardous to those with stomach-acid-related problems; these products should not be used by them; nor should they be used with aspirin or ibuprofen. Don't use for more than three weeks without consulting a physician.

Attapulgite is supposed to reduce the number of bowel movements, but its effectiveness is in dispute.

Kaolin and **pectin** (as in Kaopectate) are, respectively, a fine white clay and a plant fiber. The FDA expert panel has found them both, alone and in combination, ineffective in the treatment of diarrhea. They do *not* diminish cramping, frequency of bowel movement, or fluid and mineral loss. However they do seem to make the stools firmer and thereby decrease discomfort; this may be worthwhile since the treatment is safe.

Loperamide (Imodium is the only brand available now) works by blocking intestinal nerves, thereby reducing irritability and contractions. This is a potent drug that until recently was available only by prescription. Overuse can paralyze the intestinal muscles and cause severe constipation. Do not exceed recommended dosage. Do not use for more than two days without consulting your physician. Do not use if there is a fever or blood in the stool. Nursing and pregnant women and people taking prescription drugs should not use loperamide without consulting their doctors.

Diet Aids

None of the drugs offered as diet aids (appetite suppressants) have been proved to be effective. Taking worthless pills to treat obesity and control weight has become an American tradition. It took several decades of experience with amphetamine and its relatives for us to learn that they do not work and can be dangerous. Now we have embraced **phenylpropanolamine (PPA),** a chemical cousin of amphetamine and the main ingredient in scores of OTC diet aid products. It is a decongestant used in many cold products as well as an alleged appetite suppressant. Side effects can include headache, nausea, anxiety, palpitation, nervousness, dizziness, insomnia, and perhaps increased blood pressure. These can be aggravated by the caffeine that is an ingredient in some such products.

There is only meager evidence that the drugs help control appetite and no evidence whatsoever that they are a significant aid in the long-term treatment of obesity, the utterly fantastic claims of the promoters notwithstanding. They are explicitly not recommended for people with heart disease, thyroid disorders, depression, diabetes, or hypertension because of serious potential hazards. However, mass screenings and other surveys indicate that a third or so of those with the latter two disorders (who are among those most likely to be obese) do not know they have them. Given these facts, it is difficult to justify the OTC status and use of these drugs for weight control. We recommend against their use.

Another important problem with the widespread availability of PPA—practically anyone can buy it in bulk and go into the mail-order diet-pill business—is that it is frequently present in high doses in "look-alikes," drugs sold illicitly as amphetamine. Thousands of poisonings occur each year from the use of these drugs. Common symptoms include severe headache, vomiting, heavy sweating, tremors, seizures, and hallucinations, delusions, and other psychiatric symptoms. Suicide attempts and other violence also occur.

Benzocaine is a local anesthetic added to candies and gums to numb the taste buds and thereby decrease the appetite. There is little evidence to support this theory, however, and none at all to support the claims of significant weight reduction.

Starch blockers are extracts of certain beans that are supposed to block the digestion of starch and thereby allow more eating without weight gain. Studies indicate they do *not* work. If they did, bacterial action on the undigested starch would be expected to produce fairly severe gastrointestinal symptoms, especially diarrhea and excessive gas.

"Health food" store diet aids, such as spirulina, bee pollen, herbal extracts, glucomannan, and various amino acids, are all bogus products. None of them has been shown to work as claimed by their promoters.

Homeopathic Products

Homeopathy is a pseudoscientific system developed in the early 1800s by Samuel Hahnemann, a German physician. It's a kind of magic or alchemy disguised as science, and its tenets are completely incompatible with those of scientific medicine. Homeopaths believe that extremely small dilutions of a toxin can cure diseases whose symptoms are similar to the effects of large doses of the toxin. The greater the dilution, the more powerful the effect. For the most severe cases the substances are diluted so much that, mathematically, not a single atom is left.

How, then, does a homeopathic remedy exert its effect? By the vibrations it leaves behind in the water, alcohol, lactose, or other medium, according to the homeopaths. But if such a thing were possible there would be no chemistry as we know it. Every substance would leave its vibes for eternity on everything it ever came into contact with. There would be no pure substances that followed any knowable laws because everything would always have its unique and complex combination of vibrations depending on its unique history.

The question naturally occurs: How far do homeopaths take their theory? Do they treat, say, lead poisoning with more lead? Incredibly, the answer is yes. Bee stings are treated with more bee venom, mercury poisoning with more mercury, and so on for any kind of poisoning, be it benzene, alcohol, heroin, streptococcus, or atomic radiation.

Homeopathic theory and practice was thoroughly demolished in 1842 by Oliver Wendell Holmes in his essay, "Homeopathy and Its Kindred Delusions," and has been further refuted many times since. Perhaps the strongest evidence that its founder was slightly addled is Hahnemann's own textbook, published in 1828, in which he attributes most chronic diseases to the improper treatment of scabies infection by establishment physicians.

In spite of the absurdity of homeopathic theory and the lack of clinical evidence to support its claims, the peddling of homeopathic remedies is a booming business. Practically every kind of herb, heavy metal, and nutrient mineral one can imagine is put into pills and liquid extracts that are marketed as nonprescription remedies for every disease under the sun. Of course, if the preparations are high potency, there may not be *any* of the active ingredient listed on the label to be found in the pills—just vibrations. Why the FDA allows these rackets to continue is a major mystery. We suggest you avoid all homeopathic products and look carefully at the credentials of anyone who prescribes or recommends such products. The same goes for "glandulars," pills containing raw, powdered glands and other organs, and for "tissue salts" or "cell salts." These are offshoots of homeopathy and are equally irrational.

Laxatives

It is almost always preferable to treat constipation with high-fiber food, water, and exercise (plain walking is fine) rather than laxatives. However, when traveling, camping, or sailing, it may not be practical to eat the best foods or do enough walking, and laxatives may be a convenient occasional aid. In this event there is only one class of laxatives that is a rational choice: the bulk laxatives, which contain methylcellulose, psyllium, and other fibrous plant products. These work by absorbing water and creating bulk, just like fiber from food. It is important that they be taken with plenty of water to prevent them from drying and possibly blocking the intestine. Their sodium and sugar content should be checked by those who must restrict sodium or calories.

Not one of the other types of laxatives works like food and each is associated with certain risks. Long-term use of stimulant laxatives (such as phenolphthalein, senna, disacodyl, or danthron) actually dilates the large bowel and decreases its sensitivity to bulk so that it becomes dependent on chemical stimulation for contraction. Laxatives sold in "health food" stores are often made from stimulant herbs and are among the most hazardous.

Saline laxatives (those with magnesium) are not as good as bulk laxatives, but they do draw water into the colon and can help when bulk laxatives alone don't work. They are safe for occasional use for most people.

Pain-Fever-Inflammation Drugs

Americans spend a couple billion dollars each year on hundreds of proprietary OTCs for miscellaneous pains and fever. Only three active ingredients go into all these products: **aspirin** (and chemical sisters with equivalent actions), **acetaminophen,** and **ibuprofen.** These drugs are similar in that they all relieve certain kinds of pain very effectively and they all relieve fever. However, aspirin and ibuprofen also relieve inflammation, while acetaminophen does not. These drugs should not be combined, nor should they be taken for more than a week or while using prescription pain relievers, without consulting a physician.

Acetaminophen can reduce pain and fever, but since it cannot reduce inflammation its applications are more limited than aspirin's. Its main uses are for headache and fever. It generally has fewer side effects than aspirin, but it can cause some gastrointestinal upset. Acute overdose and chronic overuse can cause severe and sometimes fatal liver damage. The toxic dose is lower than for aspirin, so overdose is more dangerous.

Aspirin is a popular and effective remedy for common headaches, toothaches, pain due to injury and inflammation of muscles and joints, controlling fever, and dysmenorrhea and premenstrual syndrome. It has its roots in herbal remedies that contain salicylate. Other salicylates (like choline and magnesium salicylate) are essentially aspirin equivalents and they have the same effects, uses, and hazards.

Side effects of aspirin include ringing in the ears, hyperacidity, and queasy stomach. Aspirin should be avoided by pregnant women, children under sixteen with suspected viral infections like flu or chickenpox, those who are allergic to aspirin, those who have gastric acid problems like peptic ulcers, and those who take certain prescription drugs. For example, asthma is sometimes aggravated by the drug. Aspirin can promote excessive bleeding, so it should not be used in the days before or after surgery, including tooth extraction, or a month or so before childbirth.

Enteric-coated aspirin is designed to dissolve in the intestine rather than the stomach in order to avoid stomach bleeding. Because it is absorbed slowly and less reliably, it was rated ineffective by the FDA panel that reviewed it. Many physicians consider this a mistake since effective blood levels are achieved in many patients whose stomachs are spared in the process. As long as it affords relief, it would seem to be a good choice for those who must take it often.

Questionable Variations. Time-released products are more expensive than regular tablets and there is no added benefit. Aspirin chewing gum is especially not recommended for sore throat because it is irritating, causing a burning sensation in the mouth and throat. There is no reason to buy anything but plain aspirin without caffeine, antihistamines, or buffers. (If gastric distress is a problem, take an antacid a few minutes after the aspirin; buffers are not likely to help a good deal.) Nor is there any reason to buy the costly *extra-*, *mega-*, *super-*, or *arthritis-strength* aspirin or acetaminophen. You can just take an extra pill or half a pill of the cheaper and equally effective preparations. Avoid products alleged to be superior for specific types of pain. For example, Doan's Pills are marketed for back pain, and while they contain magnesium salicylate, an aspirin equivalent, and cost much more than plain aspirin, they provide no additional benefits.

Ibuprofen, like aspirin, is effective for headaches, toothaches, muscle and joint inflammation and pain, fever, and menstrual discomfort. Also like aspirin, it can cause gastric distress and should be avoided by most people with ulcers and other acid-related disorders. People allergic to aspirin should not take ibuprofen, since cross-reaction may occur.

Which Should You Use?

Aspirin and ibuprofen are more effective for pain associated with inflammation, as in sports-related injuries, arthritis, dysmenorrhea, and toothaches, but they should be avoided by those at risk for serious side effects as described above. In these cases acetaminophen may be just as effective and less risky, or it may be somewhat less effective. For most headaches acetaminophen is as effective as the others and usually preferable because of the lower risk of side effects. It is available in liquid form, which the others are not, so it is sometimes useful for young children and those who cannot swallow pills.

Sleep Aids

The active ingredients of OTC sleep aids are **diphenhydramine,** and **doxylamine,** antihistamines that also produce drowsiness. These drugs can cause dizziness, dry mouth, blurred vision, confusion, stomach problems, loss of appetite, ringing in the ears, difficult urination in men, and other side effects. They often produce insomnia and nervousness in children. They are hazardous to people with asthma, glaucoma, prostate enlargement, and other problems, and may interact dangerously with other drugs, including sedatives, alcohol, and anticonvulsants. They should not be used by pregnant or lactating women.

Skin and Other Topical Products

The marketplace offers thousands of products that are supposed to make our skin and hair more attractive, make us smell better, and deal with discomfort and disorders of the skin, eyes, ears, genitals, and anorectal area. Attempting to decide on a rational basis which if any of the products to use can try one's sanity. We cannot review individual products here, but the following comments on the major categories should help you protect your sanity by narrowing your choices somewhat.

The following categories of products are discussed: **acne products, antiperspirants and deodorants, burn products, cosmetics, ear-care products, eye-care products, fungus fighters, hair-care products, hemorrhoid products, insect repellants, itch remedies, minor wound treatments, soaps, sunburn products and sunscreens, vaginal products,** and **wart products.**

Acne Products

Some OTC acne products can aggravate the problem by clogging the pores. There are some effective products, however, that contain **benzoyl peroxide** in a non-oily base. Look for the simplest, cheapest product with this ingredient and use it carefully, according to instructions on the label.

Antiperspirants and Deodorants

The body odor and body wetness problems have probably been aggravated in recent decades by the increasing use of synthetic fabrics in clothing. Unlike cotton, these newer materials all have a strong tendency to hold moisture in, so skin bacteria and their malodorous gases proliferate. The rise of the white-collar class has helped fuel the enormous growth of the antiperspirant and deodorant industry partly because office workers' pants and shirts usually must be of the permanent-press, wrinkle-free variety. It is not a law, but a powerful tradition not often bucked. People working in the typical close quarters of modern offices clad in their several layers of synthetic fabrics would knock each other over with their body odor if they did not do something about it.

That something has been to spray, roll, smear, and bathe in tons of chemicals in hundreds of products. The main ingredients in most current products are perfumes and **aluminum hydroxychloride** (and similar aluminum salts), which cause irritation and allergic rashes in some people. The advantage of the aluminum hydroxychloride is that by stopping perspiration it not only inhibits odor development but also protects clothes from ugly stains.

For those who are allergic to effective commercial products, or who do not like the idea of inhibiting the natural function of perspiring, there are a couple inexpensive, safe, and effective deodorants. One is **baking soda.** Simply dissolve about a quarter teaspoon in a quarter cup of warm water and pat it on the offending areas. The other is plain **rubbing alcohol** applied with a cotton ball and allowed to dry. These methods will not stop perspiration, so they don't solve the problem of stained clothes, but they are quite effective in reducing body odor, apparently by inhibiting the proliferation of skin bacteria. The wetness problem can be reduced by wearing light cotton clothes and cutting down on coffee and other stimulants that promote sweating.

Burn Products

These are sprays and ointments that contain local anesthetics. They do not promote healing and even provoke allergic responses in some. The pain relief is not much more than cold water provides. In short, these are not very useful products.

Cosmetics

There are thousands of creams, lotions, foundations, blushes, lipsticks, and brush-ons marketed as beauty aids. The use of these cosmetics is primarily an aesthetic matter, a question of taste that must be decided by individuals, perhaps with the expert guidance of cosmetologists. There are, however, some health problems associated with cosmetic use, and those who would be beautiful should also be wise—or at least alert to some of the hazards discussed here.

It should be kept in mind that cosmetics are not regulated in the way drugs are. The firms that make cosmetics are not required to register with the FDA or submit their products for approval. But they must declare their ingredients in order of predominance, with the main ingredient listed first. Fragrances need not be named but they must be listed as "fragrance."

Acne is a very common result of the frequent use of cosmetics. Almost all foundations, powders, cold creams, and lotions tend to clog the pores as well as provide acnegenic oils. They can be cleaned off and the pores cleared with an astringent like rubbing alcohol, but if you put the makeup back on, the pimples will remain. This is an aesthetic judgment that most people would agree with: No makeup is so good that its benefits outweigh the acne it might cause. So if a cosmetic aggravates or causes acne, stop using it.

Allergic reactions to cosmetics and hair removers are very common. In fact, the continued application of almost anything to the skin is likely to eventually cause sensitization to the substance and an allergic reaction the next time it is applied. Sensitization can occur on the first or five hundredth application. Once it does, the substance will always cause a reaction.

Cosmetic manufacturers do extensive testing on all ingredients in order to use those that take the longest to produce sensitization. So-called "hypoallergenic" ingredients are more hype than hypo, since they have not been proved to be less allergenic than other ingredients. Manufacturers keep complaint files, and when it appears that significant numbers of people are developing allergies to an ingredient it is replaced. This is one reason that the formulas for cosmetics are continually changing, though usually imperceptibly and without a corresponding name change.

Your best defense against developing allergic reactions to cosmetics is to use them sparingly and infrequently. Be alert for reactions (like little red bumps, a rash, or itching) to anything you put on your skin, and stop using it immediately should one occur.

Irritation is a common side effect of many cosmetics and other skin products. The redness, pain, and itching are caused by the chemical reaction of the substance with the skin, not by an allergic reaction. Aluminum chlorides in antiperspirants, shaving powders, and wax hair removers are commonly irritating, more so to some people than others. Just about any solvent, like nail polish remover and some makeup removers, can cause irritation and roughness of the skin.

Photosensitization is a common problem with cosmetics and perfumes. Many of their ingredients sensitize the skin to the sun so that relatively brief exposure causes sunburn. Therefore, caution is advised in the use of these products before exposure to the sun.

Ear-Care Products

Earwax Remover. As explained in Section Two (see **Hearing Loss and Ear Infections**), earwax helps to warm and protect the ear canal. It normally works its way out slowly and should not be removed with bobby pins, cotton swabs, or other probes: These should *never* be inserted into the ear. Instead the outer ear should be cleaned with soapy water and a little finger and nothing else. On rare occasions, however, excessive wax does accumulate and needs removing. This is done by squirting warm water into the canal with a rubber syringe made for the purpose. Ask at a drugstore.

The task can be made easier, especially if the wax is impacted, by first inserting an earwax softening agent. Look for a product with **carbamide peroxide** in glycerin and use it strictly according to instructions. If irritation occurs do *not* use it again. Don't get into the habit of removing earwax; most people never have to do it. Those who do should do it only occasionally and with care not to remove wax unnecessarily; it is there for a reason. If you notice hearing impairment, don't try to treat it yourself; consult a physician.

Ear canal drying agents, ear drops for use after swimming and bathing, contain rubbing alcohol that mixes with water in the canal and causes it to evaporate more readily. This helps control swimmer's ear and surfer's ear, which are aggravated by wetness. These products sometimes irritate the ear, in which case their use should be stopped. An electric hair dryer is often more effective and less irritating, especially during a flare-up, but also for routine use by those prone to these ear problems.

CAUTION

If you also use eye drops, be very careful not to confuse them with your ear drops, which often come in similar bottles. While eye drops placed in the ear will not cause problems, ear drops placed in the eye will cause excruciating pain for several hours. The alcohol causes the conjunctiva to become very inflamed and frighteningly red. Should this accident occur you will know it immediately, so only one eye will be affected. It should be rinsed copiously for at least ten minutes and a physician should be consulted.

Eye-Care Products

Eye drops for "soothing tired eyes" and "getting the red out" are among the more questionable OTCs. There is nothing in any eye drops that can relieve eyestrain or fatigue of the eye muscles, and placing drops in one's eyes is never very soothing. If one frequently has red eyes, an eye examination is in order. The active ingredients, naphazoline and tetrahydrozoline, constrict the superficial blood vessels of the eye and thereby temporarily decrease the redness. They are generally harmless, but tolerance to their effect can develop and sometimes sensitivity occurs, causing the eyes to become even redder. The more often the products are used, the more likely this is to occur.

If you use eye drops and ear drops, read the caution above about not mixing them up. It is best not to store them together to reduce the chance of this happening.

Fungus Fighters

By far the most common fungal diseases are superficial infections of the skin and mucous membranes. A large number of topical agents are available. For the common Tinea infections (athlete's foot, jock itch, ringworm), products with **tolnaftate** or **miconazole** are very effective and generally lacking in side effects, though contact with the eyes must be avoided.

Hair-Care Products

Each strand of hair is covered by a cuticle, a protective protein coating. If it is damaged the hair will rapidly fray and become limp. As hair grows and ages, the cuticle tends to deteriorate and flake away, leading to split ends. There are factors that promote and hasten this process and factors that delay it. For example, excessive shampooing, sunlight, blow-drying, bleaching, dying, straightening, habitually pulling, brushing, and teasing can all damage the cuticle. So can hot water, chlorine, and brushing while the hair is wet. Important systemic (internal) factors that can result in unhealthy hair are poor nutrition, various drugs, and severe illness.

Keeping generally healthy, avoiding the various insults to hair, and keeping it clean with a mild shampoo generally suffice to keep hair healthy and attractive. This would seem to be a simple matter, but there are thousands of products available for cleaning, conditioning, and doing other things to improve hair. Shampoos, dandruff remedies, and conditioners are the most useful and purported baldness remedies the least. These categories of products are discussed below. Practically all the other products are potentially damaging to hair. Only the individual can determine whether the risk is worth the cosmetic benefit.

Baldness remedies, both those that are taken internally and those that are rubbed into the scalp, are frauds, in spite of all the testimonials and sophisticated advertisements. There are no nonprescription lotions, creams, vitamins, lights, massages, drugs, or other products or procedures that can make hair grow. True, there are a handful of prescription drugs and hormones that promote hair growth in some circumstances and one of them, minoxidil (Rogaine), is approved as a prescription topical (rub-on) baldness remedy. However, it must be taken continuously and is quite expensive. Only a small percentage of users benefit substantially.

Conditioners, which are applied to hair after shampooing, are of several types with different functions. Acid rinses like dilute lemon juice or vinegar are used to remove any film left by highly alkaline cleansers. They tend to flatten the cuticle and increase sheen, but they are not antistatic and will not prevent "fly-away" hair. Cream rinses are slightly acidic surfactants, substances that coat the hair, flatten the cuticle, add sheen, and neutralize static electric charges, thereby reducing "fly-away." Instant and protein conditioners are like cream rinses, but they also contain proteins, fats, oils, waxes, and other ingredients that lubricate and add luster and body. The protein in particular seems to penetrate the hair shaft and thicken it.

Dandruff Products. A certain amount of dandruff (flaking scalp) is normal and can be adequately controlled by washing with a mild shampoo. Hot water and scratching or brushing the scalp too hard can cause irritation and aggravate dandruff. A dilute vinegar rinse seems to help in some cases, probably by serving as a kerotolytic, an agent that loosens up the flaking skin. Excessive use might irritate the scalp and aggravate the problem, especially in those with dry scalp and hair.

If these simple measures do not work, an OTC dandruff product may be tried, but cautiously and in moderation because overtreatment can irritate the scalp and aggravate the problem. The most effective products contain **zinc pyrithione.** Products with **selenium sulfide** are available in low concentrations without a prescription. They often work, but sometimes not for long. Alternating the use of products with these ingredients may help. If nothing seems to work and you have severe dandruff with large flakes or very oily scalp, you should consult a dermatologist.

Shampoos contain mild detergents that are generally superior to soaps because they clean better, work well in hard water, are less alkaline, and rinse out completely. All the other ingredients in shampoos, the thickeners, colors, fragrances and so on, are not necessary for cleaning.

Conditioners are best used separately after washing.

How often and thoroughly should you shampoo? Usually two to five times a week, depending on how oily and dirty your hair gets. Unless you have acne or severe dandruff that is aggravated by oily hair, it is better to err on the side of less washing. Squeaky clean hair is a sign of excessive shampooing and using water that is too hot. This can damage the hair by weakening and removing the cuticle and promoting dryness and splitting. It cannot, however, make your hair fall out.

The choice of shampoo is mostly a personal and cosmetic matter, not a question of health. However certain health-related points should be kept in mind. Those with sensitive skin, frequently lighter-skinned people, should be alert to signs of irritation and allergic reactions. If they occur, try a different shampoo. In fact, it is a good idea for those with sensitive skin and scalps to frequently switch shampoos, and to always dilute them before applying. Almost all shampoos are only slightly alkaline, and therefore not very harsh, so claims about pH-balance are superfluous.

Hemorrhoid Products

The proper treatment and prevention of hemorrhoids involves walking and other exercise, and adequate fiber and water in the diet. There are no commercial products that promote the healing or resolution of hemorrhoids. Their use should be considered only for the temporary relief of acute symptoms. A wide variety of ingredients go into hemorrhoid products, including astringents, counter-irritants, protectants, local anesthetics, vasoconstrictors, atropine-type drugs, and vitamins A and D.

Of all these ingredients the only ones that are undeniably safe and effective are protectants such as petroleum jelly, zinc oxide, cocoa butter, and shark liver oil, provided they make up at least 50 percent of the product. All the other ingredients are unproved, irrational, or otherwise inadvisable. Local anesthetics, for example, often sensitize people to novocaine and other pain killers, so that their use in the future would cause an allergic reaction. Atropine-type agents have no effect on the swollen veins, and there is not the slightest evidence that vitamins applied to the anorectal area promote the healing or resolution of hemorrhoids.

Since we are left with protectants as the only worthwhile ingredients, essentially all the commercial preparations for hemorrhoids are eliminated. There is no reason to buy expensive products with lots of worthless ingredients. Therefore, if you feel you must put something on your anorectal area for the temporary relief of the symptoms of hemorrhoids, just use petroleum jelly or zinc oxide.

Insect Repellants

Insect repellants can help make life livable when mosquitoes and gnats threaten to drive you batty. Look for products with **diethyltoluamide (DEET)** and/or **dimethyl phthalate.** Foams and liquids are better than sprays because they have higher concentrations and are cheaper. Use these products carefully and as sparingly as you can, especially with young children. The active substances can be absorbed through the skin and prolonged use of large amounts can cause neurological symptoms such as anxiety, lethargy, confusion, seizures, and coma.

Thiamine, alias vitamin B-1, in large doses is sometimes recommended to keep bugs away, but it does not work. The same goes for brewer's yeast.

Itch Remedies

Colloidal oatmeal is a safe and effective anti-itch remedy, especially useful when large areas of the body are affected. You can soak a limb or your whole body in it. Cornstarch can also be used this way, but it is probably not quite as effective.

Hydrocortisone creams are quite effective. They should be used strictly in accordance with instructions on the label or those of your physician.

Calamine lotion is of marginal and questionable benefit. While promoted as an itch remedy, it may in fact increase itching by drying the skin.

Minor Wound Treatments

Minor cuts and scratches can be adequately treated by thorough cleaning with water and perhaps a mild soap. The wound should be covered with a bandage and kept clean. If pus appears, hot water soaks can be used to promote drainage. There is almost never any reason to apply iodine, alcohol, topical antibiotics, or other liquids or ointments. None of them offers any advantage over thorough cleaning, and some of them are painful when applied or capable of producing allergic sensitivity. Therefore, if a minor wound does not seem to be healing after a few days, and especially if an infection seems to be getting worse or spreading to other parts of your skin, consult a physician rather than trying to treat it with OTC products.

Soaps

In spite of all the claims made for various soaps, very little is really known about how they affect our skin because adequate research is not done. The advertising claims about soaps being mild or gentle are unproved and often completely without foundation. Some studies of popular brands of soap show that most of the heavily promoted, expensive, supposedly gentle soaps are among the most irritating and likely to produce chapping in sensitive people.

Bar soaps can harbor pathogenic bacteria for several hours and theoretically serve as a medium for the spread of disease. Some experts believe they do not belong in public or semipublic bathrooms or large kitchens from which many people are served. However, there is no evidence that they actually do help spread diseases, even in hospitals where germs and bars of soap are everywhere. Nevertheless, the controversy seems to be stimulating a switch to liquid soap dispensers in some institutions and even private homes.

Deodorant soaps containing antimicrobial chemicals are questionable products because they don't necessarily work as claimed, and they sometimes produce photosensitivity, that is, irritation of the skin when exposed to the sun.

Sunburn Products and Sunscreens

Dozens of heavily advertised products for relief of sunburn pain contain benzocaine, a local anesthetic. It provides only marginal relief, probably no more than cold water, and it can provoke allergic reactions. Therefore, none of these products can be recommended. Aspirin and ibuprofen are more likely to provide significant relief.

The best approach, of course, is to prevent sunburn by limiting exposure to the sun and using products with a sunscreen such as **para-aminobenzoic acid (PABA)** or **oxybenzone.** Look for a sun protection factor (SPF) of 15 or more in a water-resistant product and apply the product generously for maximum protection. The SPF numbers (2 to 21) are much more important than the specific active ingredients, so choose a product with the protective power you need that is a cream, fluid, or gel, depending on convenience, skin type, and possible sensitivity to ingredients.

Vaginal Products

The vagina is normally clean, for it is washed, lubricated, and defended against irritation and infection by its secretions. Any unusual or foul-smelling discharge should be discussed with a physician. The normal, though sometimes offensive, odor that may develop toward the end of the day is a product of sweat and normal vaginal secretions altered by exposure to oxygen and held by the pubic hair. It is easily controlled with daily washing of the pubic area. All-cotton panties and outer garments are preferable to synthetics because they allow evaporation of moisture and thereby inhibit bacteria proliferation and odor accumulation. There is no need to use "feminine hygiene sprays," which can cause irritation and allergic reactions. These products can be considered consumer frauds since they have nothing to do with hygiene, which concerns cleanliness and health.

Routine douching is also not necessary, but it is usually not harmful if done properly. Warm water, with or without a little white vinegar or baking soda, is all that should be used, unless a physician advises otherwise. The vagina should *not* be held closed while douching because water may be forced into the cervix and Fallopian tubes; this could cause infection. Also, douching should be avoided during pregnancy and the month after childbirth or abortion, unless a physician recommends it.

Wart Products

Warts are caused by viruses and usually go away by themselves. However, warts on the sole of the foot or the ano-genital area should be treated by a physician. If you want to get rid of a wart elsewhere on the skin, look for a product with **salicylic acid** and use it in strict accordance with the instructions. Products with various vitamins are nothing but placebos.

Herbal Drugs and Herbalism

Plants have been used for therapeutic purposes for thousands of years. The effects of many plants were no doubt discovered by accident when they were tried as food and when they contaminated drinking water. In other cases the origin of an herb's use is astrological or otherwise superstitious. For example, the anthropocentric "doctrine of signatures" (subscribed to by American Indians and some medieval herbalists) held that plants usually provide a clue to their medical uses. Liverleaf is vaguely shaped like a liver and was used in liver ailments; plants yielding milky juices were used to promote lactation; and seneca snakeroot, named for its shape, was used for snake bites. While usually ineffective for the purported uses, such plants were often found useful for other purposes.

The physiological effects of herbs are due to active chemicals, usually alkaloids, glycosides, oils, gums, and resins. Many of these chemicals have been isolated and purified, but some are still unidentified. In recent decades more and more drugs have been made completely synthetically rather than extracted from plants or made as analogues of plant compounds. Examples include some potent tranquilizers, anesthetics, anticancer drugs, and anti-infectives. More than two-thirds of the prescriptions now filled in the United States are for synthetics. However, more recently, as part of the "back to nature" movement, there has been a strong revival of interest in herbal medicine. This trend is gaining momentum and seems likely to continue for some time.

The problem is that a huge, unregulated drug industry has been unleashed on the public. Its promotions are often misleading, false, and dangerous. Most of the popular herbals (as the encyclopedias are called) provide little or no information on the toxicity of many of the herbs they prescribe for dozens of ailments. For example, in *Back to Eden* (written in the 1920s and republished in the 1970s) Jethro Kloss recommends mistletoe tea for epilepsy, but various mistletoes contain toxins that can adversely affect the heart and blood pressure. He prescribes American mandrake for intestinal problems, but it is a drastic purgative that can cause nausea, vomiting, and death by gastrointestinal inflammation. He recommends peach kernels for various ailments, but they contain cyanide and were used as a means of execution in ancient Egypt; a handful could do the job. All these and many more poisonous prescriptions and recipes are presented without a word of warning. (If this is Eden, we'll take our chances in Hades.)

Like *Back to Eden* most herb books, articles, and charts just list all the ailments that each herb has been used for, even if the herb has been found useless for most or all of the old purposes. Cures for every conceivable and deadly disease are touted, and naive readers are misled. They go out and buy or pick dozens of the recommended herbs (or something resembling them) and use them at every opportunity. It is irresponsible for publishers of recent editions of such outdated volumes not to warn the readers that the remedies presented are of historical interest only. It is reprehensible that more and more "health food" stores carry such misleading herbals and employ full-time herbalists, who often double as nutrition consultants, to guide customers to herbal cures and vitamin supplements.

While some herbs have important uses, **no physiologically active substance is devoid of some hazard.** Any herb that does anything carries some risk, and many herbs contain substances that the FDA would ban or allow only by prescription if they were labeled or sold as drugs in drugstores. When sold in bulk or as extracts in "health food" stores, even when labeled for therapeutic use and promoted by flyers, magazines, and books across the aisle, the FDA looks away, so the consumers must educate and protect themselves and their families.

Consumers should be especially wary of the many herb extract products on the market. These formulations take an irrational shotgun approach to symptoms. Like the herbals that list all the plants ever used for each symptom, these products contain irrational mixtures of unproved remedies for every ailment under the sun, including impotence, angina, arthritis, liver disease, hypertension, obesity, kidney disease, memory problems, and eczema.

The makers and sellers of these unproved remedies escape government regulation by avoiding drugstores and other large outlets and by clever ad copy and labeling. One pamphlet for a nationally distributed line of herbal extracts has a disclaimer in tiny print that says that none of the information is intended to recommend the medicinal use of herbs, yet the entire text is a catalogue of symptoms and ailments and the herbal extract mixtures best for them. Another way medicinal herb promoters get around the law is to give their products names which strongly hint at their intended uses, but make no explicit claims—LVR, ALRG, GBLAD, BP, and RUMART are examples.

All the quackery and potential hazards notwithstanding, there are some herbs that are still useful in their unrefined form. They are each briefly discussed below. You should not use these in lieu of consulting a physician for severe injuries or persistent symptoms. Other herbs probably aren't effective for their claimed medicinal purposes, but are generally harmless if used in moderation. Still others should be completely avoided due to toxicity.

Botanical names are given for those herbs about which there is often confusion.

Herbs That Are Probably Useful

Aloe is used in the treatment of burns and scrapes. Evidence supports only the use of the fresh plant, not juices, gels or other extracts. Aloe quackery is big business and fantastic claims are being made. Don't fall for promotions of aloe as a cure-all. Use externally only and avoid commercial products.

Arnica is used externally on bruises, sprains, and the like to decrease inflammation and pain. Be alert to possible development of contact dermatitis; discontinue use if irritation or rash develops. **Do not use internally in any form!** It may cause death due to severe hypertension and poisoning of the heart.

Chamomiles, German and English (*Matricaria chamomilla* and *Anthemis nobilis,* respectively), are used to reduce inflammation affecting skin and mucous membranes, and to treat peptic ulcers, gastrointestinal spasms, and menstrual cramps. The German variety has been studied more and is apparently much more potent than the English.

Comfrey roots and leaves are used to make a poultice to promote the healing of cuts, scrapes, burns, and other external wounds. They contain allantoin, which promotes cell proliferation and healing. **Do not use internally in any form!** Comfrey contains carcinogens and powerful liver toxins.

Echinacea (*Echinacea angustifolia* and *Echinacea purpurea* are so similar they are both simply called Echinacea), a type of daisy, was a popular commercial anti-infective a century ago. It fell into disuse in the 1930s with the advent of sulfa drugs. There is evidence that components of the plant stop the growth of some bacteria by stimulating certain immune functions. This herb is rated as *probably useful* not to encourage self-treatment of serious disease, but because further research should be done. *Possibly useful* would be more accurate. Echinacea is now being promoted as a wonder herb, but no one really knows how safe and effective it is. At least one component kills houseflies and other insects, which should alert users to potential toxicity. Much of the so-called echinacea on the market now is really another member of the composite family, *Parthenium integrifolium L.,* and no one knows what it does.

Feverfew (*Chrysanthemum parthenium*) has been used for centuries for the treatment of fever, headache, and arthritis. There is now good evidence that chewing a couple of leaves each day can reduce the severity and frequency of migraines. Other applications are being studied. If you want to try feverfew keep in mind that commercially available tablets are often inactive, so try to get fresh leaves. Long-term toxicity studies have not been done, so use in moderation and be alert for possible side effects.

Garlic has been used for centuries as a general cure-all, but recent interest has focused on its effects on the cardiovascular system. It may provide some protection against atherosclerosis, heart disease, and stroke by lowering cholesterol levels, lowering blood pressure, and inhibiting clot formation. Only the fresh product seems effective. Cooking does not reduce its effectiveness. Garlic powders, oils, and extracts have little or no active components left. Excessive consumption of garlic can burn the mouth, irritate the stomach, and cause hyperacidity, indigestion, and diarrhea. It might also aggravate peptic ulcers.

Ginger is a folk remedy for indigestion, colds, nausea, and vomiting. It may be useful to prevent motion sickness. A gram or so of the dried product appears sufficient. Very large doses may cause heart arrhythmias and other symptoms of toxicity.

Horehound is widely used as a tea and in cough remedies as an expectorant; it is said to loosen mucus in the lungs. Evidence for effectiveness of the commercial products is very weak, but the herb may be effective. Claims for other uses, like treating tuberculosis, are unsubstantiated.

Hyssop seems to be useful as an expectorant and to sooth sore throats and ease hoarseness. There is no evidence to support other claims for this herb.

Onions may have beneficial effects similar to those of garlic; it also has similar hazards (see above).

Slippery elm, also known as red elm, is a large deciduous tree that has been a favorite of herbalists since the American Indians taught the pioneers how to use it. The dried inner bark contains large amounts of mucilage and starch, and is an effective demulcent or emollient. It is soothing for coughs and sore throats and is well tolerated as a food when nothing else is. It is sometimes used as a baby food flavored with cinnamon, nutmeg, and sugar.

Valerian roots contain chemicals called valepotriates, which are apparently effective tranquilizers. In moderate doses the tea appears to be safe. The herb has been used for more than a thousand years and is popular in Europe. The commercial products, the scores of pills, teas, and liquid extracts, have highly variable pharmacologic activity because the valepotriates are volatile and easily dissipated.

Yarrow (*Achillea millefolium*) is similar to chamomile (see above).

Herbs Probably Not Effective but Safe in Moderation

Barberry, buchu, burdock, butcher's broom, catnip, chickweed, chicory, damiana, dandelion, devil's claw, evening primrose, fennel, fenugreek, fo-ti (*Polygonum cultiflorum,* caution: laxative, not recommended), gentian, ginseng (*Panax pseudoginseng, P. quinquefolius, P. notoginseng,* regular heavy use can be toxic), gotu kola (*Centella asiatica*), hawthorn, hops, licorice (caution: tea and candy may be hazardous to those with hypertension or heart disease), linden flowers, lovage, Mormon tea (*Ephedra nevadensis*),* mullein, myrrh, nettle, passion flower, pennyroyal (leaves only, not the oil extract, which is toxic), peppermint, raspberry leaf,* red clover, rose hips (good source of vitamin C), rosemary, sage, St. John's wort, sarsaparilla, savory, saw palmetto, scullcap, senna

*__Caution:__ high tannin content. Frequent use is not recommended. Tannin is a weak carcinogen. It also appears to block absorption of some B vitamins, some pain relievers, antihistamines, and other medications.

(caution: laxative, not recommended), uva ursi,* witch hazel, yellow dock* (caution: laxative, not recommended), yohimbe, and yucca.

Toxic Herbs That Should *Not* Be Taken Internally

American hellebore or false hellebore (*Vertatrum viride*), Angelica, apricot pits, arnica, autumn crocus, bayberry, belladonna, betony, black cohosh, bloodroot, blue cohosh, boneset, borage, buckthorn (*Rhamnus catharticus* and *R. frangula*), calamus, canaigre, chaparral (*Larrea tridentata*), coltsfoot, comfrey, datura or jimson weed, dong quai (*Angelica polymorpha* and *A. sinensis*), elder or elderberry (*Sambucus cannadensis* and *S. pubens*), eyebright, foxglove, goldenseal, gordolobo (*Senecio longilobus*), groundsel (*Senecio vulgaris*), henbane, jimson weed or thorn apple, lily of the valley or May lily (*Convallaria majalis*), lobelia, mandrake (*Mandragora officinarum*), May apple or American mandrake (*Podophyllum peltatum*), mistletoe (all varieties), pau d'Arco (several *Tabebuia* species), pennyroyal oil, pokeroot or pokeweed (*Phytolacca americana*), rue, sage (light use in cooking is okay), sassafras (*Sassafras albidum*), squill (*Urginea maritima*), tansy, tansy ragwort (*Senicio jacobaea*), tonka bean, wintergreen, woodruff (*Asperula odorata* and *Galium odoratum*), and wormwood.

Note on Chinese Herbal Remedies. Hundreds of herbs are used in Chinese medicine; they are gradually being tested for effectiveness and safety by the Chinese and others using modern scientific methods. Many of them show promise and their use may become widespread. However, aside from ginseng and a few others, Chinese herbs are still largely unknown and unavailable in the West. Therefore, this discussion focuses on an important hazard associated with so-called Chinese herbal remedies in pill form.

Herbal remedies, both as whole herbs and as extracts, have been imported from Hong Kong, Taiwan, Singapore, and elsewhere in the Orient for decades with no particular hazards reported. However, since the early 1970s many cases of sickness and some deaths have been associated with the pills, many of which turn out to contain various powerful drugs, such as phenylbutazone, aminopyrine, diuretics, tranquilizers, cortisone-type drugs, antibiotics, and common painkillers. It appears that some manufacturers have been cashing in on the American fascination with "natural medicines" by marketing shotgun mixtures of drugs as herbal remedies.

These drugs are smuggled into the United States and sold in "health food" stores, specialty shops, by mail, and through other outlets. Typically, a few dozen pills are packaged in a cellophane bag or glass bottle and labeling or illustrations may suggest the pills help in arthritis and similar conditions. The pills have been found to contain not only the powerful and hazardous drugs, but animal bones, horns and shells, toxic heavy metals, insect parts, and rodent droppings.

Addicting and Recreational Drugs

Since prehistoric times people have been eating, drinking, smoking, snorting, and taking rectally various plant potions and brews not for therapeutic purposes but for group ritual, inspiration, insight, stimulation, sedation, and pleasure. Here we discuss some of the most commonly used and abused nontherapeutic drugs. Our focus is on the history, physiological effects, health hazards, and means of combating abuse.

Prevention of drug abuse is especially important in young children and adolescents. Prolonged exposure to mind-altering and organ-damaging drugs from an early age can have disastrous consequences. Adolescence is hard enough for sober kids. Drug-induced delusions, mood swings, and bizarre behavior make normal family relations, socialization, and maturation almost impossible. The toxic effects of the drugs on the brain, lungs, liver, and hormones add to the problems. There are no easy answers, but important factors in prevention include parental love and guidance; opportunities for pleasure in recreation; opportunities for satisfaction in work; and an understanding of the physiological, psychological, and social consequences of drug abuse. We can only help with the last of these. Drug education should focus on physiological effects and hazards, avoiding exaggeration and sensationalism. Horror stories should be avoided unless they are well documented. Credibility must be maintained by absolute honesty and openness.

Treatment of drug abuse depends on age, degree of addiction or abuse, drugs involved, physical and mental health, and other factors. A family doctor can help with tobacco addiction, and should be consulted about possible health complications and detoxification by alcoholics as well as most other drug addicts and abusers. However effective, treatment that results in long-term abstinence from alcohol, heroin, cocaine, or amphetamines usually requires long-term treatment, support groups, and group therapy. There are many outpatient and residential treatment programs. Major programs with national recognition include Alcoholics Anonymous, Narcotics Anonymous, Habilitat, Phoenix House, and Secular Sobriety Groups. Many private psychiatric hospitals run detoxification and rehabilitation programs for all varieties of drug abusers, but they are usually very expensive. There are inexpensive outpatient programs run by states and counties in some areas. Information on the various options is available from the drug abuse division of your state or local department of health.

Alcohol

Ethyl alcohol (ethanol) was independently discovered many times by accidental fermentation of fruit juices and grains. In some cultures alcoholic beverages have been used for thousands of years as a palliative or sedative in illness, a crude anesthetic for bone setting or surgery, and a fairly nutritious drink, but the most important use of alcohol is as a psychoactive drug. In small amounts it commonly reduces inhibitions and promotes relaxation and social interactions. As the blood level of alcohol increases there is, progressively, loss of coordination, slowing of the reflexes, slurring of speech, dizziness, impairment of memory and judgment, lack of self-control, confusion, inability to walk, loss of bladder control, vomiting, loss of consciousness, coma, and death. Drinking can cause a hangover the next day with a throbbing headache, dizziness, nausea, upset stomach, and thirst.

Ignorance of the dangers of alcohol can promote its abuse. Since most Americans do drink, all youngsters should be made aware of all the hazards involved long before they start drinking.

Effects of Alcohol Abuse

Alcohol abuse is an enormous health problem in the United States and dozens of other countries. The cost in lives, limbs, and property is staggering. In brief summary, alcohol addiction and other alcohol abuse cause the following serious problems.

More than 25,000 traffic deaths a year (in the U.S.) and far more injuries are caused by drinking drivers, whether drunk or not. The combination of increased self-confidence, poor judgment, and impaired reflexes is deadly. Even one drink can impair driving ability. Two drinks can impair ability by about one-third. The National Safety Council recommends that a person **wait one hour for every drink consumed before driving.** Coffee does *not* speed alcohol metabolism and sobering up.

Brain damage and dementia are common in alcoholics. The damage is so severe that the brains of long-term alcoholics are unfit for use in anatomy classes. It may be that every episode of moderate to heavy drinking causes the death of hundreds or thousands of irreplaceable brain cells. This has not been proved, but serious intellectual impairment seems to be at least as common as liver damage, even in young drinkers. Death and brain damage can also be caused by mixing alcohol with other drugs, especially sedatives, tranquilizers, and narcotics.

Birth defects like "fetal alcohol syndrome" can be caused by drinking during pregnancy. The syndrome produces infants with small bodies, heads, eyes, and ears; their failure to thrive; heart and kidney defects; brain damage and intellectual impairment; and poorly developed limbs, fingers, and genitals. It is estimated that in the United States several thousand infants, perhaps 1 percent of those exposed to alcohol in the womb, are born each year with some or all of the defects. While it has not been proved that light drinking (the equivalent of less than two beers a day) causes obvious defects, it may cause subtle intellectual impairment. Abstention from all alcohol from conception through lactation is advisable.

Malnutrition is often caused by heavy drinking. Some alcoholics get half of their total calories from alcohol itself and most of the rest from the protein- and vitamin-poor carbohydrate of the drinks. Besides replacing nutrient-rich foods and contributing to obesity, alcohol increases the requirement, while reducing the intake, of protein, thiamine, folic acid, magnesium, potassium, zinc, and possibly vitamin C, calcium, vitamin A, and other nutrients.

Liver diseases, including fatty liver, alcoholic hepatitis, and often fatal liver cirrhosis, are notorious results of alcoholism. Alcoholism is also the cause of most chronic pancreatitis.

Homicide, suicide, child beating, and other violent crimes are often associated with drinking.

356 **Heart disease and heart failure** are common in alcoholics, not just because of malnutrition, but because of direct poisoning of the heart muscles. The resulting abnormal heart function does not respond to nutritional therapy unless alcohol is withdrawn. Even then the damage may be irreversible.

Impaired immunity is a common result of heavy alcohol use. Through its toxic and anesthetic effects, the drug inhibits mobilization of upper respiratory secretions, suppresses white blood cell production by the bone marrow, impairs white cell function, and otherwise disrupts the immune system. It is not surprising that alcoholics suffer a very high incidence of pneumonia, tuberculosis, and other serious infectious diseases.

Skeletal muscle poisoning also occurs and may cause general weakness, muscle tenderness, cramping, and muscle breakdown. This, of course, makes it more difficult to lose fat if you are obese or to stay fit if you are not.

Cancer of the mouth, esophagous, pancreas, and possibly breast are promoted by alcohol. The cancer risks of smoking are increased by drinking.

Sexual impotence is frequent among alcoholic men apparently because of direct damage to the nerves of the penis and brain, and because of liver damage that results in lower testosterone and higher estrogen levels.

Alcoholism Warning Signs (from Early to Late)

- Do you drink because of fatigue, worry, depression, or disappointment or to increase your self-confidence and lose your shyness?
- Do you drink after quarrels or friction with friends or family?
- Do you occasionally pass out or have memory blackouts?
- Is your drinking increasing? Do you lie about this, and become annoyed and defensive when family or friends ask about your drinking?
- Do you often drink alone? Are you losing interest in your family and friends?
- Do you drink almost continuously for days at a time?
- Do you get drunk on important occasions for which you should be sober?
- Do you get the shakes in the morning and try to chase them away with a drink?

If your answer is "yes" to one or more of these questions, you may have a problem and should reconsider your drinking habits and seek help.

TREATMENT OF ALCOHOLISM

Treatment is essential or the alcoholic will likely end up in a mental hospital, a jail, or an early grave. The following are useful methods, but their success is strongly dependent on an acknowledgment of the problem and a determination to solve it.

Good nutrition, including multivitamin and mineral supplementation, is essential to minimizing the damage done to the liver, brain, and muscles by alcohol. It may even decrease the urge to drink somewhat.

Support groups can help. Alcoholics Anonymous has thousands of local groups of ex-problem drinkers who have helped millions of alcoholics go on the wagon for long periods, even for life. The approach is based on group support, self-understanding and religious (nondenominational) faith. Most cities have chapters (check your phone directory). Those who prefer a nonreligious approach can ask local humanist groups about their counseling programs. A national grass roots movement called Secular Sobriety Groups (SSG) is gaining momentum. All alcoholics and their families are welcome at no charge and on an anonymous basis. SSG has been endorsed by Los Angeles courts, and chapters are opening in various cities.

Drugs can help some alcoholics who aren't helped much by counseling alone. Some are used to create an aversion to alcohol; others to ease withdrawal.

Amphetamine Group

Amphetamine, which is chemically similar to adrenalin, was first synthesized in 1887 but not recognized as pharmacologically active until 1927 when its hypertensive, bronchial dilating, and central stimulating effects were noticed. It was soon found to be useful in narcolepsy and has since been used for barbiturate poisoning, severe motion sickness, hyperactivity in children, depression, and weight control. The last application has generally yielded disastrous results and is no longer considered consistent with good medical practice. Variations of amphetamine, such as methamphetamine, methylphenidate (Ritalin), and phenmetrazine (Preludin), are very similar in their effects and controversial applications.

These drugs are potent stimulants and euphoriants with effects similar to cocaine, but longer lasting. They produce, in most people, wakefulness, alertness, elevation of mood, increased self-confidence, and increased physical activity. They were used in World War II by the armed forces of America, Britain, Germany, and Japan, and have been popular with millions of truck drivers, students, dieters, businessmen, athletes, and others. The drugs work by speeding the release of stimulant neurotransmitters across their synapses, causing enhanced electrical activity in certain areas of the brain. The problem is that the neurotransmitters are depleted by amphetamines, and the physiological and psychological effects of withdrawal are the exact opposite of those of the drug. Sleepiness, fatigue, hunger, and depression are inevitable and proportional to the dosage and duration of use.

Tolerance to amphetamines develops rapidly and doses tend to increase, often until the person must take large amounts just to feel normally alert and cheerful. Even with a constant dose withdrawal symptoms may set in. That's why many users progress to the extremes of amphetamine abuse. "Speed freaks" inject about 20 milligrams a day at first and rapidly increase dosage to several hundred milligrams several times a day.

During prolonged binges the user often develops symptoms indistinguishable from cocaine psychosis with all kinds of illusions and intense paranoia. Violence may be done in perceived self-defense. After months of amphetamine use the intellect may become severely disorganized and incompetent. Though hardly able to take care of him- or herself, the speed addict keeps shooting or swallowing the drug for fear of the profound depression that is inevitable should he or she stop. The intellectual impairment and depression may persist for several months after withdrawal. Some experts believe severe addiction leaves a residue of damage to the brain, a kind of biochemical scarring, because of which neurotransmitters in some areas never function quite normally again.

A frightening new development is the mass production and wide distribution of "ice," crystals of smokable methamphetamine. This product delivers large doses to the brain perhaps even faster than intravenous injection. It carries all the risks of crack cocaine and more because it is very long lasting; it promises to be a major scourge in the 1990s. Ice is cheap to produce and cheap to get addicted to; from then on it's very expensive financially, emotionally, socially, and medically. Kids *must* be told what this drug will do to their brains if they use it.

Caffeine Group

According to legend, the first coffee lover was an Ethiopian goatherd who noticed that his goats stayed awake all night if they ate the berries of the *Coffea arabica* tree. He tried them and passed along the practice. By about A.D. 1500 coffee was popular all over the Islamic world and making inroads into Europe. It created a prolonged scandal almost as great as the contemporary controversy about marijuana use, and many people called for its prohibition for health reasons. In the late 1600s Italian priests asked Pope Clement VIII to ban the brew, which they saw as a part of a Satanic plot perpetrated by the Muslims. He replied that the drink was too delicious to leave to the infidels, and cheated Satan by baptizing coffee.

Coffee, of course, is not the only source of caffeine, and caffeine is not the only stimulant in its class, the xanthines. Other sources of these alkaloids (caffeine, theophylline, and theobromine) are tea, cola drinks, maté (a small evergreen tree of South America), guarana (also a South American herb), kola nuts, chocolate, and over-the-counter stimulants and pain relievers. The xanthines are the most widely used drugs in the United States. The typical American starts on hot chocolate as an infant, soon graduates to colas, and continues on coffee, tea, and caffeine pills for life.

The Effects and Hazards of Xanthines

The main effect of caffeine and its relatives is to stimulate the central nervous system and the heart, relax the bronchial airways, and act as a diuretic. It is the central stimulation, the apparently greater energy level, relief from drowsiness, and clarity of mind that keep people coming back for more.

Caffeine periodically comes under fire whenever a study is released showing it to be harmful to this or that part of the body. The study is debated, doubted, and usually forgotten, but the evidence continues to grow. Now there is increasing pressure for health-warning labels and removal of caffeine from colas. The following is a brief summary of the case against caffeine (which applies to a lesser extent to theophylline and to an even lesser extent to theobromine).

Caffeine tends to aggravate gastritis and **peptic ulcers** by stimulating secretion of gastric acid. Most people with chronic acid-related problems are familiar with the intense burning sensation they get in their stomachs after drinking coffee, tea, or colas.

Caffeine can cause anxiety, insomnia, irritability, dizziness, and other symptoms of excessive nervous stimulation. Some people go through years of suffering with these problems and even go to psychiatrists for help without ever suspecting the true cause of their misery. When the caffeine is withdrawn the symptoms often disappear within a day or two.

Nutritional hazards confront heavy users. Caffeine, tannic acid, and other components of coffee and tea promote excretion of thiamine and other B vitamins. Combined with a borderline intake of these vitamins, this could contribute to the development of a deficiency. Coffee and tea can also reduce the absorption of iron, calcium, and possibly other minerals. Heavy users should consider supplements, especially if their eating habits are poor. Very heavy coffee drinkers, those who drink more than ten cups a day, run a risk of potassium depletion, which can cause fainting, weakness, muscle spasms, and other symptoms.

Diarrhea and other gastrointestinal disturbances can be caused by caffeine and its relatives. If you have unexplained chronic diarrhea, stop all xanthine intake. The xanthines can also cause pruritis ani; if your anus itches mysteriously, try stopping your consumption of caffeine and related substances.

Cardiovascular health may be affected by caffeine. There is some concern that heavy caffeine consumption may increase cholesterol levels and aggravate hypertension. However, tolerance to the hypertensive effects of caffeine develops rapidly; regular consumption apparently has no effect on blood pressure. Moreover, the evidence that caffeine causes cholesterol levels to increase is very weak.

Caffeine is addicting—the most socially acceptable addicting drug in the West. Sudden withdrawal often causes headache, lethargy, depression, irritability, and constipation.

Birth Defects? Caffeine in very large doses can cause cleft palate, missing toes and fingers, and other birth defects in animals. Some advocate a warning label on cans and packages of tea and coffee. "Warning to pregnant women: Consuming coffee or tea may cause birth defects or other reproductive problems." Most studies suggest that if there is a hazard to the fetus it is only at the very highest levels of consumption, and even then the hazard is slight. Nevertheless, moderation is in order for pregnant women.

Conclusions. The evidence that coffee and other sources of xanthines are serious health hazards is not overwhelming, but it is strong enough to warrant caution and moderation in their use. The heavy marketing to children of caffeine-containing soft drinks is especially objectionable. It is added to the drinks not as a flavoring agent, but simply as a drug, and it is the only psychoactive drug marketed so freely.

Major sources of caffeine and approximate content:

- **Coffee:** 70 to 150 mg per cup
- **Tea:** 30 to 50 mg per cup (additional theophylline adds to stimulant effect)
- **Caffeine-containing soft drinks:** 40 to 55 mg per 12-oz. can
- **Combination painkillers and cold pills:** 30 to 65 mg
- **Nonprescription stimulant pills:** 100 mg

Cocaine

Cocaine was the big scandal drug of the 1980s and will continue to wreak havoc in the nineties; movie stars, athletes, and other celebrities are in the news almost daily because of their involvement with it. Inner-city infants are born addicted to it and infected with AIDS because of it. Thousands of addicts are lined up seeking treatment; thousands are ending up in emergency rooms because of adverse reactions; and thousands are dying after snorting, injecting, or smoking the drug. The huge appetite of Americans for cocaine combined with its illegality has given rise to illicit marketing and gang wars on a scale not seen since Prohibition. Cocaine is relatively new to American culture and many people start using it without any knowledge of what it is and does. This scourge will never be controlled without wider understanding of the drug.

History

The coca plant, *Erythroxylon coca,* is an evergreen shrub that grows in western South America, especially Bolivia and Peru. It has been used at least since A.D. 500 and possibly much earlier; this is known from Indian mummies buried with coca leaves, and ancient pottery showing the cheek bulge typical of a coca chewer. During the Inca rule coca plantations were a state monopoly and use was restricted to the highest classes, with some exceptions for soldiers going into battle and workers on important projects. Coca was believed to be of divine origin, and indiscriminate use was considered a sacrilege.

The Spanish conquerors had mixed attitudes: The missionaries at first opposed coca as idolatry and a barrier to conversion, but the government found it essential for recruiting workers for the mines, farms, and forests. The Spanish also came to recognize the role of coca in Indian folk medicine—it was used to treat chronic pain and a variety of ailments. Eventually the church grew plantations of coca to sell to the workers or use as a wage. The Spanish came to control most of the coca and used it to manipulate and exploit the Indians.

In the 1880s researchers at the University of Göttingen isolated the most potent of several alkaloids in coca and named it cocaine. Shortly thereafter, Italian neurologist Dr. Paolo Mantegazza studied the effects of coca on himself and reported his findings in "On the Hygienic and Medicinal Virtues of Coca." Besides describing the physiological effects, he wrote of the "deeply joyful and intensely alive" feelings.

Dr. Freud and Cocaine

Mantegazza's report strongly influenced Sigmund Freud. Freud tried cocaine on himself and was impressed with the increased capacity for work and the improvement of mood he experienced. In 1884 he wrote "On Coca," his famous paper which extolled the "virtues of cocaine." He suggested therapeutic use of cocaine for digestive disorders, heart disease, nervous exhaustion, cachexia (wasting), morphine addiction, alcoholism, asthma, and sexual impotence; and use as a local anesthetic.

Only the last has survived medicine's test of time. Freud participated in the first application of cocaine as a local anesthetic for eye surgery; the patient was his own father. The cocaine worked well and is still used for this purpose. However, another of Freud's experiments with cocaine was a disaster. His friend Ernst von Fleischl had become addicted to morphine, using it for pain from an amputated thumb. Freud tried to free him from the morphine by giving him cocaine, but von Fleischl rapidly progressed to large intravenous doses of cocaine and deteriorated quickly. He had paranoid hallucinations similar to those of alcoholic *delirium tremens*—snakes crawling over him and insects under his skin. The cocaine addiction was worse than the morphine. It was said that he had gone from being the first morphine addict in Europe to be cured by cocaine, to being the first cocaine addict in Europe.

Other users were soon reporting similar problems. Within three years of introducing what he thought would be a major advance in medicine, Freud found himself widely accused of irresponsibility and recklessness, and charged with unleashing the third scourge on humanity (after alcohol and opiates). Freud had also contended that there seemed to be no lethal dose for humans, and that the toxic dose was very high. Shortly after this one of his patients died from an overdose Freud had prescribed. By 1900 scores of severe poisonings and dozens of deaths had been reported. European enthusiasm for cocaine waned.

In America William S. Halsted, widely consider the "father of modern surgery," developed new techniques using cocaine as a nerve block to produce regional anesthesia. However, he and some of his assistants, unaware of the problems being reported in Europe, experimented with cocaine and became heavily addicted. In an ironic reversal of Freud's suggested use, Halsted used morphine to ease the misery of cocaine withdrawal and became addicted to morphine.

The late 1800s saw a great proliferation of cocaine-containing patent medicines, tonics, soft drinks, ointments, suppositories, wines, cigarettes, and other products. They were advertised as effective in just about every disease. One of these products was Coca Cola, originally marketed as a medicine for headache, melancholy, and many other problems. In 1903 cocaine was removed from the formula and Coca Cola was advertised as simply a soft drink.

In 1914 the Harrison Narcotics Act removed most cocaine from the open market. Since 1970 cocaine has been classified as a schedule II drug, which includes drugs with recognized medical uses, but with high abuse potential. (Schedule I includes heroin, with no recognized medical uses and high addiction potential.) Only one U.S. company is licensed to import coca leaves. It produces all of the 500 or so kilograms used in medicine.

Pharmacology and Physiology

The most important thing to understand about cocaine is that, contrary to statements by government officials, educators, police, reporters, and others who should know better, it is not a narcotic, but a stimulant. It is remarkable that several years into the "war on drugs" the generals in this war still don't know what they are fighting. Cocaine enhances the activity of stimulant neurotransmitters in the brain. The peak of the effect occurs about fifteen to twenty minutes after snorting it into the nostrils; it wears off in about an hour. Injected and smoked cocaine act much faster. Oral doses are at least as potent as snorted but take about an extra hour to work. Heart rate and blood pressure usually increase and appetite usually decreases.

Initial euphoria is almost universally reported; this is undoubtedly the reason for the drug's popularity. Negative effects include restlessness, irritability, depression, anxiety, and paranoia. These effects, including the euphoria, are also common in amphetamine use. In fact, if cocaine is given intravenously to subjects familiar with both cocaine and amphetamine, they usually cannot distinguish it from amphetamine except by its shorter action.

Hazards of Cocaine

Sudden death may occur by direct suppression of respiratory centers in the brain, by stroke, or by cardiovascular collapse. Hundreds of cases have been reported, including both medical and illicit use. Snorting, injection, and smoking have all been implicated. Even healthy people are not immune to these dangers, but those at risk for heart attack or stroke and those with high blood pressure or blood clotting disorders should be especially wary of using cocaine. Contrary to the stereotypes, most victims of sudden death due to cocaine are not unemployed criminals or chronic addicts. They are mostly blue-collar and white-collar occasional and moderate users.

Permanent brain damage can be caused by cocaine. Spasm of blood vessels in the brain and hemorrhage in the brain can kill brain cells and result in severe headache, bizarre behavior, and a wide variety of neurologic and psychiatric complications.

Cocaine psychosis, similar to paranoid schizophrenia, with all kinds of delusions and hallucinations, can occur during heavy use. "Cocaine bugs," the delusion of insects on or under the skin, may be so real to the victim that the skin may be injured in attempts to remove them. Insomnia, anorexia, seizures, panic, extreme irritability, and headaches may occur.

Cocaine is extremely addicting. Monkeys, rats, and other animals given unlimited access to cocaine will self-administer it until they die, often ignoring food and water. In humans the withdrawal symptoms are not, as with opiates, a flulike sickness. The main problem is depression due to temporary depletion of the brain's neurotransmitters. If use continues at a given level of intake the pleasure diminishes, so in most cases the dose is steadily increased.

Being at high risk for AIDS, hepatitis B, and other blood- and sexually transmitted diseases is a consequence of the powerful addiction. In the face of withdrawal depression, addicts think nothing of risking sickness and death from sharing needles to shoot cocaine, or prostituting themselves to buy crack.

Decreased Libido. Cocaine is often hyped as a wonderful aphrodisiac, but the truth is quite the opposite. Long-term use by any method of administration can result in a dramatic reduction of libido. Moreover, even novice users are likely to experience decreased sex drive for hours after a dose. For those who progress to injecting or smoking the drug, the orgasmic rush they get often replaces sex in their lives.

Diminished capacity for pleasure is an ironic and tragic consequence of cocaine addiction; it may be permanent if dosage is high. Cocaine claims the brain's pleasure centers as its exclusive domain. No longer can the addict enjoy the little things in life like eating good food, making love, listening to music, reading, visiting with friends, playing with kids, exercising, and working. The drug depletes vital brain chemicals, causing depression, fatigue, anxiety, paranoid delusions, and many other symptoms. Most regular users wish they had never seen cocaine and eventually resolve to quit the drug, with varying degrees of success.

How to Kick Cocaine

Write down all the reasons you want to quit using the drug—the irritability, anxiety, depression, insomnia, nasal destruction, nosebleeds, run-down health, and risk of having convulsions or even a heart attack or stroke. Contemplate all the things you could do with the money and time you would save. Resolve firmly to refuse the drug if it is offered and to never seek it or buy it—even if you have to change the company you keep. If you cannot quit at once or within a week of tapering the dose down, you should seek help. Long-term treatment may be the best option. See discussion of residential treatment of opiate addiction, below.

Heroin and Other Opiates

Opium is the dried juice of the capsule of the opium poppy *Papaver somniferum* and it contains **morphine** and **codeine.** Morphine is a very powerful and addicting painkiller and narcotic; codeine is a weaker painkiller and not nearly as addicting. Opium is swallowed or smoked;

 morphine is snorted or injected under the skin, into a muscle, or into a vein; and codeine is injected or swallowed as a pill or liquid. All the opiates act directly on the central nervous system to produce pain relief, sedation, constipation, pupil constriction, and sometimes euphoria or dysphoria, nausea, and dizziness. Very large overdoses can cause death by respiratory depression. The synthetic narcotics oxycodone and pentazocine have effects similar to those of the opiates, and they are often similarly abused.

Heroin, diacetylmorphine, is made by heating morphine together with acetic acid. It was developed in Germany at the turn of the century as a "heroic" or super aspirin, hence the name. It was used for many aches, pains, and ailments, and for treating morphine addiction. It took about twenty years of over-the-counter sales and widespread use for it to be generally recognized that heroin has essentially the same effects and hazards as morphine, into which it is converted in the body.

Opiates in Early America

During the 1800s opium was imported into the United States as well as grown commercially in New England, California, Arizona, and some southern states. Morphine became widely available from many sources, all legal. Physicians, drugstores, grocery stores and mail-order companies provided pure products as well as hundreds of patent medicines containing opiates. They were used for all kinds of aches and pains, diarrhea, coughs, "women's troubles," and even colic and teething pain in infants.

Morphine was often used to treat alcoholism, which usually meant converting an alcoholic to a morphine addict. Morphine addiction was considered preferable because morphine was cheaper and less harmful to the mind and body. Compared to the loud, foulmouthed, often violent drunkard, the morphine addict was a model citizen. And while the alcoholic often suffered from ulcers, gastritis, malnutrition, liver disease, mental deterioration, and heart trouble, the morphine addict suffered little more than constipation and decreased libido.

In 1914 Congress passed the Harrison Narcotics Act, which effectively eliminated all legal supplies of morphine to addicts, who then typically switched to the still-legal heroin. When this loophole was closed in 1924 a new era began. Many older people who had been addicted for decades subsequent to opiate use for medical purposes suffered enormously from the withdrawal sickness, especially when it was compounded with pain from arthritis and other chronic health problems. In the following years addicts concentrated in cities where they could "score," generally with adulterated, contaminated, expensive heroin that was usually injected intravenously for economy.

The Nature of Heroin Addiction

During the last century and the first part of this century most opiate addiction occurred subsequent to the often misguided use of opiates to relieve the symptoms of various major and minor ailments and injuries. In recent decades addiction due to medical use has been rare. Most heroin users start taking the drug as a tranquilizer to relieve anxiety and tension, or for a high to relieve boredom.

A very few users (perhaps 3 percent) experience intense pleasure from the first dose and rapidly become addicted. Another small minority of users takes heroin once or twice a week for many months or years without becoming addicted. The vast majority of addicts start off as occasional users, gradually increase the frequency of use, and become addicted months after their first dose.

While many addicts who mainline (inject into a vein) heroin experience a rush of warmth in the abdomen that they perceive as pleasant, **the basis of addiction is not pleasure but pain.** The addict must take the drug three or four times every day to prevent the very severe **withdrawal sickness,** which typically includes yawning, hot and cold flashes, profuse sweating, watering eyes and nose, abdominal cramps, nausea, vomiting, diarrhea, muscle and joint aches and pains, and severe anxiety.

After an addict kicks the habit he or she is likely to suffer from a **post-addiction syndrome** consisting of anxiety, depression, poor tolerance for major and minor stresses (loud noises, heat, cold, annoyances, and inconveniences), and a craving for the drug. If a relapse occurs and the addict returns to the drug he or she is generally not motivated by a hedonistic love of pleasure but by a desperate attempt to feel normal. The post-addiction syndrome varies in severity, comes and goes in waves, and can last many months, which helps explain why relapse is so common.

Health Hazards of Heroin Addiction

The health hazards of opiate addiction depend on social circumstances, especially whether or not the drug is legally available. When it is, it can be taken regularly for many years with surprisingly mild effects on health. For example, Dr. William S. Halsted became addicted to morphine at age thirty-four, subsequent to using it to cure his cocaine addiction.

 He remained healthy, vigorous, active, renowed for his skill, and addicted until his death at seventy.

There have been many like Halsted who apparently suffer little more than constipation, decreased libido, and constricted pupils that make it hard to see in the dark. While constipation can promote hemorrhoids and possibly other problems, there is no evidence of the kind of malnutrition, brain damage, mental deterioration, and psychosis often seen in alcoholics.

The effects on women may include cessation of ovulation and, if they do get pregnant, complications like toxemia, hemorrhage, and premature delivery. It is not clear whether these effects are due to the drug or the stress and malnutrition that accompany addiction when the drug is expensive and hard to get.

The typical heroin addict who uses illicit, expensive, adulterated heroin is at risk for a host of serious health problems, including hepatitis, AIDS, and other infections; kidney failure; malnutrition and all its consequences; and injury due to violence, including murder and suicide. Sudden death may occur due to accidental overdose, especially if taken with alcohol or sedatives.

The Treatment of Heroin Addiction

Even when opiates were legal and widely used, addiction to them was viewed with alarm; few people wanted to become or remain addicted. Physicians and addicts tried various means of quitting the drugs, including gradual withdrawal, going cold turkey, taking hot or cold baths, and taking belladonna, naloxone (an opiate antagonist), and other drugs. Whatever was tried, even if the addicts got past withdrawal sickness and stayed clean for weeks, the vast majority returned to the morphine or heroin within a few months, driven by the post-addiction syndrome.

Since the 1960s some of the most successful programs for kicking heroin have involved daily oral doses of the drug methadone, a synthetic narcotic developed by opium-poor Germany during World War II. Methadone substantially reduces withdrawal sickness, so it is very useful in detoxification. Methadone maintenance programs help the addicts who can get past heroin withdrawal but always end up back on the needle within a few months. The drug quiets the post-addiction syndrome and blocks the effects of heroin should the addict take it. As long as one stays on methadone he or she can lead an essentially normal life. Many thousands of heroin addicts who would otherwise be busy stealing and fencing all day to support their habits have been freed by methadone programs to hold jobs, go to school, and otherwise function in society.

Side effects of methadone include constipation and slightly decreased libido, but the effects are generally weaker than with heroin. A large dose can kill a child and, like all drugs, methadone should be kept out of the reach of children.

Of course, curing the addiction without resorting to another addiction is far preferable to methadone regimens. The best tool for this is long-term treatment in a residential facility with lots of group therapy and occupational rehabilitation. Addicts must be taught social and work skills that will help them survive and be happy, which takes time. Because of this and the post-addiction syndrome, good programs last many months, preferably at least a year. Habilitat in Hawaii is a good example of a residential treatment program with all the ingredients for success. The program is long-term (generally fourteen to twenty months), it includes almost daily group encounters led by skilled and compassionate ex-addicts, and it emphasizes practical job training.

Marijuana

The hemp plant, *Cannabis sativa,* has been used by humans since the dawn of history. Stone Age Chinese used the fibrous weed to make fabrics for clothing, bedding, mats, nets, and the like. Before long, hemp was found useful for making ropes and sails, and it became important to all seafaring people. Just when its psychoactivity was discovered is unknown, but it was clearly a very long time ago. There is evidence of cannabis use as an anesthetic, a medicine, an aid in magic, and an intoxicant from at least a thousand years B.C. in China, Persia, and India. It was generally eaten in various ways until smoking was introduced from North America. Ironically, America, which gave the world tobacco, is one of the few places where cannabis is almost always smoked alone rather than mixed with tobacco.

Marijuana and the Body

The psychoactive constituent of marijuana is tetrahydracannabinol, THC. When marijuana is smoked the THC vaporizes and is inhaled. From the lungs it is absorbed into the blood, which takes it to all areas of the body. THC is lipophilic ("loves fat"), so it tends to concentrate in cell membranes and lipid-rich tissue such as fat, the brain, sex glands, and adrenal glands. It is metabolized, especially in the liver, and is eventually excreted, mostly in the feces and urine. A single dose may remain in the tissue for ten days or more, mostly in a slightly altered, nonpsychoactive form. Regular smokers may build up large tissue deposits.

How potent is THC? A typical one-person joint has about 10 milligrams of THC in it; 1 to 5 milligrams will get into the blood. This makes THC comparable in potency to diazepam (Valium) and similar tranquilizers. This is not to imply these drugs are equivalent. While there are similarities between them, they are substantially different. THC, for example, does tend to tranquilize the body, but most users consider it a mental stimulant; an overdose does not cause stupor and sleepiness, but anxiety and panic.

Can Marijuana Kill?

Very rarely, fatalities have occurred in India when children, probably hungry, ate large amounts of hashish, most likely on empty stomachs, assuring rapid and complete absorption of the THC. Death from smoking cannabis is practically unheard of, but one young man almost succeeded in a suicide attempt. It is estimated he had smoked about 90 grams of hashish with 5 percent THC, or 4500 milligrams, over several hours. Anything over 1 gram THC should be considered potentially lethal, especially in smaller people and those without tolerance to THC due to recent use.

The empty seed pods of sinsemilla marijuana (nonfertilized female flower tops) may have up to 10 percent THC. As domestic growers refine the art, and as entrepreneurs develop ever more potent oils, we may begin to see occasional fatal overdoses. Five grams of a potent hashish oil could be lethal. This amount could fit into about five large gelatin capsules. However, cannabis and THC will never be implicated in scores, hundreds, and thousands of sudden deaths, as are cocaine, amphetamines, and heroin.

A more likely danger is that of death and injury due to accidents caused by THC-induced fuzzyheadedness. Marijuana intoxication has been blamed for car and train wrecks and other terrible accidents. No hard figures are available, but the annual death toll could be several hundred each year.

Harmful Effects of Regular Use

Among regular users the daily dose of THC varies enormously. A very light smoker might get 1 or 2 milligrams of THC a day. A very heavy user might get one to two hundred times that. The following are possible consequences of frequent use.

Infertility in men and women, apparently by effects on pituitary hormone production and by interference with development of eggs and sperm.

Unhealthy Newborns. Since THC is known to cross the placenta, it is not surprising that there have been reports of low birth weight and symptoms similar to the fetal alcohol syndrome in infants exposed to THC in the womb; it should not be surprising if subtle learning deficiencies also occur in some of these children. Clearly, all sources of THC should be avoided during pregnancy and breast-feeding.

Cannabis smoking may cause cancer. A major group of carcinogens in tobacco and other kinds of smoke are the polynuclear aromatic hydrocarbons (PAHs). Marijuana smoke contains more than 150 PAHs, some in larger amounts than in tobacco smoke. The total tar content is about two to three times higher in marijuana than tobacco smoke. Although definitive epidemiological studies have not yet been done, cannabis has been suspected in some head, neck, and lung cancers in relatively young smokers.

Damage to the Respiratory System. As might be expected, inhaling the hot oil resin vapors and ashes of burning marijuana or hashish can cause respiratory problems. These include bronchitis, sinusitis, asthma attacks, increased nasal secretions and irritations, nasal stuffiness, frequent colds, sore throat, abnormal cells lining the respiratory tract, loss of cilia, chronic inflammation, and reduced lung capacity.

Cannabis is hazardous to those with heart disease of any kind. After smoking marijuana patients can exercise only about half as long as they normally can without heart pain. Marijuana apparently decreases oxygen delivery to the heart muscle.

Decreased Libido. Marijuana can cause decreased testosterone in the blood, lowered sperm count, and decreased sex drive, as has been reported for methadone, morphine, alcohol, and other drugs. These results are especially significant because lowered testosterone levels might affect normal development at puberty, and more and more youngsters are smoking marijuana now.

Contamination with pesticides and herbicides has always been a concern for marijuana smokers. Hashish smokers have long had to contend with aldulterants like shoe polish, camel dung, and assorted plant resins. Illness is occasionally associated with deliberate or incidental contamination of cannabis products, but the problem has always been considered minor. Now, however, the spector of mercury looms like a dark cloud over those who smoke cannabis grown in the volcanic soils of Hawaii, California, and some other states. Not only are the mercury levels of such plants often high, but smoking them leads to much greater absorption of the poison than does eating vegetables grown in the same soil.

Changes in Sleep and Memory. Marijuana has been reported to increase total sleeping time, increase napping, and reduce rapid eye movement (REM) sleep (dreaming). The decrease in dreaming may be related to marijuana's inhibition of memory. Both may be caused by THC's interference with nucleic acid and protein synthesis in the brain, processes believed to be essential steps in memory formation.

Changes in mood are common, along with lethargy, difficulty in thinking and speaking, confusion, apathy, loss of motivation, forgetfulness, irritability, suspiciousness, deterioration of time sense, emotional dullness, headaches, depression, feelings of unreality, difficulty concentrating, decreased libido, negligence to details, and loss of sense of purpose.

These changes make optimal functioning impossible. The person may become withdrawn, antisocial, and unable to relate to others or perform adequately in his or her work. Such people often seek medical help on their own or are persuaded to by concerned relatives or friends. Dozens of cases are described in the medical literature. If the person can be induced to stop smoking cannabis, the symptoms tend to subside over a period of weeks—alertness returns, thinking improves, and energy levels increase. But how easy is it for a heavy user to abstain or drastically cut down once motivated to do so? This brings us to the question of addiction.

Is Cannabis Addicting?

According to the 1972 report of the National Commission on Marijuana and Drug Abuse (the Shafer Commission), "Cannabis does not lead to physical dependence." Yet Fitz Ludlow, in his classic memoirs, *Confessions of a Hashish Eater,* lamented his enslavement to hashish and describes the agony he suffered in his efforts to free himself, which he finally did after several years of regular use. Was his dependence imaginary or a literary invention for dramatic effect? Was he mimicking Thomas DeQuincy *(Confessions of an Opium Eater)* or did the commission miss something?

Psychoactivity, tolerance, and withdrawal symptoms are the main features of addicting drugs. In the case of marijuana there is no question about the psychoactivity. Nor is there any question that tolerance develops. Very heavy smokers may smoke 10 grams of potent hashish a day and function normally (though not necessarily optimally), while one-twentieth that amount would incapacitate a novice smoker for several hours.

The last criterion of addiction is the withdrawal syndrome. Such symptoms have been detected in monkeys given THC for two weeks, starting twelve hours after the last dose and lasting five days. The withdrawal syndrome consists of loss of appetite, yawning, hair erection, irritability, hair-pulling, tremors, twitches, and photophobia. Some monkeys will learn to self-inject THC and keep themselves free of withdrawal symptoms this way.

In humans the situation is similar. Withdrawal symptoms may include decreased appetite, insomnia, restlessness, anxiety, gastric hyperacidity, irritability, seclusiveness, excessive perspiration, increased libido, and, of course, a craving for the drug. The symptoms may last for several days. The craving can last for months, but is especially strong in the first month.

Cannabinolism is the most logical term for addiction to cannabis products. *Cannabinol* is short for *tetrahydracannabinol,* and *cannabinolism* and *cannabinolic* are perfectly analogous to *alcoholism* and *alcoholic.* None of the other terms commonly used is adequate. *Pothead,* for example, would seem to apply only to the users of crude marijuana, not hashish or other cannabis products. *Hashaholic* may have a nice ring to it, but it grates on one's sense of logic; it is a nonsense word.

As marijuana use increases in this country we may see the emergence of specialists in THC addiction along with special counseling services and clinics for the cannabinolic. These clinics would likely draw on the techniques used in tobacco, alcohol, and narcotic addiction clinics—individual counseling, group therapy, exercise, aversion therapy, and so on. There is already a group called Potsmokers Anonymous in some cities. In severe cases cannabinolics, especially teenagers, might do better in long-term facilities mostly used for rehabilitation of heroin and cocaine addicts. Every effort must be made to keep youngsters off of the drug while their minds and bodies are still developing.

Signs of Incipient Cannabinolism

- lethargy and decreased motivation, activity, stamina, and libido;
- forgetfulness, losing things;

- decreased dreaming and dream recall;
- coughing, sore throat, chest pains, easily winded due to smoking cannabis, but being unable to quit;
- tolerance, as indicated by smoking more and more for the same effect.

Education is society's best defense against addiction to this drug since the hazards of cannabis are subtle, long-term, and not always obvious to the user, especially the novice.

How to Quit Smoking Cannabis

Make a list of all the reasons you want to quit—the low energy level, poor memory, wasted money and time, harm to the lungs, and so on. Concentrate on these and resolve to avoid the drug. Develop good eating and exercise habits so you'll feel good, and get involved in physical and intellectual hobbies that keep you constructively busy. If you cannot quit on your own, get in touch with Alcoholics Anonymous, Narcotics Anonymous, Potsmokers Anonymous, or another treatment program.

Nitrous Oxide

Also known as laughing gas, nitrous oxide was used for fun for at least fifty years before it was used as an anesthetic for simple surgery and childbirth. It was synthesized in the 1770s and soon became a popular recreational drug with young dentists, doctors, students, and poets. Now it is used in millions of surgical and dental procedures each year, and thousands of surgical, dental, and veterinary workers are chronically exposed to the gas from leakage. Nitrous oxide is also still a popular recreational drug. The usual source is theft from a hospital or restaurant (the aerosol is used for whipping cream). The largest group of abusers are health professionals and students.

The effect is generally described as a floating, numb, cool sensation with pleasant tingling and giddy hilarity. It only lasts about three to five minutes after inhalation stops, and has little perceivable aftereffect. However, prolonged inhalation without added oxygen can cause anoxia, brain damage, and death. Chronic abuse, even with adequate oxygen, can cause abnormal sensations, concentration and memory impairment, psychotic behavior, and a wide variety of other symptoms of nerve damage and dysfunction, as well as bone marrow toxicity. The effects mimic those of vitamin B-12 deficiency. It turns out that nitrous oxide destroys vitamin B-12, and this probably accounts for much of the long-term toxicity.

PCP

Phencyclidine, or PCP, is a synthetic drug patented in 1963 for surgical use as an analgesic and anesthetic that does not depress respiration or heart function. It was withdrawn for use in humans in 1965 because of serious aftereffects, such as confusion, disorientation, agitation, and delirium. It is now marketed as an animal tranquilizer and anesthetic.

PCP is easy to make and is sold on the black market as "angel dust," "hog," or (mixed with LSD) as "mescaline" or "psilocybin." This latter has been a very common hoax since the late 1960s. PCP is usually smoked with marijuana or parsley, though it is also snorted up the nostrils, taken in pill form, or injected. The dose is 5 milligrams or more. Tolerance develops and the dose tends to increase with continued use. Like THC, the active component of marijuana, PCP remains in the body for days, even weeks.

The desired effects are a sense of sensory deprivation, isolation, floating, and numbness, sometimes with visions, vivid "dreams," and a sense of separation from the body. The effects last about two to five hours, depending on dose and tolerance. Residual effects and a hangover may include depression, lethargy, irritability, anxiety, and confusion.

PCP abuse is one of the most serious drug problems in the United States. Severe adverse reactions send several thousand young Americans to emergency rooms every year and cause at least a hundred deaths. It is most popular with youngsters aged sixteen to twenty. There is no specific antidote for PCP. Minor tranquilizers are sometimes given, but their effectiveness is doubted; they may actually interfere with the metabolism and excretion of the PCP. Nor does reassurance, or talking a person down seem to help as it often does with marijuana and LSD overdose.

Summary of Hazards. Regular use can cause depression, lethargy, memory and concentration impairment, decreased libido, and other problems. Tolerance and dependence can develop, and withdrawal symptoms may occur. Due to impairment of reflexes and judgment, serious accidents can occur. Overdose is common and can cause a psychotic reaction with mania, severe anxiety, severe depression, catatonia, confusion, delusions, paranoia, and violent behavior. There may also be physical symptoms such as nystagmus (involuntary eye rolling), high blood pressure, vomiting, drooling, heavy sweating, loss of bowel and bladder control, and slurred speech. Coma and death may occur. Psychotic reactions may last days or weeks, with complete amnesia of having taken the drug.

Psychedelic Drugs

Practically everything about these drugs is controversial, though probably less so than in the 1960s when they were at their peak of popularity and notoriety, and their mere mention excited intense fascination or fear. Even the term *psychedelic* is disputed. It was coined by psychiatrist Humphry Osmond from the Greek for *mind revealing* or *mind manifesting* as an alternative to the misleading *hallucinogenic* and *psychotomimetic.*

LSD (lysergic acid diethylamide), mescaline, psilocybin, and psilocin are the basic or prototype psychedelics. Some would include a dozen or so methoxylated amphetamines such as MMDA ("ecstasy") and MDA ("STP"). These are chemical hybrids of amphetamine and mescaline, and their effects are generally a similar hybrid. Dimethytryptamine, DMT, is a close chemical relative of psilocybin and has some similar effects, but is much shorter acting.

LSD was synthesized in 1938 at Sandoz Laboratories in Switzerland and put aside for lack of interesting effects on animals. But five years later Dr. Albert Hofman, one of the codiscoverers, made a few milligrams and accidently ingested or absorbed through his skin a tiny amount, experiencing about two hours of fantastic kaleidoscopic visions.

Gradually researchers started to work with the chemical. By 1965 at least one hundred thousand psychiatric patients and volunteers, including many psychologists, psychiatrists, and other health professionals, had taken LSD. Many of these people effectively proselytized and got their spouses, friends, and colleagues to take it. Hofman himself, his wife, and some friends, continued to take LSD for many years in the manner of Aldous Huxley, reverently and infrequently.

In the late sixties, with the Vietnam War and social unrest raging, the mass proselytizers, like Tim Leary, inspired millions to take LSD, and illicit LSD use soon dwarfed authorized and discrete use. In February, 1968, Tim Leary, speaking to a large crowd of cheering Berkeley, California teenagers, said that "dope dealers are the real campus heroes," and he praised Orange Sunshine (a particularly potent formulation of LSD) as the purest and best "acid" (LSD) available. In the same breath he said the happiest, holiest people he knew took LSD once a week. We can only guess how many bad trips, suicides, and psychotic reactions were precipitated by this talk and the scores of others he gave in those days. Leary also promoted multidrug use and blatant hedonism.

All this has had a profound impact on the use of psychedelics, which came to be viewed as just more dope. Restrictions have ended practically all legitimate research on these drugs. Ironically, abusers can get psychedelics about as easily as cigarettes.

Mescaline is the active component of the peyote cactus. Black market products include sliced and dried peyote "buttons" and, rarely, purified mescaline sulfate extracted from peyote. Most so-called mescaline sold in tablets and capsules is really LSD and/or PCP. Mescaline is relatively weak, so the effective dose is large, nearly a third of a gram, which would be about three thousand LSD doses. It is very bitter and causes nausea and vomiting for an hour or so. The desired effects last about six to ten hours.

Peyote, an even stronger emetic than pure mescaline, contains other alkaloids, some of which are toxic. Strychnine is abundant in the hairy tufts on the cactus, and these are removed. Peyote has been used for hundreds of years by the Huicholes and other American Indians, especially members of the Native American Church, for whom it is legal (though this status is now in jeopardy). Abuse occurs with some young users who seem to suffer some degree of personality disintegration, much as LSD abusers do. However, moderate use by Church members, no more than once every few months, seems to have socially beneficial effects, somewhat like group therapy, but with rituals and chemically induced suggestibility.

Psilocybin and **psilocin** are the active components of several species of *Paneolus* and *Psilocybe* mushrooms, which grow in many areas of the world and have been used for centuries. Because they are so perishable, these mushrooms are rarely sold on the black market. Almost all illicit "psilocybin" in tablet form is really LSD and/or PCP. Psilocybin and psilocin are very powerful drugs with effects comparable to those of LSD, so it is rather astonishing that growing kits, including viable spores, are sold openly and legally through the U.S. mail. Full-page color ads have been running in *High Times* and other magazines for many years, so the enterprise must be very successful. There are apparently no plans to outlaw the spores, so psilocybin and psilocin will remain by far the most potent (gram for gram) of all recreational drugs available legally and without a prescription. They are approximately one hundred times as potent as mescaline.

378 What the Psychedelics Do

These drugs produce dramatic changes in perception, mood, emotion, and thinking, without producing (at moderate doses) major physiological changes, delirium, amnesia, or addiction. This has been their primary appeal and accounts for the fact that, far more than all other drugs combined, psychedelics have attracted poets, philosophers, artists, scientists, mystics, and other soul-searching people as well as thrill seekers. Compelling accounts of the effects of the drugs have been written by Aldous and Laura Huxley, Alan Watts, Anaïs Nin, Humphry Osmond, Weir Mitchell, and many others. Artists and musicians have also given expression to psychedelic inspiration.

LSD has been used with some reported success (and some failures) as an adjunct to psychotherapy in alcoholism and in criminal rehabilitation. It has also been used to ease pain and psychic trauma in terminal cancer patients, but severe government restrictions have almost eliminated all therapeutic use.

The Hazards of the Psychedelics

Death and maiming by accident are real possibilities when psychedelics are taken carelessly, frivolously, and in unsuitable environments. People have walked out of windows or into moving traffic while their perceptions and judgment were distorted or overwhelmed by the onslaught of sensory and emotional data.

Death by suicide during or soon after a psychedelic drug experience has been reported in a few cases of LSD therapy, but the overall incidence of such suicides is no higher than the rate among non-LSD users undergoing therapy. Suicides reported among illicit LSD users are complicated by the simultaneous use of other drugs and preexisting emotional problems. Fear of insanity and profound depression after a trip may provoke suicide. Probably the best known case is that of Frank Olson, who was slipped LSD in a drink by the head of MKULTRA, the CIA's mind-control project. Olson had a psychotic breakdown and, two weeks later, killed himself by jumping out of a tenth-story window. His lack of preparation for the experience and his consequent belief that he was insane probably played a large role in his suicide. Slipping people LSD should legally be considered similar to rape, assault, or even attempted murder.

A bad trip can be caused by an overdose, poor preparation, poor environment, mixture with other drugs, or individual susceptibility. It is dominated by fear, anxiety, remorse, paranoia, and above all a sense that one will never be normal again, that insanity and misery will prevail for life, even that the universe itself is inherently evil and hellish. Such reactions usually fade within a day or two, and the person's return to normal is almost as fast and remarkable as the descent into hell had been.

A trusted companion, friend, loved one, or health professional can greatly ease the suffering and reduce the risk of self-harm by repeated assurances that all the changes are illusory and temporary, and that everything will be all right in a few hours. It only makes things worse to react with alarm, take drastic therapeutic measures, or reprimand the person.

Chlorpromazine and other tranquilizers often help, possibly by directly inhibiting the drug activity in the brain. Niacin in large doses (up to about a half gram) may also decrease the effects of the drug and hasten return to normal, but this has not been proved. Coffee and other stimulants should *not* be taken, since they tend to increase anxiety.

Flashbacks sometimes occur. These are transient recurrences of the perceptual and emotional changes experienced while on a psychedelic. They are most likely to occur during emotional stress, fatigue, and above all marijuana intoxication. They last a few seconds to a few minutes; some enjoy the flashbacks, but some find them frightening.

Evidence of brain damage from long-term use has been sought but not found, though very heavy users (several hundred trips) sometimes do suspiciously poorly on some nonverbal abstraction tests. Frequent users tend to be eccentric, unable to hold a job, childlike, passive, and given to magical thinking, but these characteristics are often due, at least in part, to preexisting personality traits and cultural factors.

Precipitation of psychosis by chronic psychedelic use in vulnerable people has been reported but critics say too much varied drug use has been involved in the cases to pin the blame on psychedelics. Some psychiatrists conclude that psychedelic use is often an attempt, usually unsuccessful, to treat one's emotional problems, and that abuse of psychedelics is a symptom, not a cause, of psychosis.

Psychedelics tend to be "cultogenic." The charismatic person who takes a psychedelic and comes to believe he or she has seen or become God easily gathers a flock of unsettled young people made more suggestible by psychedelic use. Such communities and cults were very common in the 1960s and early 1970s. The Farm, Steve Gaskin and his followers' still-thriving community in Tennessee, is the bright side of this coin; Charles Manson's murderous cult is the dark side. Many ancient religions and cultures were inspired and heavily influenced by psychedelics. The three-thousand-year-old culture of the peyote-using Huicholes of Mexico and the Mazatecas who worship (and ingest) the Sacred Mushroom (psilocybe) are prime examples.

Genetic damage, birth defects, and **cancer** are apparently not caused by psychedelics, in spite of early fears. At least a hundred studies on animals and humans have shown no excess of these problems in users over nonusers. However, it is still considered prudent for pregnant women to avoid these and all other unnecessary drugs.

Tobacco

Tobacco use, especially cigarette smoking, is recognized by experts to be the single greatest cause of preventable illness, incapacitation, and death in the United States and many other countries. Almost 400,000 Americans die each year from smoking-related illnesses. The growing recognition of the wide array of health problems caused by tobacco and the astronomical cost of treating them has led to a significant antitobacco movement; its activities have helped reduce the percentage of people who smoke, but we still have a very long way to go.

History

We can only guess who the first tobacco smoker was, and what prompted him or her to inhale the smoke of this large-leafed member of the *Solanaceae* (nightshade, potato) family. Perhaps it was a shaman (medicine man) using the abundant smoke from the burning plant for ritual purposes. By accidently inhaling small amounts regularly he could have become addicted without knowing it, then learned to roll a dried leaf up so he could conveniently take it everywhere and smoke whenever the urge arose. Others would have been impressed with the streams and clouds of smoke. They might have believed it was the source of his power, and so imitated him. Whole populations could have become addicted this way.

In any case, Columbus and other early visitors to America were amazed at the "smoke drinking" habit of the natives. Many sailors who tried it enjoyed it and became addicted. To assure their supply, they took tobacco leaves and seeds back to Europe and around the world. Tobacco conquered Europe and Africa rapidly. By 1614 there were about seven thousand tobacco shops in London alone. The demand was so high that the dried leaf was worth its weight in silver. It was lamented that many young noblemen's estates were scattered to nothing "for the drinking of smoke," and "lost through their noses." Even the Catholic missionaries in the Americas became nicotine addicts. Efforts by the Church to prevent the use of tobacco by the public and the clergy failed. When smoking in church was banned, tobacco snuff was used.

Draconian efforts to stem the tobacco tide failed in many countries. The Sultan Murad IV banned tobacco smoking in Constantinople in 1633. Offenders were hanged, beheaded, chopped up, or tortured and maimed to death. Still, people smoked. Eventually Turkish tobacco became world famous. The Czar of Russia outlawed smoking in 1634 under penalties of fines, nostril-slitting, and severe beatings. Ironically, today the Soviet government ensures that the masses get their daily nicotine fix—and it gets the profits. The situation in the People's Republic of China is similar.

The Japanese were introduced to tobacco by the very first Europeans to land in their islands, Portuguese seamen on board a Chinese pirate vessel that took refuge from a storm in a Japanese harbor in about 1542. Within a few years the habit had become widespread. In the early 1600s tobacco smoking and cultivation were outlawed. Increasingly severe penalties, including the confiscation of all property and jail terms, were enacted. Still the habit spread. Eventually most of the military and feudal aristocracy became addicted; the laws were rescinded in 1625.

To this day, no country that has once accepted tobacco has later given it up, even in the most dire circumstances like war and epidemic heart and lung disease associated with smoking. The United States is one of a handful of modern countries to make a commitment to a smoke-free society in the forseeable future. These efforts have encouraged millions to quit, but whether the smoking population can ever be reduced to a small minority, say 10 percent of the adult population, is unknown.

Nicotine Addiction

The rapid and tenacious spread of the smoking habit around the world, in spite of the initial sickness it causes and the lack of any strongly pleasurable effects, is evidence of the power of the chemical addiction. No one should feel inferior or weak-willed because of failure to quit.

Some of the finest minds in the world have been hooked for life.

As early as age thirty-eight, Sigmund Freud was warned by his doctor to reduce his twenty-cigar-a-day habit or risk continued heart arrhythmias and possibly serious heart disease. Freud stopped once for seven weeks, but suffered depression and "severe affection of the heart, worse than I had when smoking." He renewed the habit. Later he quit again, this time for fourteen months. According to his friend and fellow psychoanalyst Dr. Ernest Jones, "the torture was beyond human power to bear." He struggled unsuccessfully against the habit for another twenty years, in spite of his own concern that the habit interfered with his psychoanalytic studies and caused increasing heart pain, "tobacco angina," whenever he smoked.

At age sixty-seven, Freud noticed cancerous sores on his palate and jaw. For the next sixteen years of his life he went through thirty-three operations, during which most of his jaw was removed. He was often in severe pain and unable to speak, eat, or work. His doctors blamed his cigars, but he continued to smoke; he died of cancer at the age of eighty-three. It seems plausible that Freud's unsuccessful struggle against his tobacco habit helped to inspire his theory of Thanatos, the opposite of Eros, the subconscious longing for the grave.

There have been millions, like Freud: victims of tobacco-induced angina unable to quit smoking; lung cancer and stroke victims puffing away on their way home from the hospital; emphysema patients reaching alternately for their oxygen masks and their cigarettes until the bitter end. Heroin addicts often say that kicking tobacco is more difficult than kicking heroin. Part of the problem is that the withdrawal symptoms can last for many months before subsiding. They include extreme anxiety, uncontrollable appetite and weight gain, depression, irritability, intellectual impairment, drowsiness, lethargy, insomnia, dizziness, and heart palpitations.

The addicting substance in tobacco is nicotine, an alkaloid that is easily absorbed by lung and mouth, acts as a sympathetic and parasympathetic nervous system stimulant, causing sharp vasoconstriction and increased blood pressure. It also enters the brain and produces changes perceived as stimulating or relaxing, depending on the person's needs at the moment. It is very short acting; the typical addict takes tobacco smoke or snuff continuously throughout the day.

Nicotine is actually a deadly poison. The amount in one cigarette, if all absorbed at once, could cause death by respiratory paralysis. It has been used as an insecticide. The body recognizes it as a poison and tries to cough or vomit it out the first few times but tolerance develops, the immediately unpleasant side effects subside, and the dose is increased. The youngster who gags on his first few puffs but persists is soon a full-fledged addict. It has been estimated that 70 percent of those who smoke more than one cigarette during adolescence will continue smoking for the next forty years. Few if any other drugs can claim such potent addicting power. Even in wartime conditions with near-starvation rations, addicts will often trade their little food for tobacco.

America's Favorite Poison

The tobacco habit is the largest single cause of disease and premature death in the United States. It is also enormously costly. The lifetime cost of the tobacco alone can top fifty thousand dollars (including interest if the money were saved instead) for one person. The cost of medical care for the many health problems caused by smoking can be even greater. Then there is the cost of fires, insurance, and lost work time. This drain on resources can greatly decrease an individual's, family's, or nation's standard of living. The total cost to Americans is one to two hundred billion dollars per year.

Below is a brief summary of the problems associated with and caused by smoking cigarettes. The degree of risk is associated with the number of cigarettes smoked, their tar and nicotine content, and the depth of inhalation. Some of the risks also apply, but usually to a lesser degree, to cigar and pipe smoking and, to a far less extent, to chronic exposure to smoked-filled air.

Atherosclerosis and Heart Attack. By promoting hardening of the arteries, increasing the clotting rate (by promoting platelet clumping), promoting blood lipid abnormalities, causing irregular heartbeat, and reducing the oxygen-carrying capacity of the blood, smoking increases the rate of heart attack about threefold. The excess of deaths from heart disease due to smoking is much greater even than the excess of deaths from lung cancer due to smoking. The risk is greatly increased by the presence of other risk factors, like high cholesterol levels. The generalized atherosclerosis promoted by smoking can also impair memory and cause hearing loss.

Hypertension and Strokes. Malignant hypertension is much more likely to develop in those with high blood pressure who smoke than in those who don't. Once this phase develops, it is more likely to be lethal in smokers. This, combined with the increased risk of atherosclerosis, makes smoking very dangerous for those with hypertension.

Peripheral Vascular Disease is promoted by cigarette smoking. The legs are commonly affected by intermittent claudication, muscle pains from exercise due to poor circulation. Diabetics are especially vulnerable because the smoking increases the blood vessel damage done by the disease. Buerger's disease, with inflammation, scarring, and clot formation in leg blood vessels occurs in a few people, mostly young Jewish men with unusual sensitivity to tobacco.

Emphysema. Tobacco smoke with its tars coats the alveoli (air sacs) of the lungs, causing them to lose their normal elasticity. The alveoli eventually disintegrate into nonfunctional scar tissue worthless for breathing. The damage is irreversible and the victim becomes a cripple for life. Smoking is by far the most important single cause of emphysema.

Lung Cancer. Tobacco smoke is full of proved carcinogens and cocarcinogens that coat the lungs of smokers. It is not surprising that smoking is by far the most important cause of lung cancer, one of the leading causes of cancer deaths. Women, who once rarely got lung cancer, have come a long way and now die of the disease with increasing frequency. One reason the cancer is so deadly is that there are often no symptoms or X-ray signs until it has spread to other organs.

Mouth and Throat Cancer. Carcinogenic chemicals from tobacco smoke enter the cells lining the mouth and tongue. Long-term exposure leads to yellowish-white, leathery plaques (leukoplakia), which frequently become cancerous. Cancer of the larynx is six times as frequent in smokers as in nonsmokers. Cancer of the esophagus is also much more common in smokers.

Chronic bronchitis is a frequent consequence of cigarette smoking. The respiratory mucosal cells produce extra mucus in response to the irritating smoke particles and chemicals. There is frequent coughing, shortness of breath, and recurring respiratory infection. Smokers and children frequently exposed to cigarette smoke are more susceptible to colds and influenza. Sinusitis is much more frequent in smokers and those living with smokers. The headache and sinus pain are caused by chronic inflammation of the mucous membranes of the sinuses.

Cancer of the uterine cervix is strongly associated with cigarette smoking, especially if the habit was taken up in the early teens or sooner. The cause is apparently the smoke carcinogens carried to the uterine epithelium by the circulation. Many young and middle-aged women die or are rendered sterile by surgery. The total number of tobacco-related deaths due to cervical and lung cancers in women exceeds the total number of tobacco-related deaths due to lung cancer in men.

Bladder cancer is more frequent among smokers because the carcinogens from the smoke enter the urine and are in continuous contact with the bladder cells for years and decades. Kidney and pancreatic cancer risks are also greatly increased by smoking.

Peptic ulcers are aggravated and sometimes caused by smoking; the nicotine increases inflammation and retards healing of the lesions. A weakened esophageal sphincter can be caused by smoking; this can lead to reflux of stomach contents and consequent heartburn.

Burns. About a third of all fatalities and serious injuries from burns are caused by fires associated with smoking.

Dental and gum disease is greatly increased in smokers, who have about twice the nonsmokers' chance of becoming toothless before age sixty. This is largely due to the contribution made to plaque formation by the tobacco tars. Mouth odor and stained teeth due to smoking are significant aesthetic turn-offs. Smoking also deadens the taste buds and decreases the pleasure of eating.

Osteoporosis. Smoking can contribute to osteoporosis, a crippling bone disease, by increasing calcium removal from the bones. This is especially hazardous to postmenopausal women.

Low birth weight, stillbirths, and serious maternal bleeding are much more likely to occur if the mother smokes during pregnancy. This is because the nicotine and carbon monoxide decrease the supply of blood, oxygen, and nutrients to the fetus. Malformations, like cleft palate, may also be more likely.

Infant and child health can be adversely affected by tobacco components ingested in the breast milk of smoking mothers or inhaled in the air. Bronchitis and pneumonia are more common in infants with smoking mothers. Infants are very sensitive to cigarette smoke and can develop aversions to foods they associate with the nausea from nicotine. Exposure to smoke can aggravate chronic ear infections in infants and children.

386 **Decreased libido** among smokers has been noted by several researchers. This may be due to the decreased testosterone production, which tends to increase within a week or two of quitting.

WHAT ABOUT LOW-TAR, LOW-NICOTINE, AND FILTERED CIGARETTES?

Cigarettes with lower levels of harmful substances have been developed by changes in growing and curing methods and by the use of various kinds of filter tips. These low-yield cigarettes are apparently slightly less dangerous to the lungs and larynx, but there is no evidence that they do less damage to the cardiovascular system than regular cigarettes. This is not surprising since filters generally do not lower the level of carbon monoxide, which does the most harm to the blood vessels and heart. Besides, smokers tend to inhale deeper and faster when they switch to a low-nicotine brand. In a sense low-yield cigarettes are the most dangerous because they are generally milder tasting and make it much easier for novices and youngsters to start the habit.

WHAT ABOUT CHEWING TOBACCO AND SNUFF?

Early American Indians not only smoked rolled tobacco leaves; a few of them preferred to sniff powdered tobacco through tubes. Many Europeans preferred this more discrete method of getting a dose of nicotine. At some point someone decided to suck rather than sniff the tobacco. Chewing tobacco, which usually has sugar and other additives, is now much more popular than snuff, but still far less so than cigarettes. Smokers enjoy the clouds of smoke and the ritual of smoking.

Smokeless tobacco has certain health advantages over the smoking varieties since it does not produce the dangerous gases (carbon monoxide, hydrogen cyanide, and nitrogen oxides) that are so harmful to the lungs and circulatory system. However, in most users there is abrasion of the teeth and recession of the gums that can lead to dental and gum disease. Even more important, nearly 5 percent of habitual users develop cancers in their mouths, often in the area where the tobacco is held. This causes several thousand deaths a year in the United States. Moreover, the nicotine in smokeless tobacco can aggravate ulcers and hypertension, and provoke heart arrhythmias. Smokeless tobacco delivers more nicotine than smoking and creates a stronger addiction; it is very difficult to quit. A new form of smokeless tobacco, tobacco gum flavored with peppermint or cinnamon, is raising serious concerns because of its appeal to young people.

How to Stop Smoking

Not everyone finds quitting as difficult as Freud did. Millions of Americans have quit smoking for long periods. Some eventually return to smoking, but many stay free of the habit for life. Success depends on a number of factors, including the level of addiction (how much smoking for how long), the motivation to quit, and the utilization of effective quitting techniques.

We can't affect anyone's level of addiction, but the above discussion should provide some motivation to quit. Here we will briefly discuss some of the methods that have been used successfully by others. No method can be guaranteed to work for everyone. It has been said that there are as many stop-smoking methods as there are ex-smokers. And some people do not need any particular method or technique. With motivation and willpower they simply quit. If this has not worked for you, some of the following suggestions might help.

Work up to quitting for a few days. When you smoke, concentrate on the harshness and the stench. Visualize the hundreds of harmful chemicals that are coating your mouth, throat, and lungs and damaging your arteries, heart, and brain. When you are not smoking, imagine yourself an ex-smoker with clean-smelling breath and clothes and a clear brain. Visualize your lungs as pink, clean, and healthy; your heart unhurried by nicotine and unencumbered by carbon monoxide; and your arteries clear and wide open. Imagine yourself declining offered cigarettes. It is important to recognize that you are not giving up or losing anything; you are gaining health, employability, reduced insurance rates, reduced risk of burning your house down, a better sense of taste, improved exercise tolerance, money in the bank, and a longer life. Write down all the most important reasons you have for quitting.

Start a regular exercise program. This will counter the withdrawal symptoms by making you feel generally better physically and mentally, helping you to relax and sleep better, and building your self-confidence. It will also help prevent fat gain, which is a problem in about a third of those who quit smoking.

Recruit at least one supporter, preferably an ex-smoker, who will accept your commitment to quit, check on your progress, and lend encouragement when you need it. Your local American Cancer Society can provide you with names of ex-smokers who volunteer for this role.

 Use oral substitutes if necessary. Carrots, cucumbers, celery, chewing gum, cinnamon sticks, ginger root, and toothpicks are favorites. (Caution: Toothpicks are the most commonly choked on items in America.) If you do gain weight, don't use this as an excuse to resume smoking. You would have to gain about a hundred pounds to equal the damage to your health done by smoking.

Avoid alcohol and caffeine since these tend to increase the urge to smoke. Avoid other sedatives and stimulants, since they tend to cloud the mind and weaken resolve. In some cases, however, the anxiety is so severe that tranquilizers may be useful in getting through the first few days.

Break up the patterns in your life associated with smoking. If you normally smoke after eating, take a walk or ride a bike instead. If you are used to smoking while you watch television, floss your teeth instead. For the first few days keep as busy as you can. Spend time in areas where smoking is prohibited. Go camping without any cigarettes.

Postpone lighting each day's first cigarette for an hour if you are tapering off. Set a schedule and stick to it. For the last week before you quit, smoke about four to six cigarettes a day. When you light up concentrate on the negative imagery developed earlier. Many smokers find that reducing their frequency below ten to fifteen cigarettes a day is especially difficult. It may be necessary to stay at this level for several weeks before cutting down to less and quitting.

Nicotine gum, available by prescription only, can be helpful by reducing withdrawal symptoms. It satisfies the craving without the carbon monoxide, cyanide, tars, and other toxins supplied by cigarettes. If you have not been able to quit smoking, ask your doctor about nicotine gum. If you do get a prescription, use the gum strictly according to instructions and keep it out of the reach of children. It is usually not recommended for those with peptic ulcers or cardiovascular disease, or for pregnant or nursing women. The gum usually must be taken for about ten to twenty weeks.

Tips on using nicotine gum: The gum works best if you are also enrolled in a stop-smoking program. You should stop smoking completely before starting the gum. Smoking and chewing could increase the level of addiction. Think of the gum as a cigarette; chew very slowly and intermittently, not all at once. Absorption should be from the mouth and throat, not the stomach.

Incidently, there are no proved effective nonprescription smoking deterrents. Don't waste your money on the myriad products containing menthol, ginger, lemon oil, cloves, silver nitrate, and other ingredients.

Formal group programs can be very helpful. Some are free and some charge up to several hundred dollars with a money-back guarantee. The American Cancer Society, Seventh Day Adventist Church, and some hospitals offer regular group sessions. Stop-smoking programs on the job have been proving quite successful and are an ideal way to improve employee health and reduce absenteeism and health care costs.

Let's Save Our Children

The initial motivation for an individual youngster to start smoking is probably similar to the motivation for our hypothetical early smokers who imitated shamans. Children associate the clouds and streams of smoke with adulthood, authority, and power. Movies and cigarette advertisements further enhance the appeal with their grossly misleading association of smoking with beauty, love, machismo, sex, fun, and health. The power of these lures is so great that adolescents accept the nausea and other symptoms to achieve the perceived status of the smoker. The prospect of heart disease or lung cancer forty or even twenty years down the road seems infinitely remote to teenagers. However, the following steps might eventually reduce the number of youngsters who take up smoking.

Parents can set a good example by not smoking, not allowing smoking in the house, and encouraging a healthy lifestyle with involvement in sports, good nutrition, and so on.

Legislatures and communities can further restrict smoking in public buildings, the sale of cigarettes to children, and the advertising of cigarettes.

Schools can "inoculate" students against smoking at an early age. Some such programs have greatly reduced the number of students who take up smoking in subsequent years. Kindergarten to seventh grade appears to be the best time to present the facts of smoking, develop an awareness of the absurd and misleading nature of cigarette ads, and provide assertiveness training and effective counters to peer pressure to smoke.

Baseball, at all levels—from high school to college, the minor leagues, and the major leagues—must ban chewing tobacco, snuff, the new tobacco gum, and all other forms of tobacco from the playing fields and dugouts.

390 Even therapeutic nicotine gum should be banned during games because it would likely be abused as a substitute for chewing tobacco. Baseball is the only sport we know of that allows players to use a dangerous and addicting drug during games. It is remarkable that during America's twenty-year "war on drugs" hardly a word has been said about this. Tobacco chewing by baseball players is so deeply ingrained in our culture that even Dear Abby once defended the practice. It helps players keep their mouths moist, she said. Funny how water works just fine for other athletes. Letters of protest from irate readers forced a retraction.

Prescription Drugs and Vaccines

Drugs that are available by prescription only are intended for use supervised by a physician who can determine the need and dosage, and monitor their effects and side effects. These drugs are generally more potent and more hazardous than nonprescription drugs. They are also more studied, tested, and reviewed, and under greater constraints to be proved effective. To provide the most benefit with the least risk prescription drugs must be used properly. The following general considerations hold for all prescription drugs.

Don't expect or ask for a drug prescription when you consult a physician. Don't be disappointed or feel cheated if you walk out of your doctor's office without a prescription. Many health problems are best treated with nondrug therapies; using drugs for them would entail a risk without providing a benefit. Many times the advice you get from your doctor about exercise, nutrition, smoking, hygiene, and *not* using drugs (recreational, nonprescription, herbs, megavitamins) is more important than any prescription he or she might give you. If it would motivate you and help you remember, ask your doctor to put all his or her advice and recommendations in writing like a prescription.

Always inform your physician about your medical history, including all reasons for medical care, all allergies and adverse drug reactions, and *all* drug use, including illicit drugs, herbs, nutritional supplements, and even topical products. You should take the drugs with you and show them to your doctor. All drugs are potentially subject to interactions with other drugs, including antacids, aspirin, birth control pills, medicinal herbs, coffee, tea, colas, marijuana, tobacco, other recreational drugs, and sometimes even food. Heed all precautions from your doctor or pharmacist.

Inform your doctor if you are pregnant or lactating. Many drugs can cause birth defects, subtle neurological damage, low birth weight, kidney damage, and other problems. Taken by the mother, they enter her milk and can cause adverse reactions in the breast-feeding infant.

Keep all appointments with your physician. Many prescription drugs require very careful monitoring of blood levels and effects to determine safety and effectiveness.

Understand why the drug has been prescribed. What is it supposed to do? How quickly is it supposed to work? Ask if you don't know.

Follow your doctor's prescriptions exactly. Take the drugs according to schedule. Know what to do if you forget a dose; in most cases the next dose is not increased to make up for the forgotten one, but sometimes it is. If in doubt and you cannot contact your doctor, call and ask a pharmacist.

Understand how and when to take the drug. Taking it with lots of water (one or two cups) is usually advisable, but do you take it with meals or between? Are there certain foods and drinks that should be avoided with the drug? Be sure all this is written down for you.

Store your drugs properly. In general, they should be kept in a cool, dry place and out of the reach of children. Refrigerators and bathroom medicine cabinets are not good places. High in a cool bedroom is usually a good spot.

Be sure you understand the side effects the drug may produce and when to consult your doctor about them. Some are common, mild, and to be expected, while others are serious threats. Ask your doctor what side effects are common and are not to be concerned about; and what side effects he or she should be called about. Have this written down for you.

Do not suddenly stop taking a prescribed drug without consulting your doctor, unless you experience severe side effects. (In that case do stop taking the drug and contact your doctor right away.) Many drugs need to be decreased gradually; sudden withdrawal can be dangerous. Other drugs, like antibiotics, may be ineffective if the entire prescription is not taken.

Never take a prescription drug not prescribed for you, or for other than the prescribed purpose. Don't diagnose yourself and then treat yourself with a drug you get from a friend who didn't finish a prescription. Do not keep unused portions of prescriptions around for later use. Prescription drugs must be prescribed specifically for you in the proper dosage and dose schedule. Similarly, *never* let others "borrow" your prescription drugs. If you stop taking a prescription drug for any reason, throw away the remaining pills. Old drugs can decompose into poisons and should never be taken.

Vaccines

In the late eighteenth century William Jenner discovered that fluid from cowpox sores could immunize people against the deadly smallpox. Since then a great deal has been learned about viruses and bacteria, and vaccines have been developed against several very important infectious diseases. Smallpox has been eradicated, so the vaccine against it is no longer necessary. This is one of the great achievements of scientific medicine and an inspiration for efforts against other deadly diseases.

The vaccines routinely given or highly recommended for children, adults, and special risk groups are listed at the end of this section. One of the newest and most important is against Haemophilus influenza type b (Hib).

Vaccines are under research and development for herpes, human papilloma viruses (HPV), hepatitis A, cytomegalovirus (CMV), malaria, tooth decay, gonorrhea, syphilis, chlamydia, traveler's diarrhea, leprosy, tuberculosis, certain urinary tract infections, infectious mononucleosis, strep throat and rheumatic fever, AIDS, viral and bacterial food poisoning, and several types of cancer. Moreover, work never stops on better versions of vaccines already in use. One of the most exciting areas of research with profound, even revolutionary possibilities is vaccination not against microbes, but against our own T-cells (a type of lymphocyte) that have gone haywire and are causing autoimmune diseases. Such vaccines could bring a flood of breakthroughs in treating such serious diseases as diabetes, multiple sclerosis, and rheumatoid arthritis.

Generally speaking, vaccines are becoming increasingly important in all our lives. When environmental and hygienic measures are inadequate or ineffective, vaccines are the ultimate weapons, the silver bullets of preventive medicine. Their role continues to grow, especially with the continuing development of strains of bacteria resistant to antibiotics. Children and adults will be immunized against more and more diseases. Even the vaccines we don't get, but others do, affect us by decreasing the pool of infected people and stopping epidemics that could cost billions and eventually engulf us too. We will all breathe a sigh of relief, for example, when an AIDS vaccine is developed, even if we don't all get the vaccine.

A vaccine consists of a dead or modified form of a disease-causing microbe or, in a few cases, cancer cells. It works by stimulating the body's production of antibodies to the organism. If the microbe should then enter the body, it is neutralized and removed before it can multiply and cause disease. Vaccines can have an impact far beyond the immediate disease in question. For example, the hepatitis B vaccine is most important as a weapon against liver cancer; future herpes and HPV vaccines will prevent some cervical cancers; and a vaccine against the Epstein-Barr virus would help prevent not only infectious mononucleosis, but some kinds of cancer (especially Burkitt's lymphoma) and perhaps rheumatoid arthritis.

Opposition to Immunization

Just as there are a few people who believe that the earth is flat, and some who doubt the evolution of species, so there are those who do not believe in vaccinations. Until recently the doubts were mostly based on religious beliefs, but the occurrence of polio and other preventable diseases among the Amish and other religious groups has prompted a change of heart in them. Now the opposition to vaccines comes mostly from health cultists and cranks who either doubt that microbes cause disease or believe that doctors and public health officials have conspired with the pharmaceutical industry to foist unnecessary and dangerous drugs on the public.

It is true that some vaccines cause side effects in a small percentage of people. Concern has recently been focused on the pertussis (whooping cough) vaccine, which has been associated with episodes of screaming, convulsions, and brain damage in a very few infants. However, when its use decreases the incidence of the dreadful disease rises dramatically. A safer vaccine will likely be available very soon, but in most cases it is certainly safer to be vaccinated than not. Nevertheless, parents should be told about the possible side effects, and children who have severe reactions should not receive more pertussis vaccine.

Summary of Available Vaccines

Vaccination against diphtheria, tetanus, pertussis (whooping cough), polio, mumps, measles, and rubella is routine in infants and children. A vaccine is now available for Hib and is strongly recommended for all children between eighteen and twenty-four months. Its use should become routine. Future Hib vaccines will be effective at an earlier age and will greatly reduce the incidence of the disease.

A good chickenpox vaccine is available for high-risk groups, and its use may become routine for all. Vaccines against hepatitis B, many bacterial pneumonias, seasonal influenzas, meningococcal meningitis, yellow fever, cholera, plague, rabies, typhoid fever, typhus, and anthrax are available for high-risk groups.

Immunizations for Children

The following is the recommended schedule for immunization of normal infants and children:

AGE	VACCINE(S)
2 months	DTP, OPV
4 months	DTP, OPV
6 months	DTP
15 months	MMR
15–18 months	DTP, OPV
18 months	PRP-D
4–6 years	DTP, OPV
14–16, then every ten years	Td

Vaccine Initials: DTP = Diphtheria, Tetanus, Pertussis; OPV = Oral Polio Vaccine; MMR = Measles, Mumps, Rubella; PRP-D = Diphtheria toxoid–Hib conjugate (This is to prevent Hib. Due to frequent improvements, vaccines against Hib will probably go through several name changes and strange initials); Td = Tetanus and diphtheria for adults.

Immunizations for Adults

Adults should have a **tetanus-diphtheria booster** every ten years at mid-decade (ages twenty-five, thirty-five, etc.). Other vaccines should be considered for adults as follows:

Influenza vaccine for those with a variety of chronic disease, healthy people over sixty-five, residents of nursing homes, and health care workers. It is given each year in the fall or early winter.

Pneumococcal pneumonia vaccine for those at high risk due to underlying health problems, as well as healthy people over sixty-five. It is given once.

Hepatitis B vaccine for those at high risk (see **Hepatitis** in Section Two). A series of three injections is given over several weeks.

Measles vaccine for those born after 1956 without either verification of immunization with a live measles vaccine on or after their first birthday, verification that measles occured, or laboratory evidence of immunity. If in doubt, it's cheaper to get the vaccine than to test for immunity.

Rubella vaccine for those without verification of immunization with a live vaccine on or after their first birthday or laboratory evidence of immunity.

Immunization for Travel

No vaccinations are required for those traveling from the United States to Europe, Canada, Mexico, or the Caribbean. Travelers to other areas should consult their physicians or the nearest Department of Health for specific requirements. The main threats in parts of Africa, Asia, and South America are yellow fever, cholera, typhoid fever, hepatitis B, and malaria. The latter is preventable by antimalarials but not yet by vaccine. For more on malaria and vaccines against hepatitis B, pneumonia, influenza, and rabies, see separate discussions of each disease in Section Two.

Appendix A

Recommended Dietary Allowances[a]

Designed for the maintenance of good nutrition of practically all healthy people in the United States

Protein						
	Age (years) or Condition	Weight[b]		Height[b]		Protein
		(kg)	(lb)	(cm)	(in)	(g)
Infants	0.0–0.5	6	13	60	24	13
	0.5–1.0	9	20	71	28	14
Children	1–3	13	29	90	35	16
	4–6	20	44	112	44	24
	7–10	28	62	132	52	28
Males	11–14	45	99	157	62	45
	15–18	66	145	176	69	59
	19–24	72	160	177	70	58
	25–50	79	174	176	70	63
	51+	77	170	173	68	63
Females	11–14	46	101	157	62	46
	15–18	55	120	163	64	44
	19–24	58	128	164	65	46
	25–50	63	138	163	64	50
	51+	65	143	160	63	50
Pregnant						60
Lactating	1st 6 months					65
	2nd 6 months					62

[a]The allowances, expressed as average daily intakes over time, are intended to provide for individual variations among most normal persons as they live in the United States under usual environmental stresses. Diets should be based on a variety of common foods in order to provide other nutrients for which human requirements have been less well defined. See text for detailed discussion of allowances and of nutrients not tabulated.

[b]Weights and heights of Reference Adults are actual medians for the U.S. population of the designated age. The use of these figures does not imply that the height-to-weight ratios are ideal.

Fat-Soluble Vitamins					
	Age (years) or Condition	Vitamin A (μg RE)[c]	Vitamin D (μg)[d]	Vitamin E (mg α–TE)[e]	Vitamin K (μg)
Infants	0.0–0.5	375	7.5	3	5
	0.5–1.0	375	10	4	10
Children	1–3	400	10	6	15
	4–6	500	10	7	20
	7–10	700	10	7	30
Males	11–14	1,000	10	10	45
	15–18	1,000	10	10	65
	19–24	1,000	10	10	70
	25–50	1,000	5	10	80
	51+	1,000	5	10	80
Females	11–14	800	10	8	45
	15–18	800	10	8	55
	19–24	800	10	8	60
	25–50	800	5	8	65
	51+	800	5	8	65
Pregnant		800	10	10	65
Lactating	1st 6 months	1,300	10	12	65
	2nd 6 months	1,200	10	11	65

[c] Retinol equivalents. 1 retinol equivalent = 1 μg retinol or 6 μg β-carotene. 1 RE = 3.33 I.U.
[d] As cholecalciferol. 10 μg cholecalciferol = 400 I.U. of vitamin D.
[e] α-Tocopherol equivalents. 1 mg d-α tocopherol = 1 α-TE.

Water-Soluble Vitamins

	Age (years) or Condition	Vitamin C (mg)	Thiamin (mg)	Riboflavin (mg)	Niacin (mg NE)[f]	Vitamin B_6 (mg)	Folate (μg)	Vitamin B_{12} (μg)
Infants	0.0–0.5	30	0.3	0.4	5	0.3	25	0.3
	0.5–1.0	35	0.4	0.5	6	0.6	35	0.5
Children	1–3	40	0.7	0.8	9	1.0	50	0.7
	4–6	45	0.9	1.1	12	1.1	75	1.0
	7–10	45	1.0	1.2	13	1.4	100	1.4
Males	11–14	50	1.3	1.5	17	1.7	150	2.0
	15–18	60	1.5	1.8	20	2.0	200	2.0
	19–24	60	1.5	1.7	19	2.0	200	2.0
	25–50	60	1.5	1.7	19	2.0	200	2.0
	51+	60	1.2	1.4	15	2.0	200	2.0
Females	11–14	50	1.1	1.3	15	1.4	150	2.0
	15–18	60	1.1	1.3	15	1.5	180	2.0
	19–24	60	1.1	1.3	15	1.6	180	2.0
	25–50	60	1.1	1.3	15	1.6	180	2.0
	51+	60	1.0	1.2	13	1.6	180	2.0
Pregnant		70	1.5	1.6	17	2.2	400	2.2
Lactating	1st 6 months	95	1.6	1.8	20	2.1	280	2.6
	2nd 6 months	90	1.6	1.7	20	2.1	260	2.6

[f] 1 NE (niacin equivalent) is equal to 1 mg of niacin or 60 mg of dietary tryptophan.

Source: FOOD AND NUTRITION BOARD, NATIONAL ACADEMY OF SCIENCES—NATIONAL RESEARCH COUNCIL. Revised 1989.

Minerals								
	Age (years) or Condition	Calcium (mg)	Phosphorus (mg)	Magnesium (mg)	Iron (mg)	Zinc (mg)	Iodine (μg)	Selenium (μg)
Infants	0.0–0.5	400	300	40	6	5	40	10
	0.5–1.0	600	500	60	10	5	50	15
Children	1–3	800	800	80	10	10	70	20
	4–6	800	800	120	10	10	90	20
	7–10	800	800	170	10	10	120	30
Males	11–14	1,200	1,200	270	12	15	150	40
	15–18	1,200	1,200	400	12	15	150	50
	19–24	1,200	1,200	350	10	15	150	70
	25–50	800	800	350	10	15	150	70
	51+	800	800	350	10	15	150	70
Females	11–14	1,200	1,200	280	15	12	150	45
	15–18	1,200	1,200	300	15	12	150	50
	19–24	1,200	1,200	280	15	12	150	55
	25–50	800	800	280	15	12	150	55
	51+	800	800	280	10	12	150	55
Pregnant		1,200	1,200	320	30	15	175	65
Lactating	1st 6 months	1,200	1,200	355	15	19	200	75
	2nd 6 months	1,200	1,200	340	15	16	200	75

Summary Table

Estimated Safe and Adequate Daily Dietary Intakes of Selected Vitamins and Minerals[a]

Category	Age (years)	Vitamins	
		Biotin (μg)	Pantothenic Acid (mg)
Infants	0.0–0.5	10	2
	0.5–1.0	15	3
Children and adolescents	1–3	20	3
	4–6	25	3–4
	7–10	30	4–5
	11+	30–100	4–7
Adults		30–100	4–7

Category	Age (years)	Trace Elements[b]				
		Copper (mg)	Manganese (mg)	Fluoride (mg)	Chromium (μg)	Molybdenum (μg)
Infants	0.0–0.5	0.4–0.6	0.3–0.6	0.1–0.5	10–40	15–30
	0.5–1.0	0.6–0.7	0.6–1.0	0.2–1.0	20–60	20–40
Children and adolescents	1–3	0.7–1.0	1.0–1.5	0.5–1.5	20–80	25–50
	4–6	1.0–1.5	1.5–2.0	1.0–2.5	30–120	30–75
	7–10	1.0–2.0	2.0–3.0	1.5–2.5	50–200	50–150
	11+	1.5–2.5	2.0–5.0	1.5–2.5	50–200	75–250
Adults		1.5–3.0	2.0–5.0	1.5–4.0	50–200	75–250

[a]Because there is less information on which to base allowances, these figures are not given in the main table of RDA and are provided here in the form of ranges of recommended intakes.

[b]Since the toxic levels for many trace elements may be only several times usual intakes, the upper levels for the trace elements given in this table should not be habitually exceeded.

Appendix B

Nutritive Values of Common Foods

FOOD, APPROXIMATE HOUSEHOLD MEASURES AND MARKET UNITS		VALUES FOR EDIBLE PART OF FOODS															
			Water	Food energy	Protein	Fat	Carbohydrate	Calcium	Phosphorus	Iron	Sodium	Potassium	Vitamin A value	Thiamin	Riboflavin	Niacin	Ascorbic acid
		Grams	*Percent*	*Calories*	*Grams*	*Grams*	*Grams*	*Milligrams*	*Milligrams*	*Milligrams*	*Milligrams*	*Milligrams*	*International units*	*Milligrams*	*Milligrams*	*Milligrams*	*Milligrams*
ALMONDS:																	
Dried:																	
In shell (refuse: shells, 60%):																	
Cup	1 cup	78	4.7	187	5.8	16.9	6.1	73	157	1.5	1	241	0	.07	.29	1.1	Trace
Pound (yields 6.4 oz., approx. 1¼ cups, shelled whole nuts).	1 lb	454	4.7	1,085	33.7	98.3	35.4	424	914	8.5	7	1,402	0	.44	1.67	6.3	Trace
10 nuts	10 nuts	25	4.7	60	1.9	5.4	2.0	23	50	.5	Trace	77	0	.02	.09	.4	Trace

Source: Selected items from Nutritive Value of American Foods Agriculture Handbook No. 456

FOOD, APPROXIMATE HOUSEHOLD MEASURES AND MARKET UNITS			Water	Food energy	Protein	Fat	Carbohydrate	Calcium	Phosphorus	Iron	Sodium	Potassium	Vitamin A value	Thiamin	Riboflavin	Niacin	Ascorbic acid
		Grams	Percent	Calories	Grams	Grams	Grams	Milligrams	Milligrams	Milligrams	Milligrams	Milligrams	International units	Milligrams	Milligrams	Milligrams	Milligrams
Shelled:																	
Whole	1 cup	142	4.7	849	26.4	77.0	27.7	332	716	6.7	6	1,098	0	.34	1.31	5.0	Trace
Pound (yield from approx. 2½ lb., in shell)	1 lb	454	4.7	2,713	84.4	245.9	88.5	1,061	2,286	21.3	18	3,506	0	1.09	4.17	15.9	Trace
Roasted (in oil), salted:																	
Cup (approx. 120 nuts)	1 cup	157	4.7	984	29.2	90.6	30.6	369	791	7.4	311	1,214	0	.08	1.44	5.5	0
Pound	1 lb	454	.7	2,844	84.4	261.7	88.5	1,066	2,286	21.3	898	3,506	0	.23	4.17	15.9	0
APPLES:																	
Raw, commercial varieties:																	
Fruit, 3-in. diam. (approx. 2½ per pound)	1 apple	180	84.4	96	.3	1.0	24.0	12	17	.5	2	182	150	.05	.03	.2	7
Pound	1 lb	454	84.4	263	.9	2.7	65.8	32	45	1.4	5	499	410	.14	.09	.5	18
APRICOTS:																	
Raw:																	
Pound	1 lb	454	85.3	217	4.3	.9	54.6	72	98	2.1	4	1,198	11,510	.18	.17	2.6	43
Dried, sulfured	1 lb	454	25.0	1,179	22.7	2.3	301.6	304	490	24.9	118	4,441	49,440	.05	.78	15.0	54
Medium	10 halves	35	25.0	91	1.8	.2	23.3	23	38	1.9	9	343	3,820	Trace	.06	1.2	4
APRICOT NECTAR, CANNED OR BOTTLED (APPROX. 40% FRUIT):	1 cup	251	84.6	143	.8	.3	36.6	23	30	.5	Trace	379	2,380	.03	.03	.5	8
ARTICHOKES, GLOBE OR FRENCH, COOKED (BOILED), DRAINED																	
Bud or globe	1 bud, medium	300	86.5	—	3.4	.2	11.9	61	83	1.3	36	361	180	.08	.05	.8	10

ASPARAGUS:																	
Raw spears (green):																	
Pound	1 lb	454	91.7	118	11.3	.9	22.7	100	281	4.5	9	1,261	4,080	.82	.91	6.8	150
Cooked spears (green) (boiled), drained: Medium, ½-in. diam. at base	4 spears	60	93.6	12	1.3	.1	2.2	13	30	.4	1	110	540	.10	.11	.8	16
Pound	1 lb	454	93.6	91	10.0	.9	16.3	95	227	2.7	5	830	4,080	.73	.82	6.4	118
AVOCADO:																	
All commercial varieties:																	
Whole fruit (refuse: seed and skin, 25%); wt., 10⅔ oz.	1 avocado	302	74.0	378	4.8	37.1	14.3	23	95	1.4	9	1,368	660	0.25	0.45	8.6	82
BACON, CURED:																	
Cooked (broiled or fried), drained:																	
Slab, yield from 1 lb., raw	4.8 oz	136	8.1	807	35.8	70.7	4.3	19	305	4.5	1,389	321	(0)	.69	.46	7.1	—
Slice, thick (approx. 12 slices per pound, raw)	2 slices	24	8.1	143	6.4	12.5	.8	3	54	.8	245	57	(0)	.12	.08	1.2	—
Slice, thin (approx. 28 slices per pound, raw)	2 slices	10	8.1	61	2.7	5.2	.3	1	22	.3	102	24	(0)	.05	.03	.5	—
BANANAS:																	
Raw:																	
Medium	1 banana	175	75.7	101	1.3	.2	26.4	10	31	.8	1	440	230	.06	.07	.8	12
	1 lb	454	75.7	386	5.0	.9	100.7	36	118	3.2	5	1,678	860	.23	.27	3.2	45
Red	1 banana	193	74.4	118	1.6	.3	30.7	13	24	1.0	1	485	520	.07	.05	.8	(13)
	1 lb	454	74.4	408	5.4	.9	106.1	45	82	3.6	5	1,678	1,810	.23	.18	2.7	(45)
Dehydrated or banana flakes:	1 cup	100	3	340	4.4	.8	88.6	32	104	2.8	4	1,477	760	.18	.24	2.8	7
BASS, STRIPED, OVENFRIED:	16⅞ oz	480	60.8	941	103.2	40.8	32.2	—	—	—	—	—	—	—	—	—	—
Yield from 1 lb., raw fillets	1 fillet	200	60.8	892	43.0	17.0	13.4	—	—	—	—	—	—	—	—	—	—
BEANS, COMMON, MATURE SEEDS, DRY:																	
White:																	
Cooked, Great Northern or navy (no residual cooking liquid):																	
Great Northern	1 cup	180	69.0	212	14.0	1.1	38.2	90	266	4.9	13	749	0	.25	.13	1.3	0
Pea (navy)	1 cup	190	69.0	224	14.8	1.1	40.3	95	281	5.1	13	790	0	.27	.13	1.3	0

FOOD, APPROXIMATE HOUSEHOLD MEASURES AND MARKET UNITS		VALUES FOR EDIBLE PART OF FOODS															
			Water	Food energy	Protein	Fat	Carbohydrate	Calcium	Phosphorus	Iron	Sodium	Potassium	Vitamin A value	Thiamin	Riboflavin	Niacin	Ascorbic acid
		Grams	*Percent*	*Calories*	*Grams*	*Grams*	*Grams*	*Milligrams*	*Milligrams*	*Milligrams*	*Milligrams*	*Milligrams*	*International units*	*Milligrams*	*Milligrams*	*Milligrams*	*Milligrams*
Pound	1 lb	454	69.0	535	35.4	2.7	96.2	227	671	12.2	32	1,887	0	.64	.32	3.2	0
Canned, solids and liquids:																	
Cup	1 cup	255	68.5	306	16.1	1.3	58.7	173	309	5.1	862	683	150	.18	.10	1.5	5
Pound	1 lb	454	68.5	544	28.6	2.3	104.3	308	549	9.1	1,533	1,216	270	.32	.18	2.7	9
Red, kidney:																	
Cooked (no residual cooking liquid):																	
Cup	1 cup	185	69.0	218	14.4	.9	39.6	70	259	4.4	6	629	10	.20	.11	1.3	—
Pound	1 lb	454	69.0	535	35.4	2.3	97.1	172	635	10.9	14	1,542	30	.50	.27	3.2	—
Canned, solilds and liquid:																	
Cup	1 cup	255	76.0	230	14.5	1.0	41.8	74	278	4.6	8	673	10	.13	.10	1.5	—
Pound	1 lb	454	76.0	408	25.9	1.8	74.4	132	494	8.2	14	1,198	20	.23	.18	2.7	—
BEANS, SNAP:																	
Green:																	
Cooked (boiled), drained	1 cup	125	92.4	31	2.0	.3	6.8	63	46	.8	5	189	680	.09	.11	.6	15
	1 lb	454	92.4	113	7.3	.9	24.5	227	168	2.7	18	685	2,450	.32	.41	2.3	54
BEEF, TRIMMED TO RETAIL BASIS:																	
Boneless chuck and chuck cuts:																	
Cooked (braised or stewed), drained (81% lean, 19% fat):																	
Yield from 1 lb., raw beef (item 218)	10.7 oz	304	49.4	994	79.0	72.7	0	33	426	10.0	138	632	130	.15	.61	12.2	—

Cup, chopped or diced pieces (not packed)	1 cup	140	49.4	458	36.4	33.5	0	15	196	4.6	64	291	60	.07	.28	5.6	—
T-bone steak, choice grade:																	
Cooked (broiled):																	
Lean with fat (56% lean, 44% fat):																	
Yield from 1 lb., raw beef with bone	10.4 oz	295	36.4	1,395	57.5	127.4	0	24	490	7.7	141	644	220	.17	.47	12.1	—
Lean, trimmed of separable fat:																	
Yield from 1 lb., raw beef with bone	5.8 oz	165	57.9	368	50.2	17.0	0	20	401	6.1	123	562	30	.13	.38	9.7	—
Ground beef:																	
Lean with 10% fat:																	
Cooked:																	
Yield from 1 lb., raw ground beef	12 oz	340	60.0	745	93.2	38.4	0	41	782	11.9	228	1,044	70	.32	.78	20.4	—
Patty	1 (3 oz)	85	60.0	186	23.3	9.6	0	10	196	3.0	57	261	20	.08	.20	5.1	—
Lean with 21% fat:																	
Cooked:																	
Yield from 1 lb., raw ground beef	11½ oz	326	54.2	932	78.9	66.2	0	36	632	10.4	193	884	120	.28	.68	17.6	—
Patty	1 (2.9 oz)	82	54.2	235	19.8	16.6	0	9	159	2.6	49	221	30	.07	.17	4.4	—
BEETS, COMMON, RED:																	
Cooked (boiled), drained, peeled:																	
Diced or sliced	1 cup	170	90.9	54	1.9	.2	12.2	24	39	.9	73	354	30	.05	.07	.5	10
Pound (approx. 2⅔ cups diced or sliced)	1 lb	454	90.9	145	5.0	.5	32.7	64	104	2.3	195	943	90	.14	.18	1.4	27
BLUEBERRIES:																	
Raw	1 cup	145	83.2	90	1.0	.7	22.2	22	19	1.5	1	117	150	(.04)	(.09)	(.7)	20
	1 lb	454	83.2	281	3.2	2.3	69.4	68	59	4.5	5	367	450	(.14)	(.27)	(2.3)	64
BRAZIL NUTS:																	
In shell (refuse: shells, 52%):	1 lb	454	4.6	1,424	31.1	145.6	23.7	405	1,509	7.4	2	1,557	Trace	2.09	.26	3.5	—
Shelled	1 cup	140	4.6	916	20.0	93.7	15.3	260	970	4.8	1	1,001	Trace	1.34	.17	2.2	—
	1 lb	454	4.6	2,967	64.9	303.5	49.4	844	3,143	15.4	5	3,243	Trace	4.35	.54	7.3	—
	1 oz. or 6–8 kernels.	28	4.6	185	4.1	19.0	3.1	53	196	1.0	Trace	203	Trace	.27	.03	.5	—

FOOD, APPROXIMATE HOUSEHOLD MEASURES AND MARKET UNITS		VALUES FOR EDIBLE PART OF FOODS															
			Water	Food energy	Protein	Fat	Carbohydrate	Calcium	Phosphorus	Iron	Sodium	Potassium	Vitamin A value	Thiamin	Riboflavin	Niacin	Ascorbic acid
		Grams	*Percent*	*Calories*	*Grams*	*Grams*	*Grams*	*Milligrams*	*Milligrams*	*Milligrams*	*Milligrams*	*Milligrams*	*International units*	*Milligrams*	*Milligrams*	*Milligrams*	*Milligrams*
BREAD:																	
White, enriched	1 loaf or 1 lb	454	35.6	1,225	39.5	14.5	229.1	381	440	11.3	2,300	476	Trace	1.13	.95	10.9	Trace
Whole-wheat	1 loaf or 1 lb	454	36.4	1,102	47.6	13.6	216.4	449	1,034	13.6	2,390	1,238	Trace	1.17	.54	12.7	Trace
BROCCOLI, STALKS (HEAD OR BUD CLUSTERS, STEM AND LEAVES):																	
Raw	1 lb	454	89.1	145	16.3	1.4	26.8	467	354	5.0	68	1,733	11,340	.45	1.04	4.1	513
Cooked (boiled), drained:																	
Stalks, cut into ½-in. pieces	1 cup	155	91.3	40	4.8	.5	7.0	136	96	1.2	16	414	3,880	.14	.31	1.2	140
Stalks, whole or cut	1 lb	454	91.3	118	14.1	1.4	20.4	399	281	3.6	45	1,211	11,340	.41	.91	3.6	408
BRUSSELS SPROUTS:																	
Raw	1 lb	454	85.2	204	22.2	1.8	37.6	163	363	6.8	64	1,769	2,490	.45	.73	4.1	463
Cooked (boiled), drained	1 cup	155	88.2	56	6.5	.6	9.9	50	112	1.7	16	423	810	.12	.22	1.2	135
	1 lb	454	88.2	163	19.1	1.8	29.0	145	327	5.0	45	1,238	2,360	.36	.64	3.6	395
CABBAGE:																	
Common varieties																	
Raw:																	
Shredded finely or chopped	1 cup	90	92.4	22	1.2	.2	4.9	44	26	.4	18	210	120	.05	.05	.3	42
	1 lb	454	92.4	109	5.9	.9	24.5	222	132	1.8	91	1,057	590	.23	.23	1.4	213
Cooked (boiled until tender), drained	1 cup	145	93.9	29	1.6	.3	6.2	64	29	.4	20	236	190	.06	.06	.4	48
CARROTS:																	
Raw:	1 carrot 3 oz.	81	88.2	30	.8	.1	7.0	27	26	.5	34	246	7,930	.04	.04	.4	6

Grated or shredded	1 cup	110	88.2	46	1.2	.2	10.7	41	40	.8	52	375	12,100	.07	.06	.7	9
	1 lb	454	88.2	191	5.0	.9	44.0	168	163	3.2	213	1,547	49,900	.27	.23	2.7	36
Cooked (boiled), drained:																	
Sliced	1 cup	155	91.2	48	1.4	.3	11.0	51	48	.9	51	344	16,280	.08	.08	.8	9
	1 lb	454	91.2	141	4.1	.9	32.2	150	141	2.7	150	1,007	47,630	.23	.23	2.8	27
CAULIFLOWER:																	
Raw:	1 cup	85	91.0	23	2.3	.2	4.4	21	48	.9	11	251	50	.09	.09	.6	66
Sliced	1 lb	454	91.0	122	12.2	.9	23.6	113	254	5.0	59	1,338	270	.50	.45	3.2	354
Cooked (boiled), drained:	1 cup	125	92.8	28	2.9	.3	5.1	26	53	.9	11	258	80	.11	.10	.8	69
Cup	1 lb	454	92.8	100	10.4	.9	18.6	95	191	3.2	41	934	270	.41	.36	2.7	249
CELERY, GREEN																	
Raw:																	
Chopped or diced pieces	1 cup	120	94.1	20	1.1	.1	4.7	47	34	.4	151	409	320	.04	.04	.4	11
	1 lb	454	94.1	77	4.1	.5	17.7	177	127	1.4	572	1,547	1,220	.14	.14	1.4	41
Cooked:																	
Diced pieces	1 cup	150	95.3	21	1.2	.2	4.7	47	33	.3	132	359	390	.03	.05	.5	9
	1 lb	454	95.3	64	3.6	.5	14.1	141	100	.9	399	1,084	1,180	.09	.14	1.4	27
CHARD, SWISS:																	
Raw	1 lb	454	91.1	113	10.9	1.4	20.9	399	177	14.5	667	2,495	29,480	.27	.77	2.8	145
Cooked (boiled), drained:																	
Leaves	1 cup	175	93.7	32	3.2	.4	5.8	128	42	3.2	151	562	9,450	.07	.19	.7	28
	1 lb	454	93.7	82	8.2	.9	15.0	331	109	8.2	390	1,456	24,490	.18	.50	1.8	73
NATURAL CHEESES:																	
Blue or Roquefort type:	1 lb	454	40	1,669	97.5	138.3	9.1	1,429	1,538	(2.3)	—	—	(5,620)	.14	2.77	5.4	(0)
	1 oz	28	40	104	6.1	8.6	.6	89	96	(.1)	—	—	(350)	.01	.17	.3	(0)
Brick:	1 lb	454	41.0	1,678	100.7	138.3	8.6	3,311	2,064	(4.1)	—	—	(5,620)	—	2.04	.5	(0)
	1 oz	28	41.0	105	6.3	8.6	.5	207	129	(.3)	—	—	(350)	—	.18	Trace	(0)
Cheddar (domestic type):	1 lb	454	37	1,805	113.4	146.1	9.5	3,402	2,168	4.5	3,175	372	(5,940)	.14	2.09	.5	(0)
	1 oz	28	37	113	7.1	9.1	.6	213	136	.3	198	23	(370)	.01	.13	Trace	(0)
Cottage cheese (cottage cheese dry curd with creaming mixture; 4.2% milk fat), large or small curd:																	
Packed	1 cup	245	78.3	260	33.3	10.3	7.1	230	372	.7	561	208	(420)	.07	.61	.2	(0)
	1 lb	454	78.3	481	61.7	19.1	13.2	426	689	1.4	1,039	386	(770)	.14	1.13	.5	(O)
	1 oz	28	78.3	30	3.9	1.2	.8	27	43	.1	65	24	(50)	.01	.07	Trace	(0)

FOOD, APPROXIMATE HOUSEHOLD MEASURES AND MARKET UNITS		VALUES FOR EDIBLE PART OF FOODS															
			Water	Food energy	Protein	Fat	Carbohydrate	Calcium	Phosphorus	Iron	Sodium	Potassium	Vitamin A value	Thiamin	Riboflavin	Niacin	Ascorbic acid
		Grams	*Percent*	*Calories*	*Grams*	*Grams*	*Grams*	*Milligrams*	*Milligrams*	*Milligrams*	*Milligrams*	*Milligrams*	*International units*	*Milligrams*	*Milligrams*	*Milligrams*	*Milligrams*
Cottage cheese dry curd (without creaming mixture; 0.3% milk fat):																	
Packed	1 cup	200	79.0	172	34.0	.6	5.4	180	350	.8	580	144	(20)	.06	.56	(.2)	(0)
	1 lb	454	79.0	390	77.1	1.4	12.2	408	794	1.8	1,315	327	(50)	.14	1.27	(.5)	(0)
	1 oz	28	79.0	24	4.8	.1	.8	26	50	.1	82	20	(Trace)	.01	.08	(Trace)	(0)
Parmesan:																	
Grated:																	
Packed	1 cup	140	17	654	59.8	43.1	4.9	1,893	1,296	.7	1,218	248	(1,760)	.03	1.22	.3	(0)
	1 tbsp	5	17	23	2.1	1.5	.2	68	46	Trace	44	9	(60)	Trace	.04	Trace	(0)
	1 lb	454	17	2,118	193.7	139.7	15.9	6,133	4,200	2.3	3,946	803	(5,720)	.09	3.95	.9	(0)
	1 oz	28	17	132	12.1	8.7	1.0	383	263	.1	247	50	(360)	.01	.25	.1	(0)
Swiss (domestic)	1 lb	454	39	1,678	124.7	127.0	7.7	4,196	2,554	4.1	3,221	472	(5,170)	.05	(1.81)	(.5)	(0)
	1 oz	28	39	105	7.8	7.9	.5	262	160	.3	201	29	(320)	Trace	(.11)	(Trace)	(0)
CHERRIES:																	
Raw:																	
Sweet:																	
Whole	10 cherries	75	80.4	47	.9	.2	11.7	15	13	.3	1	129	70	.03	.04	.3	7
Pound	1 lb	454	80.4	286	5.3	1.2	71.0	90	78	1.6	8	780	450	.20	.24	1.6	41
CHESTNUTS:																	
Fresh:																	
In shell	1 lb	454	52.5	713	10.7	5.5	154.7	99	323	6.2	22	1,668	—	.81	.81	2.2	—
Shelled	10 nuts	90	52.5	141	2.1	1.1	30.7	20	64	1.2	4	331	—	.16	.16	.4	—
	1 lb	454	52.5	880	13.2	6.8	191.0	122	399	7.7	27	2,059	—	1.00	1.00	2.7	—

CHICKEN, COOKED:																	
All classes, roasted:																	
Light meat without skin:																	
Chopped or diced	1 cup	140	63.8	232	44.2	4.8	0	15	371	1.8	90	575	80	.06	.14	16.2	—
	1 lb	454	63.8	753	143.3	15.4	0	50	1,202	5.9	290	1,864	270	.18	.45	52.6	—
	2 pieces	50	63.8	83	15.8	1.7	0	6	133	.7	32	206	30	.02	.05	5.8	—
Dark meat without skin:																	
Chopped or diced	1 cup	140	64.4	246	39.2	8.8	0	18	321	2.4	120	449	210	.10	.32	7.8	—
	1 lb	454	64.4	798	127.0	28.6	0	59	1,039	7.7	390	1,456	680	.32	1.04	25.4	—
	4 pieces	40	64.4	70	11.2	2.5	0	5	92	.7	34	128	60	.03	.09	2.2	—
Broilers, ready-to-cook, broiled, flesh only:																	
Yield from 1 lb., ready-to-cook broilers	7.1 oz	201	71.0	273	47.8	7.6	0	18	404	3.4	133	551	180	.10	.38	17.7	—
Fryers, ready-to-cook, fried:																	
Flesh, skin, giblets:																	
Yield from 1 lb., ready-to-cook fryers	8 oz	227	53.3	565	69.7	26.8	6.6	30	577	5.2	—	—	1,860	.16	1.29	20.7	—
Light meat without skin	2 pieces	50	59.5	99	16.1	3.1	.6	6	140	.7	34	217	30	.03	.13	6.5	—
Dark meat without skin	4 pieces	40	57.5	88	12.2	3.7	.6	6	94	.7	35	132	50	.03	.18	2.7	—
cut-up parts:	½ breast	94	58.4	160	25.7	5.1	1.2	9	218	1.3	—	—	70	.04	.17	11.6	—
	1 drumstick	56	55.0	88	12.2	3.8	.4	6	89	.9	—	—	50	.03	.15	2.7	—
	1 thigh	65	55.8	122	15.0	5.9	1.3	7	121	1.2	—	—	100	.03	.25	3.5	—
	1 wing	50	52.6	82	8.8	4.5	.8	3	72	.6	—	—	80	.02	.08	2.1	—
COCONUT MEAT:																	
Fresh:																	
Shredded or packed	1 cup	130	50.9	450	4.6	45.9	12.2	17	124	2.2	30	333	0	.07	.03	.7	4
	1 lb	454	50.9	1,569	15.9	160.1	42.6	59	431	7.7	104	1,161	0	.23	.09	2.3	14
Dried, unsweetened (desiccated)	1 lb	454	3.5	3,003	32.7	294.4	104.3	118	848	15.0	—	2,667	0	.27	.18	2.7	0
COD:																	
Cooked (broiled), with butter or margarine:																	
Fillet, 5 in. long, 2½ in. wide, ⅞ in. thick	1 fillet	65	64.6	111	18.5	3.4	0	20	178	.7	72	265	120	.05	.07	2.0	—
CORN, SWEET:																	
Cooked (boiled), drained:																	
Kernels, cut off cob before cooking	1 cup	165	76.5	137	5.3	1.7	31.0	5	147	1.0	Trace	272	660	.18	.17	2.1	12
	1 lb	454	76.5	376	14.5	4.5	85.3	14	404	2.7	Trace	748	1,810	.50	.45	5.9	32

FOOD, APPROXIMATE HOUSEHOLD MEASURES AND MARKET UNITS		VALUES FOR EDIBLE PART OF FOODS															
			Water	Food energy	Protein	Fat	Carbohydrate	Calcium	Phosphorus	Iron	Sodium	Potassium	Vitamin A value	Thiamin	Riboflavin	Niacin	Ascorbic acid
		Grams	*Percent*	*Calories*	*Grams*	*Grams*	*Grams*	*Milligrams*	*Milligrams*	*Milligrams*	*Milligrams*	*Milligrams*	*International units*	*Milligrams*	*Milligrams*	*Milligrams*	*Milligrams*
Kernels, cooked on cob (refuse: cob, 45%):																	
Ear, 5 in. long, 1¾-in. diam	1 ear	140	74.1	70	2.5	.8	16.2	2	69	.5	Trace	151	310	.09	.08	1.1	7
	1 lb	454	74.1	227	8.2	2.5	52.4	7	222	1.5	Trace	489	1,000	.30	.25	3.5	22
CRESS, GARDEN:																	
Raw	1 lb	454	89.4	145	11.8	3.2	24.9	367	345	5.9	64	2,749	42,180	.36	1.18	4.5	313
Cooked (boiled), drained	1 cup	135	92.5	31	2.6	.8	5.1	82	65	1.1	11	477	10,400	.08	.22	1.1	46
	1 lb	454	92.5	104	8.6	2.7	17.2	277	218	3.6	36	1,601	34,930	.27	.73	3.6	154
CUCUMBERS, RAW:																	
Not pared:																	
Sliced	1 cup	105	95.1	16	.9	.1	3.6	26	28	1.2	6	168	260	.03	.04	.2	12
	1 lb	454	95.1	68	4.1	.5	15.4	113	122	5.0	27	726	1,130	.14	.18	.9	50
Pared:																	
Sliced	1 cup	140	95.7	20	.8	.1	4.5	24	25	.4	8	224	Trace	.04	.06	.3	15
	1 lb	454	95.7	64	2.7	.5	14.5	77	82	1.4	27	726	Trace	.14	.18	.9	50
DATES, MOISTURIZED OR HYDRATED:																	
With pits (refuse: pits, 18%)	10 dates	92	22.5	219	1.8	.4	58.3	47	50	2.4	1	518	40	.07	.08	1.8	0
	1 lb	454	22.5	1,081	8.7	2.0	287.7	233	249	11.8	4	2,557	200	.36	.39	8.7	0
Without pits:	1 lb	454	22.5	1,243	10.0	2.3	330.7	268	286	13.6	5	2,939	230	.41	.45	10.0	0
	10 dates	80	22.5	219	1.8	.4	58.3	47	50	2.4	1	518	40	.07	.08	1.8	0

EGGS:																	
Chicken:																	
Medium	1 egg	50	73.7	72	5.7	5.1	.4	24	90	1.0	54	57	520	.05	.13	Trace	0
Medium	1 white	29	87.6	15	3.2	Trace	.2	3	4	Trace	42	40	0	Trace	.08	Trace	0
EGGPLANT, COOKED (BOILED), DRAINED:	1 cup	200	94.3	38	2.0	.4	8.2	22	42	1.2	2	300	20	.10	.08	1.0	6
Cup, diced	1 lb	454	94.3	86	4.5	.9	18.6	50	95	2.7	5	680	50	.23	.18	2.3	14
FARINA:																	
Enriched:																	
Regular (about 15 min. cooking time):																	
Cooked	1 cup	245	89.5	103	3.2	.2	21.3	10	29	—	353	22	(0)	.10	.07	1.0	(0)
Quick cooking (about 2–5 min. cooking time):																	
Cooked	1 cup	245	89.0	105	3.2	.2	21.8	147	162	—	466	25	(0)	.12	.07	1.0	(0)
Instant cooking (about ½ min. cooking time):																	
Cooked	1 cup	245	85.9	135	4.2	.2	27.9	189	147	—	461	32	(0)	.17	.10	1.2	(0)
Unenriched, regular (about 15 min. cooking time):																	
Cooked	1 cup	245	89.5	103	3.2	.2	21.3	10	29	.5	353	22	(0)	.02	.02	.2	(0)
FIGS:																	
Raw:																	
Medium, 2¼-in. diam. (approx. 9 per pound)	1 fig	50	77.5	40	.6	.2	10.2	18	11	.3	1	97	40	.03	.03	.2	1
FILBERTS (HAZELNUTS):																	
In shell (refuse: shells, 54%):																	
Pound (yields approx. 7⅓	1 lb	454	5.8	1,323	26.3	130.2	34.9	436	703	7.1	4	1,469	—	.96	—	1.9	Trace
oz., shelled nuts)	10 nuts	30	5.8	87	1.7	8.6	2.3	29	47	.5	Trace	97	—	.06	—	.1	Trace
Shelled:	1 cup	135	5.8	856	17.0	84.2	22.5	282	455	4.6	3	950	—	.62	—	1.2	Trace
Whole	1 lb	454	5.8	2,876	57.2	283.0	75.8	948	1,529	15.4	9	3,193	—	2.09	—	4.1	Trace
Pound (yield from approx. 2¼ lb., in shell)																	
FLOUNDER, BAKED WITH BUTTER OR MARGARINE:																	
Fillet, 8¼ in. long, 2¾ in. wide, ¼ in. thick	1 fillet •	100	58.1	202	30.0	8.2	0	23	344	1.4	237	587	—	.07	.08	2.5	2

FOOD, APPROXIMATE HOUSEHOLD MEASURES AND MARKET UNITS		VALUES FOR EDIBLE PART OF FOODS															
			Water	Food energy	Protein	Fat	Carbohydrate	Calcium	Phosphorus	Iron	Sodium	Potassium	Vitamin A value	Thiamin	Riboflavin	Niacin	Ascorbic acid
		Grams	*Percent*	*Calories*	*Grams*	*Grams*	*Grams*	*Milligrams*	*Milligrams*	*Milligrams*	*Milligrams*	*Milligrams*	*International units*	*Milligrams*	*Milligrams*	*Milligrams*	*Milligrams*
GRAPEFRUIT																	
All varieties:																	
3½-in. diam.	1 grapefruit	400	88.4	80	1.0	.2	20.8	31	31	.8	2	265	160	.08	.04	.4	74
Juice	1 cup	246	90.0	96	1.2	.2	22.6	22	37	.5	2	399	200	.10	.05	.5	93
GRAPES:																	
Raw:																	
American type (slip skin) as Concord, Delaware, whole (refuse: seeds and skins, 34%):	10 grapes	40	81.6	18	.3	.3	4.1	4	3	.1	1	42	30	(.01)	(.01)	(.1)	1
	1 cup	153	81.6	70	1.3	1.0	15.9	16	12	.4	3	160	100	(.05)	(.03)	(.3)	4
	1 lb	454	81.6	207	3.9	3.0	47.0	48	36	1.2	9	473	300	(.15)	(.09)	(.9)	12
European type (adherent skin) as Thompson Seedless																	
Whole:																	
Seedless types	10 grapes	50	81.4	34	.3	.2	8.7	6	10	.2	2	87	(50)	.03	.02	.2	2
	1 cup	160	81.4	107	1.0	.5	27.7	19	32	.6	5	277	(160)	.08	.05	.5	6
Seeded types (refuse: seeds, 5%)	10 grapes	60	81.4	38	.3	.2	9.9	7	11	.2	2	90	(60)	.03	.02	.2	2
	1 cup	160	81.4	102	.9	.5	26.3	18	30	.6	5	263	(150)	.08	.05	.5	6
GRAPEJUICE:																	
Canned or bottled:	1 cup	253	82.9	167	.5	Trace	42.0	28	30	.8	5	293	—	.10	.05	.5	Trace

HALIBUT, ATLANTIC AND PACIFIC, BROILED WITH BUTTER OR MARGARINE:																	
Yield from 1 lb., raw fillets	12⅞ oz	365	66.6	624	92.0	25.6	0	58	905	2.9	489	1,916	2,480	0.18	0.26	30.3	—
KALE, LEAVES WITHOUT STEMS, MIDRIBS:																	
Raw	1 lb	454	82.7	240	(27.2)	(3.6)	40.8	1,129	422	12.2	(340)	(1,715)	45,360	.73	1.18	9.5	844
Cooked (boiled), drained	1 cup	110	87.8	43	(5.0)	(.8)	6.7	206	64	1.8	(47)	(243)	9,130	.11	.20	1.8	102
LENTILS, MATURE SEEDS, DRY:																	
Cooked	1 cup	200	72.0	212	15.6	Trace	38.6	50	238	4.2	—	498	40	0.14	0.12	1.2	0
LETTUCE, RAW:																	
Butterhead varieties such as Boston types and Bibb:	1 cup	55	95.1	8	.7	.1	1.4	19	14	1.1	5	145	530	.03	.03	.2	4
Chopped or shredded pieces	1 lb	454	95.1	64	5.4	.9	11.3	159	118	9.1	41	1,198	4,400	.27	.27	1.4	36
Crisphead varieties such as Iceberg, Chopped or shredded	1 cup	55	95.5	7	.5	.1	1.6	11	12	.3	5	96	180	.03	.03	.2	8
pieces	1 lb	454	95.5	59	4.1	.5	13.2	91	100	2.8	41	794	1,500	.27	.27	1.4	27
Looseleaf or bunching varieties such as Grand Rapids, Salad Bowl, Simpson: Chopped or shredded	1 cup	55	94.0	10	.7	.2	1.9	37	14	.8	5	145	1,050	.03	.04	.2	10
pieces	1 lb	454	94.0	82	5.9	1.4	15.9	308	118	6.4	41	1,198	8,620	.23	.86	1.8	82
LOBSTER, NORTHERN, COOKED:	1 lb	454	76.8	431	84.8	6.8	1.4	295	871	3.6	953	816	—	.45	.32	—	—
MACKEREL, ATLANTIC, BROILED WITH BUTTER OR MARGARINE:																	
Yield from 1 lb., raw fillets	12⅞ oz	365	61.6	861	79.6	57.7	0	22	1,022	4.4	—	—	(1,930)	0.55	0.99	27.7	—

FOOD, APPROXIMATE HOUSEHOLD MEASURES AND MARKET UNITS		VALUES FOR EDIBLE PART OF FOODS															
			Water	Food energy	Protein	Fat	Carbohydrate	Calcium	Phosphorus	Iron	Sodium	Potassium	Vitamin A value	Thiamin	Riboflavin	Niacin	Ascorbic acid
		Grams	Percent	Calories	Grams	Grams	Grams	Milligrams	Milligrams	Milligrams	Milligrams	Milligrams	International units	Milligrams	Milligrams	Milligrams	Milligrams
MANGOS, RAW:																	
Whole (refuse: seeds and skin, 33%)	1 fruit	300	81.7	152	1.6	.9	38.8	23	30	.9	16	437	11,000	.12	.12	2.5	81
Pound	1 lb	454	81.7	299	3.2	1.8	76.2	45	59	1.8	32	857	21,770	.28	.23	5.0	159
MILK, COW:																	
Whole, 3.5% fat	1 qt	976	87.4	634	34.2	34.2	47.8	1,152	908	0.4	488	1,405	1,410	0.29	1.66	1.0	10
	1 cup	244	87.4	159	8.5	8.5	12.0	288	227	.1	122	351	350	.07	.41	.2	2
Skim	1 quart	980	90.5	353	35.3	1.0	50.0	1,186	931	.4	510	1,421	40	.34	1.76	.7	10
	1 cup	245	90.5	88	8.8	.2	12.5	296	233	.1	127	355	10	.09	.44	.2	2
MUSHROOMS:																	
Agaricus campestris, cultivated commercially, raw:																	
Cup, slices, chopped or diced pieces	1 cup	70	90.4	20	1.9	.2	3.1	4	81	.6	11	290	Trace	.07	.32	2.9	2
Pound	1 lb	454	90.4	127	12.2	1.4	20.0	27	526	3.6	68	1,878	Trace	.45	2.09	19.1	14
MUSKMELONS:																	
Cantaloups																	
Whole, 5-in. diam.; wt., approx. 2⅓ lb.	1 melon	1,060	91.2	159	3.7	.5	39.8	74	85	2.1	64	1,330	18,020	.21	.16	3.2	175
Pound	1 lb	454	91.2	136	3.2	.5	34.0	64	73	1.8	54	1,139	15,420	.18	.14	2.7	150
OATMEAL OR ROLLED OATS:																	
Cooked	1 cup	240	86.5	132	4.8	2.4	23.3	22	137	1.4	523	146	(0)	.19	.05	.2	(0)

OLIVES, PICKLED; CANNED OR BOTTLED:																	
Green:																	
Whole (refuse: pits, 16%):	10 olives	46	78.2	45	.5	4.9	.5	24	7	.6	926	21	120	—	—	—	—
Large, pitted	1 lb	454	78.2	526	6.4	57.6	5.9	277	77	7.3	10,886	249	1,360	—	—	—	—
Ripe:																	
Mission:																	
Whole (refuse: pits, 14%):	10 olives	46	73.0	73	.5	8.0	1.3	42	7	.7	297	11	30	Trace	Trace	—	—
Large, pitted	1 lb	454	73.0	835	5.4	91.2	14.5	481	77	7.7	3,402	122	320	Trace	Trace	—	—
ONIONS, MATURE (DRY):																	
Raw:																	
Chopped	1 cup	170	89.1	65	2.6	.2	14.8	46	61	.9	17	267	70	0.05	0.07	0.3	17
	1 lb	454	89.1	172	6.8	.5	39.5	122	163	2.3	45	712	180	1.4	.18	.9	45
Cooked (boiled), drained:																	
Cup, whole or sliced	1 cup	210	91.8	61	2.5	.2	13.7	50	61	.8	15	231	80	.06	.06	.4	15
ORANGES, RAW,																	
All commercial varieties:																	
Whole fruit, 2½ in. diam.	1 orange	180	86.0	64	1.3	.3	16.0	54	26	.5	1	263	260	.13	.05	.5	(66)
Juice	1 cup	248	88.3	112	1.7	.5	25.8	27	42	.5	2	496	500	.22	.07	1.0	124
PAPAYAS, RAW:																	
Whole, medium fruit	1 papaya or 1 lb.	454	88.7	119	1.8	.3	30.4	61	49	.9	9	711	5,320	.12	.12	.9	170
PARSLEY,																	
Chopped	1 tbsp	3.5	85.1	2	.1	Trace	.3	7	2	.2	2	25	300	Trace	.01	Trace	6
PEACHES:																	
Raw:																	
Fruit, 2½-in. diam. (aprox.	1 peach	115	89.1	38	.6	.1	9.7	9	19	.5	1	202	1,330	.02	.05	1.0	7
4 per pound)	1 lb	454	89.1	150	2.4	.4	38.3	36	75	2.0	4	797	5,250	.08	.20	3.9	28
PEANUTS:																	
Roasted in shell, whole																	
Pounds (yields approx. 10.7 oz., shelled nuts)	1 lb	454	1.8	1,769	79.6	148.0	62.6	219	1,237	6.7	15	2,130	—	.97	.40	52.0	0
Jumbo	10 nuts	27	1.8	105	4.7	8.8	3.7	13	74	.4	1	127	—	.06	.02	3.1	0
Shelled, chopped form:	1 cup	144	1.8	838	37.7	70.1	29.7	104	586	3.2	7	1,009	—	.46	.19	24.6	0
Roasted, salted	1 cup	144	1.6	842	37.4	71.7	27.1	107	577	3.0	602	971	—	.46	.19	24.8	0
	1 lb	454	1.6	2,654	117.9	225.9	85.3	336	1,819	9.5	1,896	3,057	—	1.45	.59	78.0	0

FOOD, APPROXIMATE HOUSEHOLD MEASURES AND MARKET UNITS		VALUES FOR EDIBLE PART OF FOODS															
			Water	Food energy	Protein	Fat	Carbohydrate	Calcium	Phosphorus	Iron	Sodium	Potassium	Vitamin A value	Thiamin	Riboflavin	Niacin	Ascorbic acid
		Grams	Percent	Calories	Grams	Grams	Grams	Milligrams	Milligrams	Milligrams	Milligrams	Milligrams	International units	Milligrams	Milligrams	Milligrams	Milligrams
PEANUT BUTTER MADE WITH MODERATE AMOUNTS OF ADDED FAT, NUTRITIVE SWEETENER, SALT	1 tbsp	16	1.7	94	4.0	8.1	3.0	9	61	.3	97	100	—	.02	.02	2.4	0
PEARS:																	
Raw, (approx. 2½ per pound)	1 pear	180	83.2	100	1.1	.7	25.1	13	18	.5	3	213	30	.03	.07	.2	7
	1 lb	454	83.2	277	3.2	1.8	69.4	36	50	1.4	9	590	90	.09	.18	.5	18
PEAS, GREEN, IMMATURE:																	
Cooked (boiled), drained	1 cup	160	81.5	114	8.6	.6	19.4	37	158	2.9	2	314	860	.45	.18	3.7	32
PEAS, MATURE SEEDS, DRY																	
Cooked	1 cup	200	70.0	230	16.0	0.6	41.6	22	178	3.4	26	592	80	0.30	0.18	1.8	—
PECANS:																	
In shell (refuse: shells, 47%):																	
Pound (yields approx. 8.5 oz., shelled nuts)	1 lb	454	3.4	1,652	22.1	171.2	35.1	175	695	5.8	Trace	1,450	310	2.07	.31	2.2	5
Shelled:																	
Pound (yield from approx. 1.9 lb., in shell)	1 lb	454	3.4	3,116	41.7	323.0	66.2	331	1,311	10.9	Trace	2,735	590	3.90	.59	4.1	9
PEPPERS, SWEET, GARDEN VARIETIES:																	
Immature, green:																	
Raw:																	
Chopped or diced	1 cup	150	93.4	33	1.8	.3	7.2	14	33	1.1	20	320	630	.12	.12	.8	192
	1 lb	454	93.4	100	5.4	.9	21.8	41	100	3.2	59	966	1,910	.36	.36	2.3	581

Cooked:																	
Boiled, drained:																	
Strips	1 cup	135	94.7	24	1.4	.3	5.1	12	22	.7	12	201	570	.08	.09	.6	130
Mature, red, raw:																	
Chopped or diced	1 cup	150	90.7	47	2.1	.5	10.7	20	45	.9	—	—	6,680	(.12)	(.12)	(.8)	306
	1 lb	454	90.7	141	6.4	1.4	32.2	59	136	2.7	—	—	20,190	(.36)	(.36)	(2.3)	925
PINEAPPLE:																	
Raw:																	
Cup, diced pieces	1 cup	155	85.3	81	.6	.3	21.2	26	12	.8	2	226	110	.14	.05	.3	26
Pound (approx. 3 cups, diced pieces or 5½ slices)	1 lb	454	85.3	236	1.8	.9	62.1	77	36	2.3	5	662	320	.41	.14	.9	77
PISTACHIONUTS:																	
In shell (refuse: shells, 50%)	1 lb	454	5.3	1,347	43.8	121.8	43.1	297	1,134	16.6	—	2,204	520	1.52	—	3.2	0
Shelled	1 lb	454	5.3	2,694	87.5	243.6	86.2	594	2,268	33.1	—	4,409	1,040	3.04	—	6.4	0
PLUMS:																	
Raw:																	
Damson:																	
Whole (refuse: pits and clinging pulp, 9%):																	
Fruit, 1-in. diam	10 plums	110	81.1	66	.5	Trace	17.8	18	17	.5	2	299	(300)	.08	.08	.5	—
	1 lb	454	81.1	272	2.1	Trace	73.5	74	70	2.1	8	1,284	(1,240)	.83	.12	2.1	—
Prune type:																	
Whole (refuse: pits, 6%):																	
Fruit, 1½-in. diam.	1 plum	30	78.7	21	.2	.1	5.6	3	5	.1	Trace	48	80	.01	.01	.1	1
	1 lb	454	78.7	320	3.4	.9	84.0	51	77	2.1	4	725	1,280	.18	.18	2.1	17
POPCORN:																	
Popped																	
Plain, large kernel	1 cup	6	4.0	23	.8	.3	4.6	(1)	(17)	(.2)	(Trace)	—	—	—	(.01)	(.1)	(0)
Oil and salt added, large kernel	1 cup	9	3.1	41	.9	2.0	5.3	1	19	.2	175	—	—	—	.01	.2	0
PORK, FRESH, RETAIL CUTS:																	
Ham:																	
Cooked (baked or roasted):																	
Lean with fat (74% lean, 26% fat):																	
Yield from 1 lb., raw ham with bone and skin	9.2 oz	262	45.5	980	60.3	80.2	0	26	618	7.9	148	675	(0)	1.84	.60	12.1	—

FOOD, APPROXIMATE HOUSEHOLD MEASURES AND MARKET UNITS			Water	Food energy	Protein	Fat	Carbohydrate	Calcium	Phosphorus	Iron	Sodium	Potassium	Vitamin A value	Thiamin	Riboflavin	Niacin	Ascorbic acid
		Grams	*Percent*	*Calories*	*Grams*	*Grams*	*Grams*	*Milligrams*	*Milligrams*	*Milligrams*	*Milligrams*	*Milligrams*	*International units*	*Milligrams*	*Milligrams*	*Milligrams*	*Milligrams*
Yield from 1 lb., raw ham without bone and skin	10.9 oz	308	45.5	1,152	70.8	94.2	0	31	727	9.2	178	793	(0)	1.57	.71	14.2	—
Cup (not packed):																	
Chopped or diced:	1 cup	140	45.5	524	82.2	42.8	0	14	880	4.2	79	361	(0)	.71	.82	6.4	—
	2 pieces or 3 oz	85	45.5	318	19.6	26.0	0	9	201	2.6	48	220	(0)	.43	.20	3.9	—
Lean, trimmed of separable fat:																	
Yield from 1 lb., raw ham with bone and skin	6.8 oz	194	58.9	421	57.6	19.4	0	25	598	7.4	141	645	(0)	1.24	.56	11.1	—
Yield from 1 lb., raw ham with bone and skin	8.1 oz	228	58.9	495	67.7	22.8	0	30	702	8.7	166	758	(0)	1.46	.66	13.0	—
Cup (not packed):																	
Chopped or diced	1 cup	140	58.9	304	41.6	14.0	0	18	431	5.3	102	466	(0)	.90	.41	8.0	—
	2 pieces or 3 oz	85	58.8	184	25.2	8.5	0	11	262	3.2	62	282	(0)	.54	.25	4.8	—
Loin and loin chops:																	
Cooked:																	
Lean with fat:																	
Baked or roasted loin roast (80% lean, 20% fat):																	
Yield from 1 lb., raw loin with bone	8.6 oz	244	45.8	883	59.8	69.5	0	27	625	7.8	147	670	(0)	2.24	.63	13.7	—
Yield from 1 lb., raw loin without bone	10.9 oz	308	45.8	1,115	75.5	87.8	0	34	788	9.9	185	846	(0)	2.83	0.80	17.2	—

Cup, chopped or diced pieces (not packed)	1 cup	140	45.8	507	34.3	39.9	0	15	358	4.5	84	384	(0)	1.29	.36	7.8	—
	1 piece or 3 oz	85	45.8	308	20.8	24.2	0	9	218	2.7	51	233	(0)	.78	.22	4.8	—
Lean, trimmed of separable fat:																	
Baked or roasted loin roast:																	
Yield from 1 lb., raw loin with bone	6.9 oz	195	55.0	495	57.3	27.7	0	25	605	7.4	140	642	(0)	2.11	.60	12.7	—
Yield from 1 lb., raw loin without bone	8.7 oz	247	55.0	627	72.6	35.1	0	32	766	9.4	178	813	(0)	2.67	.77	16.1	—
Cup, chopped or diced pieces (not packed)	1 cup	140	55.0	356	41.2	19.9	0	18	434	5.3	101	461	(0)	1.51	.43	9.1	—
	1 piece or 3 oz	85	55.0	216	25.0	12.1	0	11	264	3.2	61	280	(0)	.92	.26	5.5	—
PORK, CURED:																	
Light cure, commercial:																	
Ham:																	
Baked or roasted:																	
Lean with fat (84% lean, 16% fat):																	
Yield from 1 lb., unbaked ham with bone and skin	11.3 oz	320	53.6	925	66.9	70.7	0	29	550	8.3	2,395	749	(0)	1.50	.58	11.5	—
Yield from 1 lb., unbaked ham without bone and skin	13.1 oz	372	53.6	1,075	77.7	82.2	0	33	640	9.7	2,782	870	(0)	1.75	.67	13.4	—
Chopped or diced	1 cup	140	53.6	405	29.3	30.9	0	13	241	3.6	1,049	328	(0)	.66	.25	5.0	—
	2 pieces or 3 oz	85	53.6	246	17.8	18.8	0	8	146	2.2	637	199	(0)	.40	.15	3.1	—
Lean, trimmed of separable fat:																	
Yield from 1 lb., unbaked ham with bone and skin	8.7 oz	246	61.9	460	62.2	21.6	0	27	492	7.9	2,227	697	(0)	1.43	.57	11.1	—

FOOD, APPROXIMATE HOUSEHOLD MEASURES AND MARKET UNITS		VALUES FOR EDIBLE PART OF FOODS															
			Water	Food energy	Protein	Fat	Carbohydrate	Calcium	Phosphorus	Iron	Sodium	Potassium	Vitamin A value	Thiamin	Riboflavin	Niacin	Ascorbic acid
		Grams	*Percent*	*Calories*	*Grams*	*Grams*	*Grams*	*Milligrams*	*Milligrams*	*Milligrams*	*Milligrams*	*Milligrams*	*International units*	*Milligrams*	*Milligrams*	*Milligrams*	*Milligrams*
Yield from 1 lb., unbaked ham without bone and skin	10.2 oz	288	61.9	539	72.9	25.3	0	32	576	9.2	2,610	816	(0)	1.67	.66	13.0	—
	1 cup	140	61.9	262	35.4	12.3	0	15	280	4.5	1,267	396	(0)	.81	.32	6.3	—
	2 pieces or 3 oz	85	61.9	159	21.5	7.5	0	9	170	2.7	770	241	(0)	.49	.20	3.8	—
POTATOES:																	
Baked in skin (refuse: skins and adhering potato, 23%):																	
Potato, long type, 2⅓-in. diam., 4¾ in. long	1 potato	202	75.1	145	4.0	.2	32.8	14	101	1.1	6	782	Trace	.15	.07	2.7	31
	1 lb	454	75.1	325	9.1	.3	73.7	31	227	2.4	14	1,757	Trace	.34	.15	6.1	69
French fried:																	
Length, over 2 in. to 3½ in	10 strips	50	44.7	137	2.2	6.6	18.0	8	56	.7	3	427	Trace	.07	.04	1.6	11
RAISINS, NATURAL (UNBLEACHED), SEEDLESS TYPE:																	
Uncooked:																	
Package, net wt., 15 oz. (approx. 3 cups)	1 pkg	425	18.0	1,228	10.6	.9	329.0	264	429	14.9	115	3,243	90	.47	.34	2.1	4
	1 tbsp	9	18.0	26	.2	Trace	7.0	6	9	.3	2	69	Trace	.01	.01	Trace	Trace

RICE:																	
Brown:																	
Cooked, long grain:																	
Cup:																	
Hot rice	1 cup	195	70.3	232	4.9	1.2	49.7	23	142	1.0	550	137	(0)	.18	.04	2.7	(0)
White																	
Enriched:																	
Cooked (moist, soft stage), long grain:																	
Hot rice	1 cup	205	72.6	223	4.1	.2	49.6	21	57	1.8	767	57	(0)	.23	.02	2.1	(0)
Parboiled, long grain, regular:																	
Cooked:																	
Hot rice	1 cup	175	73.4	186	3.7	.2	40.8	33	100	1.4	627	75	(0)	.19	.02	2.1	(0)
Unenriched:																	
Cooked (moist, soft stage), long grain:																	
Hot rice	1 cup	205	72.6	223	4.1	.2	49.6	21	57	.4	767	57	(0)	.04	.02	.8	(0)
SESAME SEEDS, DRY, HULLED, DECORTICATED:																	
	1 cup	150	5.5	873	27.3	801.	26.4	165	888	3.6	—	—	—	.27	.20	8.1	0
	1 tbsp	8	5.5	47	1.5	4.3	1.4	9	47	.2	—	—	—	.01	.01	.4	0
SHRIMP:																	
Medium, approx. 2½ in. long	10 shrimp	32	70.4	37	7.7	.4	.2	37	84	1.0	—	39	20	Trace	.01	.6	—
	1 lb	454	70.4	526	109.8	5.0	3.2	522	1,193	14.1	—	553	270	0.05	.14	8.2	—
SOYBEANS:																	
Mature seeds, dry:																	
Cooked	1 cup	180	71.0	234	19.8	10.3	19.4	131	322	4.9	4	972	50	.38	.16	1.1	0
SOYBEAN CURD (TOFU):																	
Piece (2½ × 2¾ × 1 in.)	1 piece	120	84.8	86	9.4	5.0	2.9	154	151	2.3	8	50	0	.07	.04	.1	0
	1 lb	454	84.8	327	35.4	19.1	10.9	581	572	8.6	32	191	0	.27	.14	.5	0
SPINACH:																	
Raw:																	
(chopped spinach)	1 cup	55	90.7	14	1.8	.2	2.4	51	28	1.7	39	259	4,460	.06	.11	.8	28
	1 lb	454	90.7	118	14.5	1.4	19.5	422	231	14.1	322	2,182	86,740	.45	.91	2.7	281
Cooked (boiled), drained:																	
Cup, leaves	1 cup	180	92.0	41	5.4	.5	6.5	167	68	4.0	90	583	14,580	.13	.25	.9	50
STRAWBERRIES:																	
Raw	1 cup	149	89.9	55	1.0	.7	12.5	31	31	1.5	1	244	90	.04	.10	.9	88
	1 lb	454	89.9	168	3.2	2.3	38.1	95	95	4.5	5	744	270	.14	.32	2.7	268

FOOD, APPROXIMATE HOUSEHOLD MEASURES AND MARKET UNITS		VALUES FOR EDIBLE PART OF FOODS															
			Water	Food energy	Protein	Fat	Carbohydrate	Calcium	Phosphorus	Iron	Sodium	Potassium	Vitamin A value	Thiamin	Riboflavin	Niacin	Ascorbic acid
		Grams	*Percent*	*Calories*	*Grams*	*Grams*	*Grams*	*Milligrams*	*Milligrams*	*Milligrams*	*Milligrams*	*Milligrams*	*International units*	*Milligrams*	*Milligrams*	*Milligrams*	*Milligrams*
SUNFLOWER SEED KERNELS, DRY:																	
In hull (refuse: hulls, 46%):																	
Pound (yields approx. 1⅔ cups hulled seeds)	1 lb	454	4.8	1,371	58.8	115.8	48.7	294	2,050	17.4	73	2,253	120	4.80	.56	13.2	—
Cup (yields approx. ⅓ cup hulled seeds)	1 cup	85	4.8	257	11.0	21.7	9.1	55	384	3.3	14	422	20	.90	.11	2.5	—
Hulled:	1 lb	454	4.8	2,540	108.9	214.6	90.3	544	3,797	32.2	136	4,173	230	8.89	1.04	24.5	—
	1 cup	145	4.8	812	34.8	68.6	28.9	174	1,214	10.3	44	1,334	70	2.84	.33	7.8	—
SWEETPOTATOES:																	
Cooked,																	
Baked in skin (refuse: skin, 22%):																	
Potato, 5 in. long 2-in. diam.	1 potato	146	63.7	161	2.4	.6	37.0	46	66	1.0	14	342	9,230	.10	.08	.8	25
	1 lb	454	63.7	499	7.4	1.8	115.0	142	205	3.2	42	1,061	28,660	.32	.25	2.5	78
SWORDFISH, BROILED WITH BUTTER OR MARGARINE																	
Yield from 1 lb., raw	10.1 oz	305	64.6	499	80.3	17.2	0	77	788	3.7	—	—	5,880	.11	.14	31.3	—
TANGERINES,																	
Medium	1 tangerine	116	87	39	.7	.2	10.0	34	15	.3	2	108	360	.05	.02	.1	27
TOMATOES, RIPE:																	
Raw	1 tomato, 7 oz	200	93.5	40	2.0	.4	8.6	24	49	.9	5	444	1,640	.11	.07	1.3	42
	1 lb	454	93.5	91	4.5	.8	19.4	54	111	2.1	12	1,007	3,720	.25	.17	2.9	95

TUNA:																	
Canned:																	
In oil:																	
Solids and liquid:																	
7 oz	1 can	198	52.6	570	47.9	40.6	0	12	582	2.2	1,584	596	180	.08	.18	20.0	—
	1 lb	454	52.6	1,306	109.8	93.0	0	27	1,334	5.0	3,629	1,365	410	.18	.41	45.8	—
Drained solids:																	
6 oz	1 can	169	60.6	333	48.7	13.9	0	(14)	395	3.2	—	—	140	.08	.20	20.1	—
	1 lb	454	60.6	894	130.6	37.2	0	(36)	1,061	8.6	—	—	360	.23	.54	54.0	—
In water:																	
Solids and liquid: 7 oz	1 can	198	70.0	251	55.4	1.6	0	32	376	3.2	81	552	—	—	.20	26.3	—
	1 lb	454	70.0	576	127.0	3.6	0	73	862	7.3	186	1,266	—	—	.45	60.3	—
TURKEY, COOKED:																	
All classes, roasted:																	
Flesh only:																	
(not packed):																	
Chopped or diced	1 cup	140	61.2	266	44.1	8.5	0	11	351	2.5	182	514	—	.07	.25	10.8	—
Light meat without skin:																	
Chopped or diced	1 cup	140	62.1	246	46.1	5.5	0	—	—	1.7	115	575	—	.07	.20	15.5	—
Piece,	3 oz	85	62.1	150	28.0	3.3	0	—	—	1.0	70	349	—	.04	.12	9.4	—
Dark meat without skin:																	
Chopped or diced	1 cup	140	60.5	284	42.0	11.0	0	—	—	3.2	139	557	—	.06	.32	5.9	—
Piece,	3 oz	85	60.5	173	25.5	7.1	0	—	—	2.0	84	338	—	.03	.20	3.6	—
WALNUTS:																	
Black:																	
In shell (refuse: shells, 78%), 1 lb (yields approx. 3½ oz., shelled nuts)	1 lb	454	3.1	627	20.5	59.2	14.8	Trace	569	6.0	3	459	300	.22	.11	.7	—
Shelled:																	
Chopped or broken kernels:																	
Cup	1 cup	125	3.1	785	25.6	74.1	18.5	Trace	713	7.5	4	575	380	.28	.14	.9	—
Pound (yield from approx. 4½ lb., in shell)	1 lb	454	3.1	2,849	93.0	269.0	67.1	Trace	2,586	27.2	14	2,087	1,360	1.00	.50	3.2	—
	1 oz	28	3.1	178	5.8	16.8	4.2	Trace	162	1.7	1	130	90	.06	.03	.2	—

FOOD, APPROXIMATE HOUSEHOLD MEASURES AND MARKET UNITS		VALUES FOR EDIBLE PART OF FOODS															
			Water	Food energy	Protein	Fat	Carbohydrate	Calcium	Phosphorus	Iron	Sodium	Potassium	Vitamin A value	Thiamin	Riboflavin	Niacin	Ascorbic acid
		Grams	*Percent*	*Calories*	*Grams*	*Grams*	*Grams*	*Milligrams*	*Milligrams*	*Milligrams*	*Milligrams*	*Milligrams*	*International units*	*Milligrams*	*Milligrams*	*Milligrams*	*Milligrams*
Persian or English:																	
In shell (refuse: shells, 55%):																	
Pound (yields approx. 7.2 oz., shelled nuts)	1 lb	454	3.5	1,329	30.2	130.6	32.2	202	776	6.3	4	918	60	.67	.27	1.8	4
10 large nuts (aprox. 1-5/16-in. diam.)	10 nuts	110	3.5	322	7.3	31.7	7.8	49	188	1.5	1	223	10	.16	.06	.4	1
Shelled:																	
Halves, 1 cup (approx. 50)	1 cup	100	3.5	651	14.8	64.0	15.8	99	380	3.1	2	450	30	.33	.13	.9	2
Pound (yield from approx. 2¼ lb., in shell)	1 lb	454	3.5	2,953	67.1	290.3	71.7	449	1,724	14.1	9	2,041	140	1.50	.59	4.1	9
Ounce (approx. 14 halves)	1 oz	28	3.5	185	4.2	18.1	4.5	28	108	.9	1	128	10	.09	.04	.3	1
WATERCRESS, LEAVES INCLUDING STEMS, RAW:																	
Chopped, finely	1 cup	125	93.3	24	2.8	.4	3.8	189	68	2.1	65	353	6,130	.10	.20	1.1	99
WATERMELON, RAW:	1 lb	454	92.6	118	2.3	.9	29.0	32	45	2.3	5	454	2,680	.14	.14	.9	32

Index

www.ingramcontent.com/pod-product-compliance
Lightning Source LLC
Chambersburg PA
CBHW021843020426
42334CB00013B/163
* 9 7 8 0 8 7 9 7 5 5 8 1 2 *